Nursing in Today's World

Challenges, Issues, and Trends

Nursing in Today's World

Challenges, Issues, and Trends

Sixth Edition

Janice Rider Ellis, RN, PhD

Professor of Nursing
Director of Nursing Education
Shoreline Community College
Seattle, Washington

Celia Love Hartley, RN, MN

Professor of Nursing
Chair, Health Sciences Division and
Director, Nursing Programs
College of the Desert
Palm Desert, California

Illustrations by Kari Berger

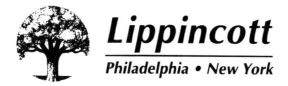

Lippincott

Philadelphia • New York

Acquisitions Editor: Lisa Marshall
Sponsoring Editor: Sandy Kasko
Project Editor: Erika Kors
Production Manager: Helen Ewan
Production Coordinator: Patricia McCloskey
Design Coordinator: Nicholas Rook

6th Edition

9 8 7 6 5 4 3 2 1

Library of Congress Cataloging-in-Publications Data

Ellis, Janice Rider.
    Nursing in today's world : challenges, issues, and trends / Janice
Rider Ellis, Celia Love Hartley. — 6th ed.
        p.   cm.
    Includes bibliographical references and index.
    ISBN 0-397-55428-1 (alk. paper)
    1. Nursing.   2. Nursing—Practice.   3. Nursing—United States.
I. Hartley, Celia Love.   II. Title.
    [DNLM: 1. Nursing—United States.   2. Education, Nursing—trends—
United States.   3. Legislation, Nursing—United States.   4. Ethics,
Nursing—United States.   5. Delivery of Health Care—United States.
6. Collective bargaining.   WY 16 E47n 1998]
RT82.E45   1998
610.73--dc21
DNLM/DLC
for Library of Congress   97-22036
                                                              CIP

Care has been taken to confirm the accuracy of the information presented and to describe generally accepted practices. However, the authors, editors, and publisher are not responsible for errors or omissions or for any consequences from application of the information in this book and make no warranty, express or implied, with respect to the contents of the publication.

The authors, editors and publisher have exerted every effort to ensure that drug selection and dosage set forth in this text are in accordance with current recommendations and practice at the time of publication. However, in view of ongoing research, changes in government regulations, and the constant flow of information relating to drug therapy and drug reactions, the reader is urged to check the package insert for each drug for any change in indications and dosage and for added warnings and precautions. This is particularly important when the recommended agent is a new or infrequently employed drug.

Some drugs and medical devices presented in this publication have Food and Drug Administration (FDA) clearance for limited use in restricted research settings. It is the responsibility of the health care provider to ascertain the FDA status of each drug or device planned for use in their clinical practice.

Preface

Nursing in Today's World has always represented a conscientious and diligent effort on our part to present, in a stimulating and engaging format, content that will assist the new graduate to participate effectively in the discipline of nursing. The rapidly progressing body of nursing knowledge, the phenomenal technological advances that have reshaped nursing care, and the colossal changes that have occurred in the health care delivery system continue to demand that the new graduate possess a sound understanding of nursing theory, the ability to think critically, and a command of the psychomotor skills that collectively comprise both the art and science of nursing.

New graduates entering the work world must bring with them a sound understanding of nursing—its heritage, history, trends, struggles, controversies, studies, and contributions. Each of the previous editions had approached this content from the traditional "in the beginning" chronological format. As we deliberated about the sixth edition, we asked ourselves how to present its information to students most effectively, how to assist instructors in squeezing a tremendous amount of material into class hours that always seem too short, and how to facilitate the process of transition from school to career. After considering all these issues, it seemed to us that it was time for a radical update in format. How can students begin to function in today's health care system unless they have some understanding of how that system came to exist and function as it does today? What are the financial factors that are influencing and driving the development and operation of health care delivery? What social and political phenomena and powers are invading health care?

Thus, the sixth edition of *Nursing in Today's World: Challenges, Issues, and Trends* takes a bold and progressive approach to the information one typically finds in "Trends" or "Issues" courses. Unit I introduces students to the health care delivery system, its financing, and the politics that impact upon it. Chapter 1 discusses the various types of institutions and agencies that provide care, from traditional acute care hospitals to community-based clinics and offices. This chapter further addresses the role of our colleagues in the health care system, discussing the contribution of traditional, alternative, and supportive health care providers. Central to all is the role of the nurse. Chapter 2 addresses the financing of health care, describing the various systems for payment from personal out-of-pocket payment to government-supported and managed programs. Cost-containment measures are explored and factors that affect the financing of health care are outlined. Chapter 3 looks at political influences on the health care system, with a special emphasis on the role played by the various nursing organizations. Ways in which nurses can be politically effective, either individually or as a member of an organization, are highlighted.

Unit II brings to the student an understanding of the development of nursing as a profession. Chapter 4 explores nursing's origins starting with health care in ancient cultures and progressing to the modern health care practices of today. Chapter 5 discusses the development of nursing as a profession, including content related to the characteristics of a profession, the differentiation between the terms profession and professional, the image of nursing, and studies about nursing. The chapter concludes with a section devoted to the traditions that have helped make nursing what it is today. We hope that students will gain an appreciation for the struggles in which nursing has been engaged and the controversies that have existed and continue to exist regarding the profession. Not all questions are answered, nor are they likely to be in the near future. Our challenge is to present this content in a format that will provoke the students' curiosity and provide an incentive for further exploration of the many issues surrounding the nursing profession. Chapter 6 outlines the educational preparation for nursing, discussing the role and preparation of the nursing assistant and the practical (vocational) nurse, as well as the many avenues to preparation for registered nurse roles. Similarities in programs are discussed and alternate forms of education described. The chapter also includes content related to factors that have influenced nursing education, differentiated practice, and forces for change in nursing education.

Unit III of the textbook focuses on legal and ethical accountability. Chapter 7 discusses the various types of credentials found among health care providers and traces the history of credentialing in the United States. The laws governing nursing are reviewed and the role of the boards of nursing are outlined. The chapter concludes with a discussion of the future of credentialing. Chapter 8 explores the legal considerations that impact the practice of nursing, through discussion of both the law in general and the application of legal principles to the profession of nursing. Chapters 9 and 10 discuss the ethical and bioethical issues that impact the practice of nursing. Chapter 9 outlines basic ethical concepts and theories and describes factors that influence ethical decision making. The chapter also explores the application of ethical issues to the profession of nursing and includes a discussion of the chemically impaired professional. Chapter 10 explores the major bioethical concerns with which health care providers wrestle.

Unit IV, the final unit of the textbook, focuses on today's health care world of work. Chapter 11 provides students with information about seeking and securing employment and includes helpful hints about preparing a letter of application and resumé and interviewing for a position. Examples are included that can be adapted for personal use. Chapter 12 discusses the new graduate's participation in the workplace, provides information about the structure of health care organizations, and describes the various patterns of nursing care delivery. The chapter concludes with a discussion of collective bargaining and the issues it presents to the nursing profession.

Each chapter begins with a set of objectives to guide the learning experience followed by a list of key terms that will be used throughout that particular chapter. Each chapter is summarized with key concepts, and critical thinking activities provide students with the opportunity to apply the content of the chapter to typical situations encountered in the health care environment. The cartoon-like illustrations have been a hallmark of the text since the first edition, and through them we hope you will gain a varied visual introduction to nursing issues that will provide some humor, as well as gratification, to your commitment to nursing.

As we have worked on refining the sixth edition, we have appreciated the comments and constructive suggestions offered by fellow educators throughout the country and by the reviewers who made recommendations regarding the content. We will be anxious to hear from you regarding this new edition and its structure. We thank the many educators who continue to select *Nursing in Today's World: Challenges, Issues, and Trends* as the textbook for your class. We know there are many texts from which to choose. In this very competitive market we appreciate your support and strive to bring to you the book that will best meet your needs.

We must certainly list among our acknowledgments appreciation to our respective husbands, Ivan and Gordon, both of whom encourage and support our efforts and allow the book to take first place on the agenda when that is necessary. Their willingness to take on extra household duties, post express mail, do the shopping, and assist with a myriad of other duties has allowed us to meet publication deadlines. And last, but not least, we wish to thank the editors at Lippincott–Raven for their help and assistance with the text.

Janice Rider Ellis, PhD, RN
Celia Love Hartley, MN, RN

Table of Contents

UNIT III Legal and Ethical Accountability for Practice 229

Economic and Political Aspects of Health Care Delivery

Health care in any country is part of the economic and political life of the nation. It reflects much of what is best about life but also serves to point out those areas where serious problems exist.

In this unit we provide a basic overview of the health care delivery system in the United States. The complexity of the system cannot be completely explained in one short unit, but we have tried to focus on the aspects that will best help you put health care issues into context. We have started with the part of the system with which you are probably most familiar: the health care settings that employ nurses. The specific characteristics of these settings—their role in health care, the roles of nurses in these settings, the colleagues with whom nurses work, and alternative health care resources—are the focus of the first chapter in this unit. From there we move to an overview of the financial aspects of the health care delivery system. Understanding the various players in the system will help you analyze specific financial issues as they arise; issues related to access to the system are addressed, as are issues of power and control. Finally, we move to the issue of the political process and how it affects nursing. The political process relates both to government and to the functioning of organizations. Our hope is that you will find an understanding of these various aspects of the health care delivery system relevant to your professional life.

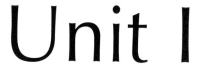

Unit I

1

Understanding the Health Care Environment

Nurses are experts on reality. No one has roots that penetrate so deeply into our health care institutions. No one sees so much, nor understands so thoroughly. (Joel, 1996)

Objectives

After completing this chapter, you should be able to

1. Discuss the three ways that health care agencies are classified.
2. Describe the various health care settings including the types of services offered and the roles that registered nurses perform in each.
3. Describe the health care delivery provided in ambulatory care settings and in community agencies.
4. Discuss the roles and interrelationships of the various health care providers in the health care system.
5. Analyze the various issues related to individual health care occupations.
6. Describe the various avenues to alternative health care and analyze their relationship to traditional medical care.

KEY TERMS

Acute care facility
Alternative health care
Community mental health centers
Complementary therapy
Herbal medicine
Homeopathy
Long-term care facility
Naturopathy

Nonprofit
Nursing home
Osteopathy
Primary care provider
Proprietary agency
Subacute care
Tertiary care hospital
Transitional care

It is an exciting but somewhat anxiety-provoking time to be a nurse. The entire health care system reverberates with change. One of the questions you may have is "Where will I work?'' Another may be ''What kind of work do I want to do?'' Still another may be ''Will there be a job for me?'' As a new graduate you will want to function within some type of health care agency or organization. An understanding of the various health care agencies and their services, the roles that nurses perform in those agencies, and of the colleagues in other disciplines with whom you will work, will help you to assume your role as a beginning nurse more effectively. As we discuss each type of health care agency, we will point out the roles that nurses play in that agency as well as the type of services it provides. As alternative health care practices grow in popularity with the public, those in the traditional health care system are challenged to understand alternative approaches to health care and to work effectively with clients who choose those resources. In order to help you with this task, we have included a discussion of alternative as well as traditional health care options (Fig.1-1).

TYPES OF HEALTH CARE AGENCIES

For many years, nursing education focused the attention of students on the acute care hospital because that was where most were employed after graduation. Those planning to move

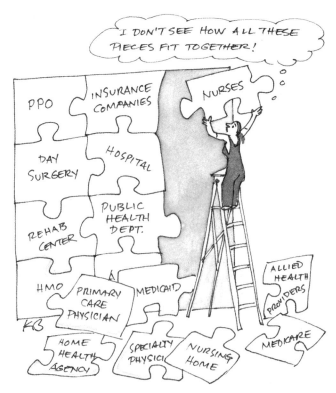

FIGURE 1-1
The many aspects of health care in the United States are not coordinated into a single system.

to other fields were expected to spend a minimum of a year or two in acute care first. By limiting experience almost exclusively to the acute care hospital as a learning environment, the educational process itself ensured that graduates would feel most comfortable seeking employment in the acute care setting.

However, the situation has changed dramatically. As health care has made revolutionary changes, more and more care has moved to settings outside the acute care hospital. The number and variety of long-term care facilities has increased dramatically and now includes rehabilitation centers, nursing homes, assisted-living settings, group homes, and adult care homes. Nursing roles in long-term care are increasingly complex and require a high degree of autonomy. Nursing education has also changed and many of you may have had the opportunity to work in long-term care settings as part of your nursing educational experiences.

Agencies within the community such as home care providers, clinics, offices, and other ambulatory care settings are growing in number. Home care nursing now encompasses a much wider spectrum of client care needs than previously. Caring for some home care clients requires a high degree of skill, but these clients represent a relatively stable population who are able to maintain their status at home as long as adequate support is available. Some clients have acute problems requiring high-intensity services. For example, hospice care enables dying persons to remain at home. Home infusion therapy allows those with complex medication needs to avoid hospitalization. Home care as part of public health has long been included in baccalaureate nursing programs. As home care has changed in focus, more nursing education programs are including experiences in the care of the individual client in the home setting.

Many ambulatory care settings are recognizing that the effective use of registered nurses may provide high-quality care at a cost lower than that provided when the physician does not have the support of professional nurses in addressing the needs of clients. Therefore, more educational settings are providing experiences in ambulatory care for nursing students.

Businesses are recognizing that nurses may fill many roles. The role of the occupational health nurse in providing information on health promotion and preventive care receives increasing emphasis. Experienced nurses are employed by insurance companies as case managers and care reviewers. Many companies that market client care supplies and equipment seek nurses as sales representatives or as staff educators.

Although many nurses continue to be employed in acute care hospitals, an increasing number of nurses employed by hospitals are working in ambulatory care areas. Day surgery, day treatment, special teaching clinics, and other outpatient services are now commonly part of the acute care hospital. Some hospitals have had rehabilitation services for years, but now are moving into what is called ''transitional care,'' that is, care during the convalescent or recovery period between acute care hospitalization and discharge home.

CLASSIFICATION OF HEALTH CARE AGENCIES

Because the health care industry is so large, so diverse, and so complex, it is difficult to understand (Fig. 1-2). Generally, agencies providing care are classified in one of three ways: according to length of stay; according to type of service; or according to ownership (Display 1-1). You need to understand that any one of these classifications is somewhat arbitrary and

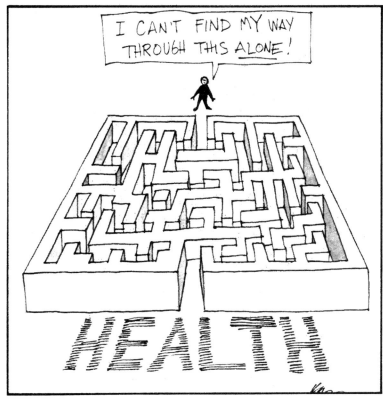

FIGURE 1-2
Clients often need assistance in finding their way through the modern health care system.

that any agency may be placed in more than one classification. With the systemic changes that are occurring, one agency may now include multiple lengths of stay, different types of service, and may combine many segments with different ownership patterns under one large entity. Nevertheless, these categories are useful because they are still used to describe institutions.

Classification According to Length of Stay

One way of classifying agencies is according to length of stay. Short-stay, traditional acute care, and long-term care are terms that reflect the length of stay in a facility. Short-stay facilities provide services to patients who are suffering from acute conditions that usually require less than 24 hours of care. In some areas the average length of stay for a person having an appendectomy is now less than 24 hours. Short-stay may take place in separate units in a hospital or in free-standing, short-stay centers.

DISPLAY 1-1
Classifications for Health Care Agencies

Length of Stay
  Short-stay
    Traditional acute care
    Long-term care
Type of Service
  General vs. specialty
  Community vs. tertiary

Subacute care/transitional care
In-home care
Ambulatory care
Type of Ownership
Governmental
Proprietary/for profit
Nonprofit

Traditional acute care takes place in hospitals. In general, acute care encompasses patients staying more than 24 hours but fewer than 30 days. However, the average length of stay for all inpatients regardless of diagnosis has been declining steadily over the past few years and has become significantly shorter since the implementation of diagnosis-related groups (DRGs) in 1983. (DRGs are discussed in greater detail in Chapter 2.) In many hospitals the average length of stay after general surgery is 3 to 5 days. Thus the distinction between the short-stay and the traditional acute care inpatient has blurred.

Long-term care facilities include those that offer services to patients with major rehabilitation needs, chronic disease, functional losses, or mental illness. The average length of stay extends from several months to years. State institutions for the mentally ill are usually considered long-term hospitals although they may have units designated for shorter, acute care stays. Some hospitals have long-term rehabilitation as their only focus. Long-term rehabilitation may also be located on one unit of an acute care hospital. Nursing homes typically care for those who will remain residents for the remainder of their lives, but many also serve people who need a period of convalescence and rehabilitation before returning to their homes. Assisted living facilities and group care homes for the developmentally disabled and the dependent elderly are designed to be permanent residences for clients. In these settings, managing the living environment is as critical as managing health-related concerns.

Classification by Type of Service

Health care agencies may also be classified according to type of service provided. The most common facility is the *general hospital* that offers medical, surgical, obstetric, emergency, and diagnostic and laboratory services. *Specialty hospitals* offer only a particular type of care, such as that provided by psychiatric hospitals, women's hospitals, or children's hospitals. Specialty hospitals tend to be less common than general hospitals.

A term frequently used when referring to hospitals is *community hospital*. Community hospitals provide general hospital services for a specific community. The majority of hospitals in the United States fall into this category.

Tertiary care hospitals are those serving as referral centers for clients with complex or unusual health problems. These hospitals have the facilities for specialized types of care such as burn centers, bone marrow transplant centers, and research-based oncology centers, as well as resources for general care. They serve a wide geographic area in addition to their own community. Tertiary care hospitals are usually associated with a university or are part of a large medical center.

Long-term care facilities offer a variety of different services. The majority of nursing homes care for the elderly who have deficits in multiple areas of daily living and need what has traditionally been termed custodial services. Some long-term care facilities now focus on individuals with continuing high-intensity needs, such as those who remain permanently dependent on a ventilator or individuals with the multiple problems of advanced AIDS. Residential facilities for young adults with severe disabilities such as cerebral palsy may focus on life skills development and occupational training. Inpatient hospices focus on respite care, symptom management, and terminal care. Rehabilitation centers focus on individuals with needs related to restoration of function, daily living abilities, and may also assist in vocational rehabilitation.

Subacute care is a growing type of service that may be offered in a special unit of a hospital (where it is sometimes termed *transitional care*) or may be provided in a long-term care setting. This care is seen as a ''middle-ground'' between the high acuity care provided to those in the acute care hospital and the care provided to more traditional long-term care clients. Typically, stays in short-term subacute units are up to 30 days in length. Some units focus on intermediate lengths of stay that usually range from 31 to 90 days, during which time clients may recover enough to move into a home setting or stabilize their conditions so that their needs can be met in a nursing home. Still other subacute units offer care that can extend for up to 2 years (Burns, 1993). The units that primarily offer medical services, where discharge is rapid, are most commonly located in hospitals; those that provide rehabilitative services are more commonly located in long-term care facilities (Taylor, 1994).

Community health care agencies offer in-home care by a variety of health care professionals including nurses, physical therapists, respiratory therapists, social workers, and home health care aides. This care may be short-term, to provide teaching and monitoring immediately after hospitalization; intermediate-term, to assist an individual until self-care is possible; or long-term, for those with ongoing health problems. Teaching family and caregivers is a large part of the home care professional's responsibility. The traditional public health department focuses on the provision of health promotion and health maintenance services to whole groups of the public as well as to individuals.

Classification According to Ownership

The final method of classifying health care agencies is according to ownership. Agencies may be classified as governmental or public, proprietary, or nonprofit.

GOVERNMENT-OWNED FACILITIES

Public or government agencies, which receive some tax support for capital and/or operational costs, may be owned and operated by federal, state, or local governments. The federal facilities usually serve the needs of a special group of individuals such as veterans, military personnel, Native Americans, or inmates in federal prisons. State mental facilities and hospitals operated by the state are also governmental institutions. Cities, counties, and hospital districts may operate acute care and long-term care agencies and public health departments.

PROPRIETARY AGENCIES

Proprietary agencies (also known as private or for-profit) are investor owned and operated. Proprietary agencies are commonly part of a corporation owned by stock holders. Some small nursing homes or group homes are owned by an individual. In these agencies, the original capital costs were provided by the owners and investors. Profits from a proprietary institution provide a return on the money invested by the stock holders or individual owners. Historically, some proprietary hospitals were owned and operated by a small group of physicians, but over the years many of these have been sold to community groups or to corporations. In the past few years there has been a significant trend toward the acquisition of health care enterprises by investor-owned corporations and the formation of multiunit, for-profit systems. Examples include Columbia/HCA Healthcare Corporation, which is based in Nashville, and Humana, Incorporated of Louisville. Each of these groups owns more than 80 hospitals and operates a number of others. Not all investor-owned institutions are general hospitals. In the long-term care field, Beverly Enterprises and Hillhaven Corporation are examples of corporations that own and operate many nursing homes across the country. The majority of the nation's nursing homes are proprietary.

NONPROFIT AGENCIES

Voluntary or nonprofit agencies are those operated by nonprofit groups such as religious bodies, fraternal groups, and community boards. More than 50% of the nation's short-term hospitals and most of the large medical centers fall into this classification. Original capital costs are obtained in a variety of ways, but most often through donation. Community fund-raising campaigns often raise donations for building, capital start-up costs, and special projects. One current concern is the purchase of nonprofit agencies by profit-making corporations. Communities often believe their interests and contributions are discounted in these large business mergers.

The term *nonprofit* may be somewhat misleading, because all facilities must make a sufficient income to maintain facilities and services, to plan for capital improvement and development, and to meet current costs of care provided. However, those facilities that are classified as nonprofit must put any profit to work in the facility rather than distribute it to stockholders.

UNDERSTANDING TODAY'S HOSPITAL

The modern hospital may be viewed as the hub or center of the health care delivery system. Hospital facilities are central to the health care of a community. They also provide education to a wide variety of health care workers and, in many cases, are centers for research and its dissemination. Hospitals are using their status and position in health care to enter into cooperative agreements and alliances with other types of providers, insurance companies, and even other hospitals. To better understand the hospitals of today, you will find it useful to look at their history and development in Chapter 4.

Inpatient Versus Outpatient Services

Two terms used frequently in today's modern hospitals are *inpatient* and *outpatient*. Individuals are termed "inpatient" when they have been admitted for the purpose of staying 24 hours or longer. The person admitted for surgery is an inpatient when the expectation is that the individual will remain in the hospital postoperatively. The woman admitted in labor becomes an inpatient because the stay is expected to be at least 24 hours in total and may extend longer if needed. Inpatient care is acute in nature, and the emphasis is on providing specific services not available elsewhere or services that can only be provided when a patient is staying in the hospital. As previously mentioned, lengths of stay in hospitals are now very short, averaging 3 to 5 days for many diagnoses.

The outpatient is an individual who comes to the hospital for services but is expected to stay less than 24 hours. Many diagnostic and treatment procedures, surgeries, and emergency health needs are treated as outpatient care. The outpatient goes through an admission process, has a procedure performed or care delivered, is determined to be ready for home care, and subsequently is discharged.

Sometimes an outpatient is retained for observation beyond the standard 24 hours. Although this individual may be moved to a conventional hospital room, admission as an inpatient may never occur and the person may be discharged as an outpatient with an extended stay. The distinction between the categories of inpatient and outpatient is important in regard to both billing and discharge to a nursing home. Both Medicare and Medicaid are billed differently for outpatient care than for inpatient care; there is no limitation on the amount that can be charged to the patient for outpatient care as there is with inpatient care. Medicare payments for nursing home care after hospitalization require that the person be admitted as an inpatient with a minimum hospital stay. When these conditions are not met, Medicare payment is denied. Older patients and their families may not understand this difference and how it affects the bills they receive and their eligibility for some types of reimbursement. Nurses must understand this difference as they help patients to plan for needed care after discharge.

Types of Services

Hospitals of today offer a wide variety of services. Not every hospital offers each of the mentioned services but more are becoming part of a corporate entity that provides all of these services (Display 1-2).

ACUTE CARE SERVICES

Hospitals provide inpatient care in a variety of different departments, that are commonly designed around the acuity or seriousness of the patient's condition. Nurses work in all of these service departments, coordinating the nursing care for individual clients, managing the care environment, and providing direct skilled care. These units comprise what most people think of when they use the designation "acute care hospital."

DISPLAY 1-2
Types of Hospital Services

- Acute care:
    Intensive care units
    Coronary care units
    Step-down units
    Medical–surgical units
    Mother–baby units
    Surgery suites
    Emergency rooms
- Diagnostic services:
    Diagnostic imaging
    Endoscopic centers
    Laboratory services
- Day surgery centers:
    Pre- and postoperative care
- Medical treatment (outpatient):
    Physical & occupational therapy
    Respiratory therapy
    Dialysis
    Chemotherapy

    Parenteral nutrition
    Antibiotic therapy
- Rehabilitation (inpatient & outpatient):
    Nursing care
    Physical & occupational therapy
    Vocational & personal counseling
- Transitional care
- Hospice inpatient care
- Hospitality units
- Home care:
    Medical services
    Hospice home care
    Infusion therapy
    Postpartum visits
- Health professional education:
    Schools of nursing
    Respiratory therapy programs
    Dietetics
    Medical residency programs

Most hospitals have units designated as *critical or intensive care units* where the most seriously ill patients, such as trauma and heart attack victims, receive sophisticated technological monitoring and care by a highly trained nursing staff who can respond to life-threatening health problems. These units are technologically complex and very expensive to create and maintain. The staff-to-patient ratio is very high to ensure the close monitoring that will prevent or identify crisis situations. Some hospitals are large enough to have several critical care units, with each unit serving different types of clients. A coronary care unit may care only for patients with medical cardiac problems. A cardiac surgery intensive care unit may care only for those who have just had cardiac surgery. A general surgery intensive care unit may care for patients with other complex postsurgical needs.

Step-down units are designed for individuals who no longer need the intensive intervention available in critical care areas but who may still need special monitoring and the resources for immediate intervention. Cardiac step-down units typically provide telemetry monitoring that allows the patient to be more ambulatory while still being closely assessed.

Traditional *medical–surgical units* are designed for the care of the person hospitalized for more routine medical or surgical inpatient care. The need for round-the-clock skilled nursing care is a major reason for inpatient care. In a medical–surgical unit, a physician visits daily and emergency care is available. Other treatment services, such as respiratory, physical, and occupational therapy, are available as needed by the hospitalized patient.

Mother–baby units in hospitals provide services attuned to the needs of the whole child-bearing family. Entire families, including siblings, are welcomed into the setting. Birthing rooms, where the atmosphere is home-like rather than institutional, and where there is the ability to labor, deliver, and recover in the same room, are currently recognized as beneficial both for patient care and hospital marketing. Amenities such as jacuzzi tubs enhance the atmosphere. Care may include the services of a lactation specialist and the opportunity to consult with childcare specialists. Because stays may be very short, home care or telephone follow-up by nurses has become part of more hospital mother–baby services.

Emergency rooms provide care for serious, acute problems of sudden onset. With the resources to manage multisystem trauma, major burns, and life-threatening cardiac conditions, the modern emergency room has altered survival for many individuals. A problem in the system occurs when clients do not have other resources for primary care and use the emergency room for this purpose.

Surgical units provide the environment and equipment for the highly specialized surgical procedures to occur. Lasers, microscopes, lithotriptors, closed circuit televisions, and sophisticated monitoring devices are just some of the high-cost equipment added to traditional surgical instruments.

DIAGNOSTIC SERVICES

Hospitals are the center for the most sophisticated *diagnostic services* available. When these costly services are available in one place, they can be used by many physicians. Many of the units providing these services have no nursing staff, but others have one or two nurses to work with the specific procedural needs of patients. Diagnostic imaging departments offer more than traditional x-rays. Magnetic resonance imaging (MRI), computerized axial tomography (CAT), sonography (ultrasound), and positron emission tomography (PET) are some of the sophisticated studies available. Endoscopic centers provide the resources to do gastro-esophago-duodenoscopy (EGD), cystoscopy, colonoscopy, and arthroscopy. Laboratories may be able to perform DNA studies and to test for cell surface antigens as well as perform the standard blood, urine and tissue tests. These diagnostic services are used for outpatients as well inpatients; in some instances, the majority of patients are outpatients.

DAY SURGERY

Day surgery centers provide an ever-increasing percentage of all surgical procedures. Presurgical care is provided as well. On the day of surgery, the patient arrives at a scheduled time (sometimes at 6:00 am) for preoperative care prior to surgery. The pace in these units is very rapid with patients being admitted, transferred to the operating room, and discharged in a continuing process throughout the day.

MEDICAL TREATMENT SERVICES

Medical treatment services originally established for those in the hospital have gradually expanded to include services for outpatients. Physical therapy, occupational therapy, respiratory therapy, and other treatments support health care for whole segments of the community. Special outpatient units provide chemotherapy, dialysis, parenteral nutrition, antibiotic therapy, and other medical treatments. Lanigan and others (1994) suggest that these new units offer opportunities for nurses to be creative and innovative in meeting client needs.

REHABILITATION SERVICES

Rehabilitation units are a part of some hospitals. These units focus on clients with major rehabilitation needs such as spinal cord injury and stroke. Even rehabilitation stays are shortening. Inpatient rehabilitation services may be provided for only a brief period of time, followed by outpatient rehabilitation services. Included in both inpatient and outpatient rehabilitation services are nursing care, physical and occupational therapy, vocational counseling, and personal counseling services.

TRANSITIONAL CARE

Many hospitals have had empty beds because of shortened lengths of stay and the shift to outpatient procedures. In an effort to use costly resources effectively to generate income, hospitals have developed transitional care units that provide long-term care services. Reimbursement is based on long-term care guidelines and the care must meet long-term care standards. A transitional care unit allows a hospital to discharge an individual from acute, inpatient care in a timely fashion because the next level of services is guaranteed to be available.

HOSPICE INPATIENT CARE

Another needed service is *hospice inpatient care*. Individuals who have chosen hospice care for their terminal illness may need temporary inpatient care for symptom management (ie, pain or nausea) or may have family caregivers who need respite from the demands of care. Some individuals wish to have care that functions according to the hospice philosophy, but do not have caregivers with the ability to provide ongoing home care. These individuals may be admitted to a hospice inpatient unit to stay until they die. Units planned for hospice care usually operate under long-term care guidelines rather than acute care guidelines.

HOSPITALITY UNITS

Day procedures and early discharge for inpatient care, may present travel difficulties for individuals who live a long distance from a major care center. In order to facilitate care for these individuals and their families, some hospitals have developed hotel-like services, often termed *hospitality units*. The patient scheduled for day surgery may plan to arrive the day before and stay overnight at a hospitality unit in order to be present for the morning surgery appointment. A family member may stay in the unit during the individual's hospitalization. After discharge, both the patient and the family member may stay one or more days before traveling home. Although the cost of staying in a hospitality unit is usually not covered by insurance, staying at a nearby hotel or motel might not be as convenient. Additionally, if an emergency occurs, the patient in a hospitality unit has care immediately available.

HOME CARE SERVICES

The number of hospitals offering *home care services* including hospice home care is growing. Home services may operate as independent departments, or in conjunction with other services. Examples include home infusion therapy that is connected to a medical treatment center and home postpartum visits that are administered through a mother-baby unit. Sometimes home care is provided by a hospital; in other instances it is provided through a contractual relationship with a home care agency.

THE EDUCATION OF THE HEALTH CARE PROFESSIONAL

The *education of health care providers* is an important function of many hospitals. Although the number of hospital-based schools of nursing offering diplomas has been decreasing steadily, a large number are still in place. There are also hospital based programs for respiratory therapy, dietetics, and other health-related occupations. A large number of hospitals serve as clinical laboratory sites for individuals enrolled in colleges and universities that provide education for health care professionals.

A physician in a residency program is considered to be in an educational program. Residents receive a salary from the hospital, and are responsible for providing services in return. In addition to augmenting the services of primary physicians, residents often provide medical services for individuals who are part of the medically underserved in a community. As pressure mounts to reduce the number of specialists and increase the number of primary care physicians, there is speculation about what will happen to some medical residency programs. At this time, part of the funding for these programs comes from Medicare reimbursement policies. These policies allow hospitals to identify educational costs and receive "pass-through" money (that is, money not related to specific individual patient care needs) from Medicare to support educational programs. If these funds were withdrawn or designated to be used for primary care preparation (such as family practice), many residency programs would not be sustained at their current size. This would also have profound effects on the function of hospitals that rely on resident physicians for day-to-day, twenty-four hour services.

THE LONG-TERM CARE FACILITY

Long-term care provides assistance with activities of daily living and health care for people of any age who are physically or mentally unable to provide adequate self-care. These conditions may extend over a limited period of time (such as during recovery from a major surgery) or may last a lifetime (as with a developmental disability). Care involves coordination of the entire multidisciplinary team to provide counseling, nursing care, rehabilitation, nutritional support, social services, and sometimes special education programs. Long-term care facilities include nursing homes, chronic disease hospitals, psychiatric hospitals, tuberculosis hospitals, and psychiatric and mental retardation facilities. The majority of long-term care facilities are nursing homes that care primarily for the elderly.

The Nursing Home Today

The nursing home is the care facility most often associated with long-term care. Although nursing homes today suffer from negative images of the past, they offer a far different environment than they did even 10 years ago. Nursing homes in the United States provide care and a positive living environment for individuals who have the greatest number of deficits in activities of daily living and who need ongoing skilled nursing care. Just as in the acute care hospital, the nursing home is expanding services beyond those traditionally associated with nursing home care.

WHO ARE THE RESIDENTS?

Although the vast majority of the elderly live in community settings, many will spend will spend their last years in a nursing home. Approximately two-thirds of the residents are women, reflecting the longer lifespan of women and the greater likelihood that a woman's spouse will precede her in death (Lipowski & Bigelow, 1996). Nursing home residents range in age from 65 to older than 100, with an average age of about 84.

HEALTH SERVICES IN NURSING HOMES

The majority of residents in nursing homes remain there because of major deficits in self care abilities and the need for ongoing care that is custodial rather than treatment oriented in focus. Maintenance of function, independence, autonomy, and rehabilitation are all goals for nursing home residents. Residents are concerned with the living environment as well as the health care environment.

Units designed for the cognitively impaired provide special facilities without barriers to mobility and without the need for restraints. Special designs and alarm systems prevent residents from wandering out of the facility. A unit for the cognitively impaired will have special approaches to care delivery that decrease stress and reduce the potential for catastrophic reactions such as hostile, angry outbursts. Reality orientation is used for those who might benefit from this therapy. Validation therapy and reminiscence are also planned to provide a supportive and rich environment. Staff development assists caregivers in responding appropriately to the special challenges of working with the cognitively impaired.

Some nursing homes have entire wings for individuals receiving posthospital convalescent care in subacute units. These individuals are admitted with a specific planned stay of 14 to 30 days. During this time the individual is aided in restoring functional abilities and planning for self or family care. Rehabilitation may be a major focus of some subacute units. This might include physical therapy for the person with a hip replacement or speech therapy after a stroke. The goal is to enable residents to return to independent living in the community.

The level of autonomy expected of nurses in nursing homes where physicians visit monthly is often surprising to those who have always worked in acute care hospitals where physicians visit patients daily. In nursing homes the individual may be a permanent resident and the nurse may be charged with managing quality of life as well as quality of care. Additionally, nurses in these settings must manage care conducted by a variety of assistive personnel and work effectively with an interdisciplinary team.

FUNDING NURSING HOME CARE

The cost of nursing home care is a concern for many because it often exceeds $3,000 per month, depending upon the care needs of the individual and the geographic location of the nursing home. Medicare only pays for a limited number of days for individuals who meet specific criteria regarding hospitalization and who need rehabilitative rather than custodial care. A few individuals have long-term care insurance that will pay some of their costs. Because this type of insurance is fairly new and quite expensive, few residents have purchased policies. The personal financial resources of most individuals will be exhausted by a prolonged nursing home stay. State administered public assistance in the form of programs such as Medicaid and Medi-Cal pays for nursing home care when an individual's personal financial resources have fallen below a certain state-determined level. As the number of elderly individuals requiring nursing home care has risen, these costs are becoming a serious budget concern in most states.

Assisted Living Facilities

A more recent development is the assisted living facility which provides care for those needing help with up to three activities of daily living. In an assisted-living arrangement, the resident can maintain maximum independence and use a shared decision-making model to decide when additional help or support is needed (DeYoung, Just, & VanDyk, 1994). As the costs of nursing home care have risen, those who are able to perform any activities of daily living are seeking the less costly and more flexible living found in assisted living.

CARE IN ASSISTED LIVING FACILITIES

In an assisted living facility all instrumental activities of daily living such as shopping, cleaning, meal preparation, and laundry are provided. A resident is expected to have some mobility (even though it may require a walker or a cane) and to eat in a dining room. Residents are also expected to manage their own medication and health needs. Assistance is provided with bathing, dressing, and other personal care as needed. Most care is provided by unlicensed assistive personnel. Nurses may be employed in a supervisory capacity and may plan for care.

When the ability to perform activities of daily living is lost, transfer to a nursing home is required by regulation. For some individuals, the transitions from independent living to assisted living and from assisted living to nursing home care are smooth ones. This is particularly true when multiple levels of care are available in the same setting. When the individual must move from the assisted living ''home'' to a nursing home, the same difficulties with transition may occur as when the individual must leave independent living for an institutional setting.

FUNDING ASSISTED LIVING

Assisted living is not supported with Medicare funds and therefore does not have to meet the stringent regulatory standards of federal legislation (Hawryluk, 1995). In some states, assisted living facilities have very little regulation. Public assistance, in the form of Medicaid, Medi-Cal, or other programs may provide some support for assisted living when the alternative would be expensive nursing home care for which the state would be responsible. However, this is not true in all jurisdictions. Most assisted living is paid for by the individual or family.

Retirement Communities

Recent years have witnessed the development of several forms of retirement communities. These communities may be self-contained towns, retirement villages, retirement subdivisions, retirement residences, or continuing-care retirement communities. The basic retirement complex is designed to provide easy care and may support independence longer than would a regular house or apartment. Home care services are provided to those in retirement communities in the same way that they are provided to those in regular homes or apartments.

Continuing care retirement communities (CCRC) provide a variety of levels of independent living and care to residents based on each resident's need. Most residents enter the community to reside in a retirement apartment. The community also maintains an assisted living section and a convalescent or nursing home center. Services such as occupational therapy, physical therapy, and dental care may also be available as home care or for those in the convalescent center. The aim is for people to reside in the setting that provides maximum autonomy and independence while assuring that needs are met. There is data to suggest that residents of continuing care retirement communities maintain better health and require less nursing home care than the general population. (Sloan, Shayne, & Conover, 1995). A major limiting factor is the cost of such communities to the individual residents. There is no governmental financial assistance available in these residences.

Rehabilitation Centers

Rehabilitation centers typically focus on a specific health care problem just as rehabilitation units in acute care hospitals do. For example, there are centers for those with spinal cord injuries and other centers focusing on head injuries or cerebral vascular accidents. Although many of these agencies prefer nurses who have taken advanced courses in rehabilitation nursing, many also employ nurses with different backgrounds such as those who have worked in a nursing homes focused on rehabilitation principles.

AMBULATORY CARE SETTINGS

Ambulatory care has long been provided in offices, clinics, and the day procedure units of hospitals. Some ambulatory care is provided in settings where people work and go to school. Providing care where people routinely spend their days rather than requiring them to go to a different site for health care often results in more effective use of health care services. All ambulatory care settings rely heavily on the skills of registered nurses.

Primary Care Offices

The health care provider contacted initially by clients who seek health care is considered a primary care provider. Today the federal government considers general practitioners, family practice specialists, pediatricians, internal medicine specialists, and obstetricians primary care physicians. Physicians' assistants and nurse practitioners are also recognized as primary care providers. The primary care provider has been the traditional mainstay of basic care for most individuals.

One of the major changes in health care has been the decrease in the number of solo practice offices and the growth of group and organizational practices. According to a recent report, in 1996, for the first time, more physicians were employed in group practice settings than in solo practice offices. Advanced practice nurses and physicians' assistants are also working in many of these group practice settings. Other registered nurses in these settings may have responsibility for answering questions on the telephone as well as teaching and providing care for patients in the office. Nursing roles in ambulatory care are expanding as the need for cost-effective use of physician time is modifying practice patterns.

Walk-in Clinics

Walk-in clinics treat clients with emergent conditions that do not require the high technology resources of the emergency room. Walk-in clinics may be referred to as immediate care facilities or as emergent care centers and are usually open during extended hours that include evenings and weekends as well as the traditional Monday through Friday office hours. Walk-in clinics have grown in popularity as people have found it increasingly difficult to gain access to traditional health care settings because of time constraints on their personal lives. Many walk-in clinics have gradually added services such as sports physical examinations for school-age children, pelvic examinations, Pap tests for women, and routine immunizations. As these clinics mature, some are beginning to act as primary care settings, advertising the willingness of staff doctors to become ''family doctors.'' Walk-in clinics have relatively small nursing staffs, often employing only one registered nurse during a shift; therefore each nurse must have a wide variety of skills and be able to function with a high degree of autonomy. Some settings do not use nurses in direct care; nurses are hired in these setting only to supervise other clinic staff members.

COMMUNITY AGENCIES

Agencies providing care in the community include public health agencies, traditional home care agencies, and home hospice care (Display 1-3).

Public Health Agencies

Public health departments are operated as agencies of the government. In general, the focus of health departments has been on broad community issues, communicable disease, and infant and child health. Although public health nurses originally did a great deal of individual family visiting, today fewer funds for visits require that public health nurses focus on individuals who are high risk and whose health affects the entire community. Public health nurses responsible for community health issues are required to have a baccalaureate degrees in nursing; however, some agencies operate a variety of clinics (such as immunization clinics) in which registered nurses with an associate degree or diploma provide teaching and direct care services.

DISPLAY 1-3
Community Agencies

- Public health departments
- Home care agencies
- Hospice home care

- Community mental health centers
- Day care centers for the older adult
- Ambulatory care dialysis centers

Traditional Home Care Agencies

Home care agencies, such as the traditional visiting nurse services and the proprietary home health care companies, provide a broad spectrum of care that may include nursing care, personal care assistance, minor housekeeping, and physical therapy for individuals in their homes. Some home care agencies focus on providing short-term visits for clients who need assistance after a hospital stay or acute illness. Others focus on clients who will need ongoing home care for years, such those requiring dialysis or ventilator support in the home. Some agencies provide nursing care for 8 to 12 hour shifts in the home in an effort to provide support and respite for family caregivers. Others provide episodic visits that last from fifteen to sixty minutes.

Hospice Home Care

Hospice care has gained great momentum as a way to provide maximum quality of life to terminally ill people. Multidisciplinary teams may include physicians, nurses, clergy, occupational and physical therapists, home health aides, social workers, and volunteers. The goal of hospice care is to assist the individual in living as he or she wishes until death. The members of multidisciplinary teams work with both the hospice patient and the family. Nurses provide special skills in symptom management for problems such as pain, nausea, anorexia, constipation and psychosocial support for end-of-life events and issues.

Community Mental Health Centers

Community mental health centers were established to allow individuals with psychiatric problems to remain in their communities. Evidence supports the belief that psychiatric clients who remain in their communities on an outpatient basis, with family and community ties intact, have more successful treatment outcomes. For those who must be hospitalized, the community mental health center provides follow-up care that facilitates early discharge. Another advantage of community mental health centers is that people seek help more readily when it is available within the community. These centers usually employ a variety of mental health workers including psychiatrists, clinical psychologists, social workers, marriage and family counselors, psychiatric nurses, and community workers. Services may include individual counseling and therapy, group or family counseling, evaluation, and referral.

In actual practice, community mental health centers have not been adequately funded to meet the many and varied needs of individuals with mental health problems. Mentally ill clients often are not eligible for care that can maintain their health but are eligible for care only when they have become acutely ill. Some people are not eligible for help because of the complex rules and regulations governing funding. Some do not continue with prescribed treatment and thus relapse; legal constraints do not allow involuntary treatment. Although this recognition of the rights of the mentally ill has been important, there also is concern that society expects mentally ill people to make rational decisions about their own best interests when they are not mentally capable of understanding the consequences of their actions. The entire area of community mental health has many problems and challenges.

Day Care Centers for the Elderly

Day care centers have been established for elderly people who can not safely be alone throughout the day. Clients are transported to the center each day by family or by a van operated by the center. While at the center, clients receive a variety of social and health services that enable them to continue to live in their own home or a family member's home. Various maintenance and rehabilitative services usually are available, including exercise classes, medication education and supervision, recreational activities, mental health care, and an opportunity to interact with other people. Some centers provide "drop in" or intermittent services for clients who need only one aspect of the program. Other centers provide care each day for clients who need continuing supervision while family members are at work or school. The nursing role in these settings may vary considerably. Some settings have advanced practice nurses who plan care and work with families. Others have nurses who provide medication supervision, assessment for ongoing health problems, and who may lead groups in reminiscence, reality orientation, or validation therapy.

Ambulatory Care Dialysis Centers

Individuals with chronic renal failure who need ongoing renal dialysis may be managed by home dialysis or by dialysis performed in a dialysis center. A dialysis center provides an environment where the individual who does not have a family care provider or a home dialysis assistant can go two to three times a week for dialysis. Nurses in dialysis centers must have high-level skills because clients with renal failure who need in-center dialysis usually have the most complex problems and coexisting illnesses.

COLLEAGUES IN HEALTH CARE

Many different groups deliver health care. Various providers exist because they meet the needs of our society in some way. Some groups are believed to provide a valuable service; the services of others are of questionable benefit. There is a short supply of qualified individuals in some areas. In other areas there are enough qualified providers, but the providers tend to be of a single gender or ethnic background. This may pose difficulties for both the client and the care provider when the two are unable to communicate effectively. Many programs are in place that strive to increase diversity among health care providers to better

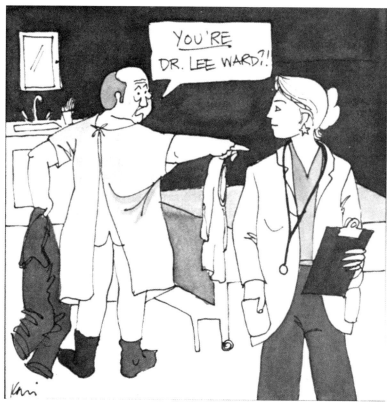

FIGURE 1-3
As the health care workforce has changed, some clients must adapt their perceptions.

meet the needs of all clients. As the health care work force changes, some clients must alter their perspectives to adapt to a wider diversity in health care providers (Fig. 1-3).

More than 230 types of health care workers have been identified within the United States. It is not within the scope of this book to discuss each of these occupations individually, but we do attempt to outline the general categories of health care providers with whom you may be working. Table 1-1 provides an overview of the education and licensure for some of the more common health care providers.

Primary Health Care Providers

The primary health care provider furnishes entry into the health care system. This person is consulted by the client for routine health maintenance, as well as for care of episodic illnesses. This health care provider has traditionally been a medical doctor, osteopathic physician, or dentist. These professionals are licensed in all states and are authorized to treat illness and prescribe drugs.

The planned cornerstone of health care reform has been an increased emphasis on the primary health care provider as the "gatekeeper" for the system. The primary provider

implements health maintenance activities that prevent the need for more expensive care. This individual provides referral to more specialized care when that is needed. Lack of access to primary care has been one of the health care problems for individuals residing in rural areas, economically disadvantaged areas in large cities, and those on welfare programs. The lack of access often has resulted in delaying care until the problem is more complex and requires greater resources to resolve. In urban areas the lack of access to primary care has often resulted in the inappropriate use of emergency room services for routine illnesses. To meet the needs of society, there is pressure to increase the number of professionals who are authorized to deliver primary care.

PHYSICIANS

The term physician refers to the doctor of medicine or the doctor of osteopathic medicine. The differences between traditional (allopathic) medicine and osteopathic medicine are becoming less distinct. Historically, the philosophy of care and remedial techniques of osteopathic physicians included treatments such as back manipulation and nutritional counseling, while allopathic physicians prescribed more drugs and performed more surgery. Osteopathic physicians and allopathic physicians practiced entirely independently of each other and used separate hospitals; a visible antagonism between the two groups was often apparent. The current environment has resulted in greater cooperation, with physicians from both backgrounds practicing side by side in clinics and hospitals. The osteopathic group is considerably smaller, has far fewer specialists, has fewer resources for research, and is less well known. However, the educational patterns for both are the similar.

Undergraduate medical education may vary in focus, but a strong biological science background is required. This is followed by 4 years of medical school. During these 4 years, formal education is stressed, with client contact occurring most often during the latter part of the program. Some medical schools are beginning to provide client contact earlier in the educational process. After completion of medical school, licensing examinations are taken.

Once individuals are licensed as physicians, they must participate in a residency program to prepare for autonomous practice. Although licensed to practice, a physician will not be accepted into any group practice or be awarded privileges at a hospital without having completed a residency. Residency programs are developed by hospitals or health care delivery systems and primarily focus on extensive experiences in providing medical care. The length of these programs varies depending on the specialty. The resident is paid a salary by the sponsoring health care agency. In state, county, and city hospitals the resident physician may serve as the primary physician for some patients, with senior staff physicians or medical school professors providing oversight. For patients who are responsible for their own medical bills (either directly or through insurance), the admitting personal physician usually remains in charge and the resident serves a supporting role in the patient's medical care. At the end of the residency, the resident physician is able to practice independently, in a group practice, or as an employee of a health care agency.

After residency training is completed, the physician is prepared to write examinations to become certified in a specialty. The person who successfully passes the specialty examination is termed *board certified*. It is not legally required that a physician be board certified to practice in a specialty area; certification in family practice increasingly is being considered a requirement for general practice.

Subspecialty training occurs after specialty training is completed. Given this pattern of education and training, a physician may have a total of 10 or more years of postsecondary education and training before beginning to work independently.

PODIATRISTS

Podiatrists (formerly called chiropodists) are educated in the care and surgery of the foot. They care for corns, bunions, and toenails; prescribe and fit corrective shoes and arch supports; and perform surgery on the feet, such as correction of deformities, removal of bunions, and removal of small tumors. A podiatrist does not prescribe systemic medication or care for any generalized disease condition. With an aging society and an increase in sports-related foot problems, the work of podiatrists is receiving more recognition.

NURSE PRACTITIONERS

As demands on the system have increased, additional professionals have been added to the group of primary care providers. Nurses working in specialized roles as primary care nurses and nurse practitioners are examples. These nurses have obtained education in addition to that required for basic licensure (most commonly in a master's degree program) and have earned certification in a particular specialty. Nurse practitioners may work with a physician in an office or clinic, or they may function independently in nursing clinics. Some states grant nurse practitioners who meet special guidelines the authority to write prescriptions. This prescriptive authority is the subject of heated debate in states not providing this option. In some areas, acute care nurse practitioners are being educated to provide medical support in hospitals that historically has been provided only by resident physicians.

Supporters suggest that the increased utilization of the nurse practitioner as a primary care provider is one of the major thrusts of health care reform. They point to geographic availability and cost savings as critical elements. In keeping with this approach, the majority of federal money available for nursing education has been allocated to advanced preparation.

PHYSICIANS' ASSISTANTS

Another primary caregiver is the physician's assistant. This person, sometimes called the *medex*, often has medical and emergency training, perhaps from military service or other health care occupations, and has completed a university program. Physician's assistant programs vary from 1-year programs to 4-year baccalaureate programs. Physicians' assistants must work under the direction of a physician at all times.

Physicians' assistants usually see clients with commonly recurring health problems such as colds, flu, fractures, and cuts needing suturing. Physicians' assistants may also provide some primary health care such as routine physical examinations. If the client needs referral to a specialist or hospital admission, the physician's assistant first refers the client to the physician with whom he or she works. In some instances the physician's assistant may work with a specialty physician such as an orthopedic physician and have responsibilities related to that specialty: applying and removing casts, for example. Some physicians' assistants work with surgeons in the role of surgical first assistant.

The use of physicians' assistants is sometimes controversial. Some clients believe that they are receiving less than quality care if they are treated by a physician's assistant instead of seeing the physician. The appropriateness of physicians' assistants writing prescriptions and orders on the charts of hospitalized clients has been questioned among health care workers. Nurses have been concerned because their own licensure laws sometimes state that they can administer medications only on the order of a licensed physician, osteopath, or dentist, yet, in some instances, nurses are asked to give medications on the order of a physician's assistant.

Another area of concern has been whether nurses working in expanded roles should be classified as physicians' assistants and be governed by the Board of Medicine rather than the Board of Nursing. Some nurses have enrolled in and completed the regular physician's assistant programs and are working in this capacity. Other nurses strongly believe that the nurse in primary care should be considered an independent nurse rather than a physician's assistant. The American Nurses Association (ANA) has supported the position that the nurse in primary care is better prepared to address the whole person's health needs than a physician's assistant.

OTHER PRIMARY CARE PROVIDERS

Social workers and *clinical psychologists* have historically performed a primary care role by providing client entry into the mental health care system, serving as counselors and supervisors of care, and furnishing referrals as needed. Because social workers and psychologists are not able to treat physical problems, they often work in cooperation with physicians or nurse practitioners who are able to manage this aspect of care. Within most health plans, clients can see these mental health workers only on referral from a primary physician.

Social problems, including lack of a social support network and the financial resources for care, create major barriers to accessing health care for many people. Clinical social workers are prepared at the master's degree level and are employed within health care agencies to provide services upon referral. Social workers work with family and significant friends in arranging for the various types of support that permit early discharge and facilitate home care. Social workers sometimes face a difficult task in obtaining financial support for the services they can provide. Some institutional providers and third-party payers are recognizing that social supports may play a very large role in an individual's movement from expensive acute care environments to home care and therefore are increasing their willingness to reimburse social workers for care.

Optometrists provide vision testing and prescribe glasses, contact lenses, and corrective exercises for eye problems. They have a general background in the assessment of eye diseases and can screen clients and refer them to an *ophthalmologist* (a physician who specializes in eye diseases) when diagnosis and treatment are needed. The scope of practice of optometrists is being expanded in some states to enable them to provide more comprehensive eye care. Because ophthalmologists and optometrists offer some of the same services, there is some disagreement between them as to the proper scope of practice for each group. Whether eye examinations and corrective lenses for vision should be part of basic health care is another area of debate in health care reform legislation.

Dentists provide for primary care of the teeth and mouth. Many dentists are beginning to provide general health screening, such as examining the mouth and throat for tumors or disease and taking blood pressure during their basic examination. A client is referred to a physician if an abnormality is noted. Dentists have an educational background similar in length to that of the physician—4 years of baccalaureate education followed by dental school. There is no residency period, and dentists begin independent practice after passing state licensing examinations. Dentists are empowered to prescribe medications in addition to providing care for the mouth and teeth. There are specialty areas in dentistry, such as orthodontics (the application of devices to change the occlusion of the teeth), just as there are in medicine. Education for specialties occurs in universities that have dental schools. After the student has graduated, the diploma indicates competence in the specialty. There is no legal requirement for advanced education to practice a dental specialty, although strong professional constraints exist.

Dental care is one of the basic health care concerns being debated. Certainly dental health is a part of overall health. However, some voices suggest that for health care to be economically viable, we must limit demands and not try to cover every aspect of health for all individuals. The expanded use of the dental hygienist has been suggested as one avenue to broadening the availability of preventive dental services while restricting costs.

Allied Health Care Workers

The Allied Health Education Directory (1995) lists twenty-nine different allied health occupations. Most allied health care professionals (eg, the clinical laboratory technician) provide diagnostic and treatment services that are related to a medical plan for care. Some professionals, such as those who work with records, serve in roles to support the system but do not have direct care responsibilities. Many allied health professions evolved in response to demand for individuals trained to manage complex technology; an example is the perfusionist who manages the cardiopulmonary bypass machine used in cardiac surgery.

Table 1-1 (p. 22) outlines the educational background required of some of these professions. You will notice that some professions require education ranging in length from 1 year (certificate programs) to 4 years (baccalaureate programs). This reveals that education is not standardized in many health professions. The five organizations listed in Display 1-4 provide accreditation for programs preparing these providers.

DISPLAY 1-4
Organizations Providing Allied Health Accreditation

1. Accreditation Council for Occupational Therapy Education
2. Commission on Accreditation of Allied Health Education
    Programs (CAAHEP has 17 separate committees on accreditation that each focus on a different allied health area.)
3. Joint Review Committee on Educational Programs in Nuclear Medicine Technology
4. Joint Review Committee on Education in Radiologic Technology
5. National Accrediting Agency for Clinical Laboratory Sciences

In addition to the allied health programs listed in Table 1-1, new allied health occupations are being added by health care facilities. Over 240 different titles for allied health personnel are found in health related literature. The stated goals of developing new occupations are to provide technical expertise, decrease costs, and offer the expertise of professionals to more clients. Many health professional groups are joining nurses in expressing concern about the trend toward adding assistive personnel who function without education or credentials. For example the American Speech Language and Hearing Association established a task force on support personnel (American Speech . . . , 1995) This task force examined the various issues related to training, credentialing, use, and supervision of assistive personnel in the field of speech pathology, and has made recommendations to the profession regarding these issues.

Below we provide you with information regarding some of the major allied health professionals with whom you may be working on an interdisciplinary team (Fig. 1-4).

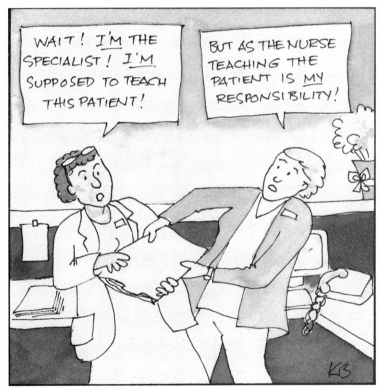

FIGURE 1-4
Overlapping roles and unclear boundaries between health care occupations can lead to conflict.

LABORATORY AND DIAGNOSTIC SERVICES

Included in the category of laboratory and diagnostic technologists and technicians are those who work in the clinical laboratory, such as the medical technologist (MT) and medical laboratory technician (MLT), as well as those who work in specialized diagnostics fields, such as the nuclear medicine technician, the electroencephalograph (EEG) technician, and the radiologic technician (RT). These people assist with all of the tests that are now used to diagnose and monitor the progression of illnesses. As new sophisticated diagnostic technology is introduced, new technicians are created to operate and monitor the equipment. Some occupations, such as the medical technologist's, require a baccalaureate degree. Others, such as the radiology technician's (RT) and medical laboratory technician's (MLT), usually have 2-year associate degrees. Still others, such as the electrocardiographic (ECG) technician's, may be learned on the job.

ADMINISTRATIVE AND BUSINESS PERSONNEL

As health care facilities have become more complex, the administrative and business aspects of health care have become more demanding. Many people are needed to maintain and retrieve information from medical records. These workers include health information administrators, health information technicians, and medical secretaries. The positions of hospital administrator and assistant administrator are changing. In the past these appointments might have been filled by a physician, an attorney, or a nurse. Because the health care system now has such specialized demands, the administrative positions are increasingly being filled by those with a baccalaureate or master's degree in health care administration. A special certification is required for those who administer nursing homes.

COMMUNITY HEALTH CARE WORKERS

As a growing field, community health has required an increasing number of workers. The major focus of community health care is the promotion of health rather than care of illness. Some workers, such as the health educator and community health visitor, work directly with individual clients. Others, such as the sanitarian, are engaged in assisting the community as a whole toward better health through maintenance of standards related to cleanliness and infectious disease control.

Other community health care workers are those who help individuals with health and personal care after discharge from the hospital. Although some of these positions are held by registered nurses who provide skilled care, many more are held by home health aides who assist with nontechnical aspects of care and may even help with household tasks and shopping. Education for home health aides, which in the past was conducted as on-the-job training, now also takes place in courses leading to certification.

MAKERS OF PROSTHETIC AND ASSISTIVE DEVICES

With technological advances, the number of different prostheses and assistive devices increases. Those who make and fit devices such as eyeglasses, braces, and artificial limbs need specialized education. They do not usually have licenses. Most are employed by health

Issues Related to Primary Health Care

One of the problems in U.S. health care is the maldistribution of primary care providers. Urban areas have proportionately more health care workers of every kind than do rural areas. Within large cities, care providers are concentrated in the more affluent areas. Many programs have attempted to provide incentives to establish practices in areas that are insufficiently served. In some of these programs, educational loans are forgiven or canceled if a person works in an underserved area after completing a course of study. In other instances schools have tried to recruit students from underserved areas, hoping that after graduation the students would return home to practice. Some schools incorporate into their programs learning experiences in rural or poorly served areas with the hope that graduates will be attracted to these areas and return later to work.

Despite these efforts, insufficiently served areas still exist for several reasons. Physicians prefer to practice where there is access to specialized medical centers and where opportunities for consultation are readily available. The tremendous physical strain involved in being the only care provider is another factor that deters physicians from practicing in rural areas. The rural physician often receives little respite from 24-hours-a-day, 7-days-a-week availability to the community. The income of a rural physician also tends to be lower than that of a physician in an urban area. Nurse practitioners increasingly are providing health care to underserved populations and have been more willing to relocate to rural or impoverished areas.

Another matter of concern is the number of physicians prepared as specialists relative to the number who act as primary care providers. In the United States approximately 60% of physicians practice in specialties and 40% practice in some area of primary care such as general practice, family practice, pediatrics, and obstetrics/gynecology. This has resulted in too few primary care providers and an excess number of specialists in some areas. Part of the health care reform legislation being introduced provides for incentives and support for those entering primary care practice.

The trend in private medical practice is toward group practices. Several specialties may be represented within a group. Although each client may have a private physician, group practice clients also may receive care from other members of the group. Group practice ensures the individual physician of more time for personal and family life.

Care in private practice is usually based on fee for service. Although some physicians attempt to make adjustments for clients with less ability to pay, one of the serious health care problems of our day is the cost of health care for even middle-class individuals. Insurance may pay for some outpatient care, and it funds most of the care given during hospitalization, but increasing numbers of people are underinsured or have no insurance.

Accreditation of Health Professional Education Programs

Specialized accreditation of programs providing education for health professionals has created nationwide standards when individual state licensing laws have differed greatly. State laws, in most instances, do not require that schools have national accreditation; in some states, however, national accreditation has been accepted in place of individual state monitoring of programs. The various organizations that provide accreditation seek to remain abreast of current practice and to be nondiscriminatory in their decision making.

The Commission on Recognition of Postsecondary Accreditation (CORPA) was a national, nonprofit, private organization that reviewed and approved specific educational accrediting agencies. This organization determined standards for accreditation policies and procedures. Through this national organization, accreditation standards across the United States became more uniform. Although this organization is being discontinued, organizations approved by CORPA will continue to have national approval until they are due for renewal. They then must apply to the Department of Education for approval.

Within the U.S. Department of Education there is now an office that reviews accrediting agencies and associations and publishes a list of those that the Department of Education recognizes as reliable authorities concerning educational quality. Although the Department of Education does not control the organizations offering accreditation and cannot create or eliminate them, the Department's approval confers recognition of standards being met. This federal office began operation a few years ago and is gradually reviewing organizations against their criteria for accreditation. Because application of the Department of Education's standards is new, some organizations are finding that they must make changes in their accreditation systems. A serious concern is that federal requirements are moving away from a system based on the overall professional judgment of colleagues about the quality of programs toward one that uses specific checklists of measurable data that may or may not really measure excellence.

The Pew Reports

The Pew Health Professions Commission supported a series of studies and reports regarding the need for the health professions to meet public needs for health care (Pew Health Professions Commission, 1995; O'Neill, 1993; Shugars et al., 1991). Much of what was reported supported trends others had identified. However, these three reports have generated discussion and controversy among health professionals, educators, and regulators. The final report (Pew Health Professions Commission, 1995) identified four major concerns regarding the future of health professional education and licensure (Display 1-5).

SKILLS NEEDED IN THE FUTURE

The first issue that the Pew Commission addressed was the redesigning of the health care work force. The Pew Commission suggested that the development of excellent generalists

---

DISPLAY 1-5
Pew Commission Recommendations

1. Redesign the health care workforce.
2. Develop an interdisciplinary focus in health professional education.
3. Examine and alter health professional regulations to make them more standardized, accountable, flexible, effective, and efficient.
4. Right-size the health professions, which will include the closure of some nursing and medical schools.

rather than narrow specialists is urgently needed. The trend of much of health care has been toward the development of more highly specialized individuals with extraordinary skills in a narrow field. Although this may provide excellence in certain areas, it does not provide for the overall health support of the nation. There will be an increasing demand for generalists who look at the whole person and focus on prevention and health maintenance.

THE NEED FOR AN INTERDISCIPLINARY FOCUS

The Pew Commission also focused on the consumer's need for interdisciplinary care and on the need for a more organized system perspective. The Commission strongly recommends that educational programs emphasize these needs in the education of all health care professionals.

CHANGES IN REGULATION OF HEALTH CARE PROVIDERS

The regulatory system for both health professional education and for practice settings represents another barrier to effective delivery of care according to the Commission (1995). They set goals that all regulation be standardized, accountable, flexible, effective, and efficient. These regulations affect issues such as entry into practice, the need for demonstrating continued competence on the part of practitioners, and the need for effective systems to handle complaints and discipline. With regard to nursing, the Commission identified the multiple entry and exit points as a strength, but recommended clear differentiation of competencies at each level to guide both educators and employers and to establish clear avenues of articulation among levels.

THE SUPPLY OF HEALTH PROFESSIONALS

For many years, the federal government has supported a variety of efforts to increase the supply of many health professionals. In the 90s, changes in the way health care is delivered have raised questions about whether we need to increase the supply of health professionals or whether we might already have an oversupply in some areas. As hospitals have restructured, nurses have been laid off and are finding it difficult to replace their acute care positions with ones that offer comparable salaries and benefits. Whether this is a matter that requires minor readjustment of the work force or whether it indicates a need for drastic change has been questioned (Fig. 1-5).

According to the Pew Commission (1995), right-sizing the professions will require closing some schools for health care professionals, including some medical schools and nursing programs. The Commission encouraged the closing of whole programs rather than downsizing existing programs in order to attain the greatest cost savings. Within nursing, they recommended the closing of some associate degree and diploma programs in order to reduce the total number of graduates. Some nursing leaders have suggested that the Pew Commission's predicted need for health professionals was based on the current system and has not taken into consideration the real health care needs of the entire population. Finally, the Pew Commission recommends ensuring that foreign nationals who train in the United States return to their own countries after graduation. While addressing over-

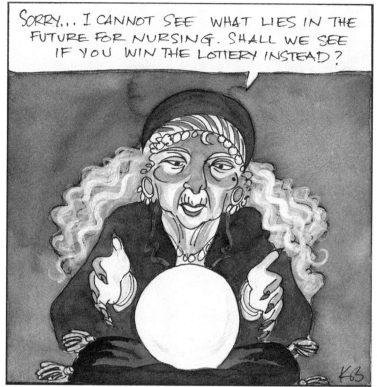

FIGURE 1-5
Exactly what the future holds for nursing is unclear but it will certainly contain change.

supply, the Commission emphasized the need to focus on delivering high quality care while reducing costs.

ALTERNATIVE HEALTH CARE

Professionals in health care often ignore the many alternative avenues of health care that people use, such as health foods, vitamins, chiropractors, and faith healers. When professionals consider these alternatives at all, they often dismiss them as quackery, with little understanding of why people turn to these resources. Increasingly, people are using what were formerly termed alternative therapies in addition to traditional medical care. In these situations, alternative therapies are often referred to as complementary therapies. According to the British Medical Journal (1996) the increase in the use of complementary therapies is a world-wide phenomenon.

Major Types of Alternative Care

The major types of alternative care available are briefly described in the following sections and summarized in Display 1-6.

DISPLAY 1-6
Alternative Health Care Resources

Chiropractic care	Massage therapy
Ethnic/religious traditions	Naturopathy
Health foods	Reflexology
Herbal medicine	Stress reduction techniques
Homeopathy	Visualization techniques
Hypnosis	

THE HEALTH FOOD MOVEMENT

The health food movement in the United States is extraordinarily popular. Countless books are written and innumerable products are produced for this market. One of the appeals of this approach to health care is that it focuses on everyday, natural resources as opposed to science and technology. Poor dietary practices are common in the United States, with many individuals eating far more fat than is recommended and neglecting fruits, vegetables, and whole grains. Many people achieve better health by paying attention to good nutrition.

Medical research is beginning to identify some benefits of using food and vitamins in therapeutic ways. We have long known that many individuals who develop Type II Diabetes later life may be able to manage their blood sugar through dietary control. The role of antioxidants in decreasing cell damage and the effect of certain phytochemicals contained in cruciferous vegetables in preventing bowel cancer are just two examples of the therapeutic benefits of nutrients.

There are hazards in this approach to health care. Megadoses of vitamins may prove toxic. Some nutrients interact with medications, decreasing their effectiveness. Individuals who choose to avoid all traditional medical care and rely on unsubstantiated claims about the therapeutic effects of nutrients may suffer a deterioration in health.

All health care professionals need to support and encourage healthy dietary practices. Often it is possible to assist clients who rely on the use of various nutrients for health care by accepting what they believe helps them, as long as it is not detrimental to their well-being. When you are willing to acknowledge their philosophy and values, these clients may be willing to consider using traditional medical care as well as nutritional approaches.

CHIROPRACTIC CARE

Many people seek medical help from chiropractors. Chiropractic care is a method of treatment based on the theory that disease is caused by interference with nerve function. It uses manipulation of the body joints, especially the spinal vertebrae, in seeking to restore normal function. The chiropractor may also use a variety of other treatments commonly associated with physical therapy, such as massage and exercise. There are definite differences among chiropractors. One group recognizes that there are illnesses that they are not competent to treat and do recommend that certain clients seek medical care. Another group believes that all illnesses may be treated by chiropractic methods and do not refer clients for medical care. A major concern is that some clients may have more serious illnesses that may be missed altogether or not recognized in time to be given optimal medical attention. Another problem with chiropractic care is the use of chiropractic treatments on infants and young children in place of immunizations and other well child services.

Many people with joint and muscle strain and tension find that chiropractic treatments relieve discomfort and support effective functioning. The Agency for Health Care Policy and Research recommends chiropractic treatment as a useful option in specific circumstances for relieving pain and discomfort in acute back pain (ACHPR, 1994).

NATUROPATHY

Naturopathy gets its name from the natural agents used in treating disease, such as food, exercise, air, water, and sunshine. The naturopathic physician treats people by recommending changes in lifestyle, diet, exercise, and the use of vitamins and herbs. For many this is a successful form of treatment. Naturopathic physicians follow a prescribed course of study that includes clinical experiences with clients and results in the doctor of naturopathy (N.D.) degree. Naturopathy is licensed in some states.

HERBAL MEDICINE

The herbalist treats illness by prescribing a wide variety of natural herbs. Many herbalists in the United States are Asian Americans who received their training in herbs during an apprenticeship with an experienced herbalist. As stated previously, naturopathic physicians may also use herbs.

We know that plants often have active ingredients that affect the human body. Digitalis, for example, was originally a dried leaf of the foxglove plant. (Digitalis drugs are now synthesized in a laboratory.) It was indeed a potent and effective medication when it was used as an herb, but dosage was not accurate and there was little scientific information regarding its effects. As research into plant products continues, our understanding of the efficacy of herbs is increasing.

It is wise to recognize the potential problems as well as the potential benefits inherent in the use of herbal medicines. Individual plants may vary in their concentration of active chemicals. This makes accurate and stable dosage of herbs very difficult. Sometimes the active ingredient may have potent side effects. For example, many individuals have used herbs that contain ephedra. Ephedra acts as a stimulant, dilates bronchioles, and decreases appetite. Therefore, it has been used for the herbal treatment of fatigue, asthma, and obesity. It also raises blood pressure, increases pulse rate, and creates feelings of tension and anxiety in some individuals. These side effects have been severe enough to precipitate stroke and cardiac problems in some individuals.

Many herbs are imported from around the world. Rules and regulations regarding labeling and content purity may not be as strict in some countries as they are in the United States. This means that some herbs that are sold may contain contaminants. Serious illnesses and even deaths have been traced to contaminants in herbal medicines.

Clients taking herbal medicines should be encouraged to share this information with their health care provider. They should also be encouraged to question carefully the sources of the herbs that they take. These actions might help clients avoid potentially harmful interactions with prescribed medications, or other adverse effects.

HOMEOPATHY

Homeopathy is based on the belief that exposure to extremely small quantities of either the substance causing an illness or a related substance will stimulate a cure. Of course, this principle is also the basis for immunization and allergy desensitization procedures. The application of this principle to other diseases has not been accepted by the medical community. The dilutions used in many homeopathic remedies are so great that a dosage may contain only a few molecules of a substance. Homeopathy was popular near the beginning of this century, but fell into disrepute as standard medical research advanced. There is currently a resurgence of interest in this approach to therapy and some new research is being done. Homeopathic practitioners are reemerging as an alternative to standard medical care. Some naturopathic doctors also use homeopathic remedies.

ETHNIC AND RELIGIOUS HEALTH CARE TRADITIONS

Native Americans, Hispanic Americans, Asian Americans, and many other ethnic groups have traditional health care resources that are still used by many people. Often termed *folk medicine*, these traditions are usually handed down by word of mouth and are used to treat common health problems. Treatment often involves the use of herbs and foods as well as traditional ceremonies. Little is understood about many of the herbs used, but some have demonstrated therapeutic effects. Within an ethnic group there may be people who are designated as healers or people with special knowledge and ability in regard to illness. The advice of such a person may be sought instead of the advice of a physician. In order to work most effectively with a client who uses folk medicine, you will need to investigate the specific beliefs and resources that he or she is using.

Every major religion of the world responds in particular ways to those who are ill. A well-established way for caring religious persons to support an ill person and for an ill person to seek support from others is through prayer. Nurses recognize that spiritual distress has a significant impact on a client's ability to move toward wellness. Supporting the individual's quest for spiritual solace and healing has been a part of the mission of many health care agencies that were established by religious bodies. The separation of prayer and spiritual care from other health care is a very modern phenomenon.

STRESS REDUCTION MECHANISMS

Relaxation and stress reduction are also examples of alternative approaches to health care. Relaxation exercises, breathing techniques, meditation, and visualization are used to reduce anxiety, reduce blood pressure, and lessen the body's response to stressors. These techniques are designed to prevent stress-related problems from developing; for many people, they are part of a plan to increase health and well-being. The use of these techniques is also suggested for the management of specific health problems.

OTHER ALTERNATIVE THERAPIES

There are a wide variety of other alternative therapies in use. Managing low back pain through a carefully developed exercise program and a reduction in life stress may provide

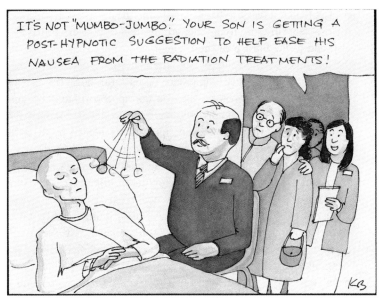

FIGURE 1-6
Alternative health care is moving more and more into mainstream practice.

longer lasting relief of pain than medication. Some individuals with migraine headaches use biofeedback control over circulation to abort migraine attacks rather than using medications. Such approaches may be used in conjunction with traditional medical treatment.

Massage therapy causes relaxation, raises endorphin levels, and is believed to enhance circulation. Reflexology, or massage of the feet, is used to enhance the body's immune system and stimulate effective physiological functioning throughout the body. Visualization may be used to help children manage painful medical procedures. Suggestions regarding healing and postoperative recovery are now used in the operating room by some anesthesiologists and surgeons. The anesthesiologist may talk to the patient who is still anesthetized, suggesting that pain will be minimal, nausea will not occur, and recovery will be rapid. This is similar to posthypnotic suggestion. Hypnosis has been used in other illnesses for symptom relief. (Fig. 1-6).

Understanding the Use of Alternative Health Care

For many clients with chronic conditions, traditional health care has offered few options. Long-term treatments often produce their own set of iatrogenic health problems, some of which are as troubling to the individual as the original disease process. A common response to these problems has been to add more medications and more treatments, each with their own potential adverse effects. Traditional health care providers often give little attention to the problems of daily living that are of greatest concern to the individual. Stress and anxiety also add to the burden of these clients.

For clients with acute health care conditions, certain treatments or medications that are prescribed may produce unpleasant or harmful side effects. Clients are often looking for alternative treatment methods that do not appear to have the same potential for harm.

Some alternative therapies have been available for many years and there are people who believe that they have been significantly helped by these alternative approaches. Unfortunately, traditional health care providers have often dismissed these therapies without investigating them thoroughly. Few alternative therapies have been formally researched, and proponents rely on undocumented reports of effectiveness.

Part of the appeal of alternative health care is the caring and personalized response that clients often receive. People who have been intimidated by businesslike clinics, and made to feel unimportant by impersonal professionals, may find that the warm, concerned, accepting atmosphere of the nonconventional setting meets many personal needs. The fact that stress and anxiety play a major role in any health problem may help explain why many people are helped by therapies that may not be based on sound scientific knowledge.

Research into alternative therapies is now being supported by the federal government, but only in a small way compared to other research. Increased attention is being paid to the responses of individuals. Concern about the role of stress in illness has prompted an increased openness to nonmedical methods of managing stress. The possibility of alternative care practices working in a complementary fashion with traditional medical care is gaining wider acceptance. Often these complementary therapies are used in order to address the whole person and not simply the disease.

Assisting Clients Who Choose Alternative Health Care

Many people who support conventional methods of health care have long ignored or repudiated the value of unorthodox health care traditions. We must recognize that alternative health care practices have persisted because people have found them to be valuable. Acknowledging health care alternatives and working cooperatively with them is usually much more productive than trying to oppose them.

One problem that clients face in seeking complementary or alternative health care is the lack of assurance that a practitioner they consult is well trained and ethical, because there are usually no universally accepted alternative health care standards (Lynn, 1996). Traditional health care providers have an obligation to assist their clients in formulating questions that reveal a practitioner's background, education, and training. We must help our clients to identify and avoid those alternative care providers who engage in unethical or harmful practices.

Many health care providers now support the use of various complementary therapies. According to Norton (1995) such issues as client choice, informed consent, and the ethical principles of beneficence and nonmaleficence (see Chapter 9) must all be considered in relation to alternative therapies. As alternative and complementary therapies move into the mainstream, greater accountability to the public is essential.

KEY CONCEPTS

- Many different types of agencies provide health care services; examples include long-term care settings, acute care hospitals, ambulatory care centers, home care agencies, and health care businesses among others. There are a wide variety of nursing roles in these different settings.
- Health care agencies are classified according to length of stay, type of service provided, and ownership of the agency.
- Long-term care facilities provide many types of care. Nursing homes provide care for those without the ability to manage activities of daily living and who need ongoing care. Assisted living centers provide fewer services. Rehabilitation centers assist the individual in returning to a maximum level of independence.
- Ambulatory care settings provide care on an outpatient basis. This care may range from simple office calls for common illnesses and health promotion activities such as immunizations to the performance of ambulatory surgery.
- Community agencies offer a wide variety of care services that may include traditional public health services, high intensity skilled care in the home, and rehabilitation services. Home care agencies offer services within the home that assist individuals in avoiding institutional care settings when they are unable to complete their own activities of daily living.
- Changes in the health care delivery system are creating a number of problems that affect health care workers. Among these, as presented by the Pew Commission, are issues related to primary care, accreditation of health professional education programs, and the future of health professional education and licensure.
- Alternative health care is growing in popularity. Some types of alternative care are being used along with traditional medical care as complementary therapies. Understanding the different types of alternative health care services, why people choose alternative health care, and how you may assist people who seek this care will form a foundation for more effective relationships with clients.

Critical Thinking Activities

1. Investigate a hospital or nursing home in your community. Find out about its average length of stay, the types of services it offers, and its type of ownership. Analyze its overall contribution to health care in your community.
2. Identify an agency in your community that offers home health care. Investigate the services offered by this agency. Compare these with the list of possible services offered by home care agencies mentioned in this chapter. If the lists do not match, analyze the factors in your community that may be responsible for the difference.
3. Choose an allied health profession other than nursing. Investigate the current education requirements for that health profession in your state. Identify the usual responsibilities associated with this profession. Provide a carefully supported argument for or against legal licensure for this health profession.

text continued

and 1974 provided the impetus to start new HMOs. Health maintenance organizations orig-inated as an alternative to traditional insurance plans. Although traditional insurance plans paid for care when subscribers were ill, health maintenance organizations were the first to provide payment for care aimed at preventing illness. Health maintenance organizations provided well child care, prenatal care, immunizations, pelvic examinations, and other pre-ventive services when insurance companies did not. A flat charge per month covered routine preventive health care, care for illness, hospitalization and, in some instances, prescription costs, outpatient care, and other services. Currently, HMO-enrolled individuals are respon-sible for some type of copayment (meaning the client pays a part of the bill). Copayments support part of the cost of care and give the consumer an incentive to use services wisely.

HMOs are characterized by different patterns of finance and governance. Some are operated by insurance companies, some are private profit-making organizations, some are nonprofit organizations, and still others are consumer owned and operated. Many newer HMOs operate as business entities that manage the financial aspects of health care and, through financial management, access to services. Consumer Reports magazine (1996) has reported that there is greater consumer satisfaction with nonprofit HMOs. As financial and governance patterns have changed over the years, there are fewer distinctions between HMOs and managed care plans provided by insurance companies.

HMOs are also characterized by different patterns of providing health services. Primary health care providers may be employed by an HMO and receive a fixed salary. In some cases, a group of primary health care providers, termed an independent practice association (IPA), may contract with an HMO to provide services for a preset fee per individual in the program. HMOs may also employ many other health care workers, including nurses. In some HMOs clients have a choice of care providers; in others they do not. HMO plans that allow an individual to choose to go outside of the plan for services that the plan does not or will not provide are called *point-of-service* plans. Usually the subscriber is eligible for some reimbursement of costs in these plans, but at a greatly reduced rate. Two examples of HMOs are described in Display 2-2.

Because the HMO receives the same income (except for modest copayments) whether a client requires extensive care or very little care, there is a built-in incentive to emphasize preventive care and avoid costly hospitalization. HMOs usually require that care be au-thorized or approved for payment before it is provided. Clients identify the required HMO approval of any type of care as a major problem. An HMO may not approve or pay for care that it considers nonessential. If a health care provider and an HMO consultant disagree about which type of treatment is appropriate, the client often feels caught in the middle. This situation frequently occurs in emergency care.

In some HMO plans, a subscriber who needs emergency care and is outside of the appropriate service area is subject to what is called the standard of the ''prudent consumer.'' This means that if a prudent lay person would consider the symptoms an emergency, the plan will pay for care. Thus, if a person with chest pain goes to an emergency room, the plan will pay even if the chest pain turns out to be esophageal reflux. In other HMO plans, the standard is more rigid and relates to the final medical diagnosis. A plan with more rigid standards would pay an individual who visited the emergency room with chest pain only if the final diagnosis were myocardial infarction, but would not pay if the final diagnosis were esophageal reflux.

Some HMO plans require that an individual travel to a designated hospital when an

DISPLAY 2-2
Health Maintenance Organizations

THE KAISER FOUNDATION HEALTH PLAN

This nonprofit organization began in California and Oregon owns and operates its own hospitals. The physicians are members of a group that contracts with the organization to provide medical services. The fee for membership covers almost all health care costs, including both outpatient and inpatient costs. Kaiser Health Plans are now available in many states.

GROUP HEALTH COOPERATIVE OF PUGET SOUND

Located in Washington State, this HMO is a consumer-owned and operated cooperative that owns and operates its own clinics and employs physicians and other health care providers. For most of its history it also operated its own hospitals but is gradually closing down inpatient services, maintaining a birthing center and outpatient surgery services, and contracting for most other hospital care. People who join the cooperative as members pay a monthly fee for comprehensive health care, which includes both outpatient and inpatient services. The membership elects the governing board; members serve on policy-making committees; and a vote of the entire membership decides some issues. In addition, Group Health Cooperative contracts with employers to provide comprehensive, prepaid coverage for employee groups. Members of the employment groups are not members of the cooperative unless they pay a separate membership fee. The employer may pay the monthly fee directly or the employee may pay the fee through payroll deduction.

These two organizations are currently exploring joint operations in order to provide multi-state health care coverage.

emergency is not life-threatening. Thus, one consumer was denied payment for a fractured ankle sustained while skiing because it was not life-threatening and because the injury was treated in the skiing community rather than back home in the consumer's designated hospital.

Because HMOs have lower health care costs than conventional fee-for-service systems, the federal government has subsidized the creation of new HMOs and has encouraged employers to offer HMOs as alternatives to traditional health insurance plans. This has speeded the development of new HMOs. Federal subsidizing of HMOs also helps to contain costs in all health plans as a result of competition. People on Medicare now have the option of joining HMOs. Under such circumstances, Medicare makes capitated payments directly to the HMO. This may limit the flexibility of the individual to seek care outside the HMO, although some HMOs are offering plans with higher copayments that allow the individual to seek care from any desired provider.

State-Administered Health Plans

States may operate a variety of health care resources for residents. All states manage some type of insurance plan for workers injured on the job. These workers' compensation plans may be managed as a state monopoly or may be contracted to private insurance companies.

Employers are required to pay premiums based upon statistical information about covered injuries and hazards in various job categories. An individual injured on the job is assured of receiving care paid for by the workers' compensation plan.

Some states administer health insurance plans. Hawaii assures universal health care coverage for residents of that state. Minnesota has been a leader in attempting to provide health services for all of its residents. The State of Washington has developed an insurance plan called the Basic Health Plan for working individuals who earn too much money to be eligible for tax-supported health care, but who do not have incomes high enough to be able to afford regular insurance. Although this plan cannot accommodate all who are eligible, it is a significant development.

The federal government also provides funds through the Medicaid programs that are administered by the states and matched with state funds. Included in this funding are the costs of nursing home care for those who have exhausted their personal financial resources.

Most states support state mental hospitals and public health services. Further public health services may be provided through county and city governments. Hospitals designed to provide care for those who are indigent may be operated by the city (such as the New York City hospitals) or by the county (such as Cook County Hospital in Chicago)(Figure 2-1).

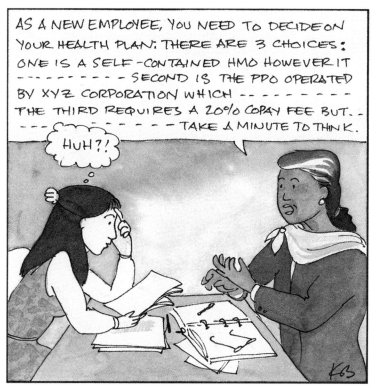

FIGURE 2-1
Health care insurance plans are complex and often confusing to the ordinary consumer.

Federal Government Programs

The federal government in the United States has been deeply involved in health care financing. Federal programs cover the elderly, the poor, federal workers, the military, veterans, and Native Americans and Native Alaskans. Some individuals are concerned about governmental involvement in our health care system; when all of these programs and agencies are considered together, it is clear that, for good or ill, the federal government already controls many aspects of health care.

MEDICARE AND MEDICAID

In 1965, after years of effort and testimony by many health-related groups (including the ANA), and with widespread public support, an amendment of the Social Security Act was passed. Title XVIII of the act, which was termed *Medicare*, provided payment for hospitalization (Part A), and insurance that could be purchased to meet physicians' fees and outpatient costs (Part B), for people over age 65 and certain others who were receiving social security payments. Medicare is administered through a federal agency called the Health Care Financing Administration (HCFA–pronounced ''hik-fah'') which uses contracted companies termed *Medicare intermediaries* to process claims.

The complexity of filing claims with Medicare and also with an insurance company designed to supplement Medicare coverage is confusing for many people. Some providers process all paperwork, but others do not. Even when claims are filed by the provider, they may be denied payment if they do not conform to specific rules and regulations. Often elderly people accept an initial denial of payment for the claim as the final decision and do not pursue the matter further. There is a high rate of reconsideration when denials are appealed; therefore, it is often wise to encourage clients to appeal a denial of payment.

Many HMOs and insurance companies are seeking the business of those on Medicare. The plans they provide supplement what Medicare pays and often cover all health care. This usually comes with a loss of choice for the consumer, a feature some individuals do not understand when they sign up for such plans.

Title IX of the Social Security Act, which was termed *Medicaid*, provides funds for health care for those dependent on public assistance. Each state is responsible for administering Medicaid: the state determines eligibility and level of coverage. Payments from the federal government to the states are administered by HCFA. Benefits vary greatly among states. California's plan, called Medi-Cal, has historically been one of the most comprehensive. As health care costs have risen, there has been great pressure to cut this program. A few states have not participated in the Medicaid program in order to avoid federal control. Some states have requested waivers from HCFA's usual regulations governing Medicaid and Medicare to allow experimentation with different plans that might help to control costs.

Medicare and Medicaid are important health care resources, but they have not been without problems. Costs have been much greater and have been rising faster than anticipated. There has been a great deal of publicity about instances of abuse, and even fraud, associated with these two programs. The goals of providing cost-effective health care to the elderly and the indigent through these programs have yet to be achieved.

Impact on Nursing. The Medicare bill contains many provisions that have made a significant impact on nursing. A definition of skilled nursing care in the original bill was narrow and excluded many important aspects of care necessary to maintaining the health of clients. Through later efforts and testimony, nursing organizations were instrumental in getting legislators to recognize that the definition of skilled nursing was a critical matter; as a result, a Senate subcommittee asked the ANA to study skilled nursing care to provide background data for the Senate. Amendments to the Medicare/Medicaid Act of 1972 encouraged study of alternative ways of providing health care in order to contain costs. These alternatives included the use of nurses in expanded roles and the use of HMOs.

Cost-Containment Initiatives. Amendments to the Medicare/Medicaid Act were also responsible for mandating review and evaluation of health care. This was done in the interests of cost containment. Institutions must review records of Medicare/Medicaid clients and compare them with specific criteria for care.

In 1982, the 97th Congress revised Medicare to prevent the serious financial deficits in the system that escalating costs could potentially create. The revisions increased the premium for Part B of Medicare (the optional portion that provides for out-of-hospital and physician care) and also increased the deductible that the individual must pay for covered service. The system of payment was changed to prospective payment based on diagnosis-related groups (DRGs). (See the discussion on patterns of payment later in this chapter.) The planners who revised Medicare also included a new mechanism for reimbursing hospice care.

In 1993, more changes, restrictions, and controls were instituted in the Medicare system: the payroll deduction for Medicare increased; the length of stay was further shortened; and rehabilitation and convalescent services moved from acute care environments to newly created subacute units in long-term care facilities and in hospitals. Many procedures that previously required an inpatient stay became outpatient services.

In 1996 the news media again began predicting serious financial problems for the Medicare system in the near future. The growing numbers of elderly, the rising costs of medications, supplies, and wages, and the widespread use of costly, highly technical therapies have all contributed to escalating health care costs. Despite all of these concerns, Medicare and Medicaid have provided health care dollars and services to many people who would otherwise have done without.

MILITARY HEALTH CARE

The military branches of the Defense Department operate hospitals and clinics for service members and their families, and also finance health care through civilian health providers in an extensive program known as CHAMPUS. The latter program allows individuals to select care providers in their community who are reimbursed in much the same way that insurance reimburses for care. Both active and retired military personnel and their dependents are covered by this comprehensive federal program, which includes inpatient, outpatient, preventive, and diagnostic services and also provides for prescriptions.

OTHER FEDERAL HEALTH CARE PROGRAMS

The Public Health Service has historically operated hospitals for merchant seamen and the Coast Guard. These facilities are also available to veterans and certain government employees. Many of these public health hospitals have been closed in recent years and the care transferred to community resources. Individuals are then covered by an insurance reimbursement plan.

Within the Department of the Interior, the Bureau of Indian Affairs has operated hospitals and clinics on Indian reservations and in native villages in Alaska. Care in these settings is sometimes minimal, limited by a low budget.

The Department of Veterans' Affairs operates many hospitals and nursing homes for veterans. These are found all across the country. For those who are eligible for care from the Veterans' Administration, benefits are comprehensive.

MANAGING THE RISING COSTS OF HEALTH CARE

Two of the major problems facing the health care system are rising costs and accessibility for all individuals. These two issues are related in that cost is one of the factors that can limit access to health care.

Understanding Increasing Costs

Many factors contribute to the rising costs of health care (Display 2-3). One important factor in cost increase is the price of new technology. New and more sophisticated diagnostic and treatment devices are being invented each year. The rising cost of technology affects every area of the health care field from the cardiac care unit to the laboratory.

An increasing population needs a greater number of facilities, and the construction of new care facilities also contributes to rising costs. In addition, existing facilities often require modifications. More space is needed for various new technologies both at the bedside and in many hospital departments. Computer systems are used more often for the documentation of care. Bedside computers that enable documentation to be done at the point-of-care decrease the amount of time required for "paper-work." More offices and conference rooms are needed. The regulations governing hospital construction have also become more stringent, requiring more fire safety and infection control measures, and protection against environmental hazards. All of these factors combine to make the "per bed" cost of new hospital construction or remodeling increasingly expensive. Additionally, the decrease in the length of hospital stay and the move to outpatient services have left many hospital beds

DISPLAY 2-3
Contributing Factors in Rising Health Care Costs

- Price of new technology
- Construction of new facilities
- Higher survival rates leading to greater need for costly intensive and/or long-term care
- Growing population of elderly adults requiring health care
- Rise in salaries for health care workers
- High costs of drugs and health-related equipment

unused. Unoccupied hospital beds create a major drain on organizations, because large sums of capital investment are tied up and not returning any income.

The average length of hospital stay for standard diagnoses has been steadily decreasing. The typical client in today's hospital is rapidly discharged to convalesce at home or in a long-term care facility, leaving behind only the very acutely ill. Many clients who would have died quickly in earlier years live through a crisis but require long and intensive care. All of these factors make the acuity level of a client today much greater. This in turn requires more intensive observation and care and the use of more specialized equipment.

The population as a whole is growing older and, statistically, the elderly have an increased incidence of all chronic illnesses. A greater percentage of the population requires health care on a regular basis and may depend on medications, treatments, and therapies for continued functioning.

Until recently, the salaries of health care workers (except for physicians) were far below those of the general society. To remedy this, for a time salaries of health care workers rose more rapidly than the general inflation rate. Physicians also had an increase in income greater than the relative inflation rate until the mid-nineties, when changes in the system began to affect income levels for physicians.

Companies that manufacture health-related devices and drugs reportedly have some of the highest profits in industry. These companies have justified their profits as appropriate relative to the risk and cost involved in their research and development activities; however, some critics think that these companies have taken advantage of the public's dependence on their products.

Lack of competition in the health care field is one factor that may contribute to higher costs. Although physicians continue to be primary gatekeepers in the system, the advent of other primary care providers, such as nurse practitioners and nurse midwives, has offered alternate and less costly care for many routine problems, and for normal life processes such as pregnancy and childbirth. However, there has been opposition to allowing these practitioners to operate in collaborative rather than dependent or subsidiary roles.

One attempt to increase the availability of nonphysician care has been the movement to obtain legislation requiring that government agencies and third-party payers (eg, insurance companies) pay the nonphysician (eg, the nurse practitioner) who provides primary care service. The traditional pattern required that payment always be made to a physician, who in turn paid the nonphysician provider. Progress has been made in regard to third-party reimbursement for nurses in primary care; however, this continues to be a problem and a major thrust of political pressure by nurses (American Medical Association, 1995).

As health care costs have continued to rise, third-party payers have used a variety of methods to control costs, including changing patterns of payment and controlling the actions of providers (Fig. 2-2).

Changing Patterns of Payment

Understanding the various methods of paying for health care services will help you understand what is happening in the various organizations and agencies involved in the health care system.

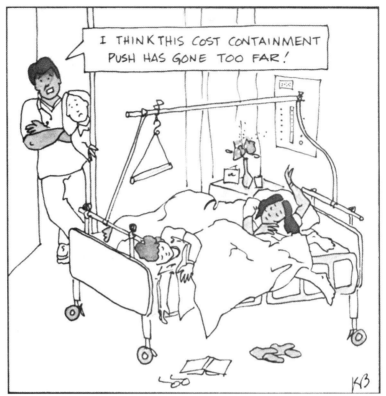

FIGURE 2-2
Federal legislation is encouraging hospitals to stop the rapid rise of health care costs.

FEE-FOR-SERVICE PAYMENT

Fee-for-service payment means that each time a service is provided, a fee is generated and then billed to the recipient of care. The more services provided, the more fees charged. This can be compared to ordering each dish in a restaurant separately and having each appear as a separate charge on the bill. This is the traditional method of charging for health care in the United States. Initially, fees were almost all paid by private individuals. When insurance companies began assisting with payment, the individual's bill was sent to the insurance company as well as to the client. The insurance company then paid its share (for example, 80%) and the client was required to pay the rest.

As costs rose, insurance companies began setting a standard rate of reimbursement. Under this system, if a policy stated that a company reimbursed at 80%, this meant 80% of a fee that the insurance company determined was reasonable. If the provider charged more than the reasonable fee, the client was responsible for the excess, in addition to 20% of the "reasonable" fee. Insurance companies usually set these fees based on statistical analysis of prevailing fees in a geographic area. In a time of rapid inflation, providers complained that there was often a serious discrepancy between the fee used for calculating benefits and the actual fees being charged.

PROSPECTIVE PAYMENT

A *prospective payment* is a reimbursement amount for a procedure or illness that has been determined in advance of the provision of service. This predetermined amount is paid without regard to actual costs in individual situations. Unlike fee-for-service payment, which reimburses each individual item of service provided, prospective payment is based on a fixed reimbursement amount for major illness or procedure categories such as "uncomplicated myocardial infarction" or "hip fracture." The third party payer determines the reimbursement amount based on statistical analysis of costs and a determination of the average length of hospital stay. If the costs are less than the prospective reimbursement, the hospital will make a higher profit, and if the costs are greater, the hospital will lose money. This form of payment is designed to provide an incentive for hospitals to control costs. Another advantage to payers in a prospective payment system is that costs are predictable. This system transfers the burden of risk (the chance that an individual may require extraordinary services) from the payer to the provider. This system can be compared to a fixed price for a dinner at a restaurant that includes appetizer, salad, main dish, dessert, and beverage. If you choose not to have the dessert, you will still be charged the same amount. For the person who wants all four items, the fixed price typically is cheaper than paying for each item separately.

DIAGNOSIS RELATED GROUPS

The major change in the method of payment for health care services began on October 1, 1983, when the federal government stopped using a fee-for-service reimbursement system for Medicare, and introduced a prospective payment system using *diagnosis related groups* (DRGs) to determine the payment for each person admitted to the hospital. This change was designed to stop the spiraling costs of Medicare and to correct inequities that made the costs of care in one facility very different from those in another facility.

Calculation of Costs. The method of determining the rates to be paid in the Medicare prospective payment system—the creation of DRGs—resulted from a computerized analysis of costs that had been billed for hospitalized individuals in the past. This analysis led to the formation of categories of medical diagnoses that require similar treatment, and for which costs are similar. Each category (or DRG) has a name and number; for example, DRG 236 is "fracture of the hip and pelvis." In addition, a decision was made to increase the payment for care when another illness or condition is present. This second condition is termed a *comorbidity*. Thus a person with heart failure whose basic DRG is "fractured hip" is designated "fractured hip with congestive heart failure." A hospital receives greater reimbursement for providing service to this person because care is more complex and costs higher. Hospitals also receive additional amounts for cases that are determined to be "outliers." An *outlier* is a case in which the client stay significantly exceeds the average. The number of days needed to qualify a case as an outlier is predetermined. For example, the average length of stay for DRG 236,"Fractured hip and pelvis," is 6.2 days, but the stay must reach 29 days for the case to be considered an outlier.

Most hospital costs are included in the DRG reimbursement. The actual DRG reimbursement amount is calculated each year by HCFA through a complex formula that considers the area of the country in which the care was provided (Northwest, Southeast, etc.), the urbanization of the area (rural, suburban, etc.), and the type of care required. Some hospital costs are still being reimbursed separately. In the past, these included costs for medical education and research conducted by the hospital; however, pressure is mounting to stop this separate payment. The goal is to include all costs in one reimbursement figure. Physician costs are also being paid separately, but some suggest that these should eventually also be included in the single rate.

Most of the controversy surrounding the implementation of DRGs has not concerned the incentives for cost control, or the prospective reimbursement system itself, but rather how the payment amounts are determined and how the system is being administered. There are conflicting studies regarding whether the DRGs adequately reflect the intensity of nursing care required (Halloran & Halloran, 1985; McKibbin et al., 1985; Yasko & Fleck, 1995). Another concern is that clients are reportedly discharged after much shorter stays, when they are still in need of care (this is the "quicker and sicker" concern—clients are discharged quicker and feeling sicker). Some alterations and modifications of the system will continue to be made but the basic prospective plan probably will remain in place.

Implications for Nurses. There are a variety of implications for nurses in the current DRG system. The availability of documents that reflect the acuity level and multiple problems of a client when records are audited for compliance is essential. The need for discharge planning is always present but is more critical as the length of stay becomes shorter. A longer length of stay significantly increases the costs to the hospital; therefore, nursing actions that prevent complications, that avoid inappropriate scheduling, and that facilitate early discharge are important. Nurses in home health agencies and long-term care facilities are caring for clients with complex nursing needs. A major concern is whether the DRG reimbursement system provides adequate funds for quality nursing care to be delivered, and whether hospitals, in their attempt to cut costs, will cut quality of care as well.

In addition to Medicare, many states are adopting systems similar to DRGs, and some private insurance carriers are now using these basic concepts in their cost-control efforts. Therefore, DRGs will continue to be an issue of concern to nurses.

CAPITATION

Capitation is yet another way of determining payment. In a capitated system a fee is paid to a provider organization for each person (each "head," thus the term) whether or not that person uses any health care services. This shifts an even greater share of the risk of providing health care from the payment organization to the provider organization. Providers in a capitated system have an incentive to guide individuals to low-cost outpatient services or other care environments rather than to the acute care hospital. A goal of this payment system is to encourage preventive services that may make high-cost interventions unnecessary. Thus, in a capitated system you may find that services such as mammograms, immunizations, stop-smoking clinics, and back-injury classes do not have any copayments attached, or the copayments may be quite low. A criticism of a capitated system is that when the provider is at risk for providing care, there may be an unconscious (or even deliberate) attempt to deny needed care to keep costs down. In some capitated systems consumers have complained that they were unable to obtain services they believed were appropriate. Health maintenance organizations were the original capitated systems.

Controlling Health Care Providers

Third-party payers and government and public agencies have all used different approaches to try to restrain rising health care costs.

CERTIFICATES OF NEED

To add new high-cost equipment or additional client care facilities, a health care institution may be required to apply for a certificate of need. This establishes that there will not be unnecessary duplication of services in an area and that a need for them exists. For example, if every hospital purchased magnetic resonance imaging (MRI) equipment that was used to only one fourth or one third of its capacity, the cost per use would have to be higher to cover the investment and maintenance costs than if the device were used to capacity.

In many states nonprofit hospitals must make application for rate increases. In their applications, they must document all the factors contributing to the need for an increase. Hearings are held, and permission for rate increases is given only when the evidence indicates that all possible economies are being observed. Private, profit-making hospitals are not held to these rules.

PREFERRED PROVIDERS

In an attempt to contain costs, third-party payers such as insurance companies, HMOs, and managed care organizations sometimes negotiate with providers of health care to provide certain kinds of care at an agreed-upon, usually lower, price. The third-party payers then provide incentives for clients to use these "preferred providers." These incentives may include the waiver of all or part of copayments by the insured, or coverage of additional conditions or situations.

Preferred provider organizations (PPOs) may be hospitals, nursing homes, corporations employing care providers, or groups of care providers who have cooperated to negotiate more successfully with third-party payers for these special contracts. The advantage to the provider is the assured number of clients and the guaranteed income. In a time of competition in health care, this may be a significant advantage. Each PPO operates independently without government regulation; therefore, the exact structure and contractual arrangements are independently determined.

MANAGED CARE

Managed care refers to any system in which the use of health care services is carefully controlled and monitored to ensure that policies are followed, that neither too much nor too little care is provided, and that costs are minimized. Owens (1995, p. 5) identifies managed care more specifically as "a system to control the cost of health care by using a select group of providers who have agreed to a predetermined payment, with the clinical interventions being managed via utilization and/or a case management process." A managed care plan can be controlled by the payer (such as an insurance company), may include both payers and providers, or may be a business entity that serves only as a go-between. HMOs have always acted as managed care systems.

In a managed care system there is always someone assigned to the role of "gatekeeper." This person monitors and restricts the use of services by the client. In most managed care plans the primary physician is expected to serve as the "gatekeeper." The physician sees the client first and then determines whether referral or diagnostic services are needed. In some managed care systems, the primary physician has decision-making authority. However, in many managed care systems, the actual gatekeeper is a plan manager who must be consulted regarding the use of services. A written request for referral may be required before the client receives permission for a referral. This may delay or deny needed care and is one source of consumer dissatisfaction with some managed care plans. Physicians express dismay over a mechanism that allows a nonphysician who has never seen a client to make critical decisions about the care needed.

Managed care controls extend to such matters as the medications that can be prescribed. There may be a specific formulary of drugs for which a managed care company has negotiated purchase at very low prices. For many conditions, there are clear therapeutic equivalents and medication restrictions are not a concern. For the person with a chronic health condition who has been stabilized on specific medications, however, moving into a managed care plan may pose a very real threat to health maintenance if the plan will not approve the client's current drugs.

CASE MANAGEMENT

Case management is a technique used in some managed care systems to efficiently move an individual requiring major health services through the system. According to the Case Management Society of America (CMSA), case management is "a collaborative process which assesses, plans, implements, coordinates, monitors, and evaluates options and services to meet an individual's health needs through communication and available resources to promote quality cost-effective outcomes." (CMSA, 1995) Case managers are most commonly assigned to high-risk clients, such as those with chronic illnesses or major traumas, who will require rehabilitation. In some settings, the case manager specializes in a particular group of high risk clients, such as those with diabetes, and is referred to as a "disease manager."

The case manager is an experienced health professional with knowledge of available resources who oversees or monitors a case to ensure that necessary care is instituted promptly and is provided in the most cost-effective setting. Nurses have often assumed the role of case manager. In this role, the nurse monitors the care as it is provided, ensures that appropriate referrals are made, that changes in the plan of care are instituted appropriately, and that the care follows established standards. Because of their understanding of the whole person, both physiological and psychosocial, and their understanding of how the system works, nurses are particularly well-suited to this role. The CMSA provides a system for certifying professional case managers.

Case managers may operate within only one part of the system—for example, managing cases from admission through discharge in a hospital. These managers are often referred to as *internal case managers*. Some may manage cases across all phases of care from outpatient through hospitalization, rehabilitation, and back to outpatient. These individuals are termed *external case managers*. At their best, case management systems ensure that there are not delays in patient transfer or breaks in communication, and that costs are minimized through efficiency. Case managers often act as advocates for clients in the system. Physicians sometimes object to what they see as the interference of the case manager in a decision-making process that used to include only the client and the physician.

VERTICALLY INTEGRATED HEALTH CARE SYSTEMS

Organizations contracting to provide managed care are also expanding their own control through the development of *vertically integrated systems*, that is, those that provide every level of health care service. A vertically integrated system may have contracted physicians, laboratories, a hospital, a subacute facility, a rehabilitation facility, and a home care agency. This allows the contracting organization to offer managed care corporations a package that provides care at all levels for each enrolled member of the managed care plan for a capitated fee. The contracting organization then has an incentive to control costs through decreasing the use of high-cost services and more effectively using low-cost alternatives. It is also in a better position to negotiate with the managed care system in regard to reimbursement. As large systems develop in this manner, hospitals become a cost center rather than a revenue center. This merging of systems is resulting in the closure of hospitals in many communities.

USING ACUITY MEASURES TO DETERMINE COSTS

Health care providers who are negotiating contracts and planning care need very accurate data regarding the specific cost of each type of service. One way of trying to understand and control these costs is through the development of *acuity* measures. Acuity in this context refers to how acutely ill a person is and how much skilled care is required.

Various ways of measuring acuity in both general hospitals and psychiatric settings have been devised. Most systems use categories that reflect the different types of care needed. Each of these categories is assigned a numerical value on a scale of 1 to 4 (or on a similar scale). All applicable category values are then summed and compared with a standard. For example, an acuity measuring system might have one category reflecting the need for assistance in personal hygiene. As a person needs more assistance, more points are assigned. Another category might reflect the amount of time needed for monitoring vital signs: the more time required, the more points assigned. Each category is assigned an appropriate number of points, and the total is computed. The points identified for an individual client are then compared with a standard and the client is assigned an acuity level. Clients with the fewest points are level 1 and require the least care. Those with the most points are level 4 and require the most care. Each system in use has its own scale for determining acuity. Acuity values are sometimes called "intensity measures" because they reflect the intensity of care needed.

In some settings acuity levels or intensity measures are being used as a mechanism for determining the staffing needs of a client care unit. Acuity levels are also used as a means of billing for the level of nursing care needed, and are reflected in a variable rather than flat charge for the nursing portion of a client's room charge. It has also been suggested that prospective reimbursement might be based on acuity level rather than on medical diagnosis because acuity levels reflect the real impact on resources more accurately than do medical diagnoses (DRGs Reflect Nursing Resources, 1985; Biordi, 1995).

Other Cost-Containment Measures

In many medical facilities, personnel are now being asked to become cost conscious. Cost consciousness involves such ordinary measures as being conservative with telephone use, canceling meal trays when clients are discharged, and using expensive supplies with care. Nursing personnel must also be aware of the tremendous cost of any complication or additional length-of-stay. Preventing complications and getting clients ready for early discharge has become a major focus of care. Care pathways are specifying care and identifying outcomes for each day of hospitalization with the goal of assuring that resources are used wisely. Physicians are being asked to judge carefully the necessity of diagnostic studies and costly procedures. Some diagnostic studies must be preapproved by the managed care organization. In some hospitals physicians are asked to consult with pharmacists before prescribing certain high-cost drugs to determine whether a low-cost therapeutic alternative exists. Although the latest aminoglycoside antibiotic might be effective, for example, an inexpensive first generation cephalosporin antibiotic might also be effective and cost 90% less. When all medication costs must be covered by a prospective payment, the hospital has a strong incentive to limit physicians' choices. Many physicians are upset about these cost-containment measures because they may interfere with the physician's independent decision-making.

Hospitals with a large population of extra-high-risk clients (eg, the very elderly or poor) have expressed concern that discharging a client for convalescence in a home with a caring family, good food, and a clean environment is very different from discharging a client to an impoverished environment. Many believe this should be considered when determining regulations for length of stay. The proponents of shortened stays point out that shortened stays have been very effective cost-containment measures. They argue further that a client's lack of a support system is a social problem and that hospitalization cannot be used to solve social problems.

The federal government has sought to control costs for Medicare and Medicaid by establishing higher deductibles (the portions that individual clients must pay) and by limiting the fees that the government will pay. Because the elderly and the poor are often unable to pay these deductible amounts, they become liabilities for health care providers, who cover these costs by collecting higher fees from those who do pay their bills. Medicaid costs have also been contained by tightening eligibility requirements, which shuts more people out of the health care system.

All of these efforts at reducing costs have affected the health care system in areas other than cost containment. They have affected decision-making processes, power structures, the kinds of care provided, and the ways that individual health care providers practice. It is important to recognize the full impact that cost containment has had.

ACCESS TO HEALTH CARE

Access to health care refers to the ability of the individual to obtain and utilize needed services. Access can be an economic issue, a geographic issue, or a sociocultural issue (Fig. 2-3).

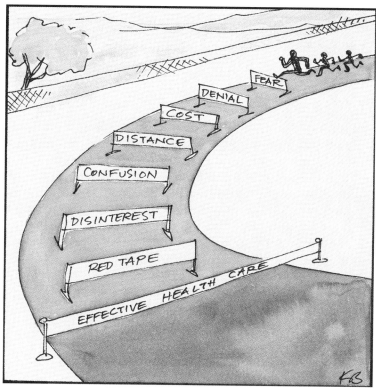

FIGURE 2-3
Despite the many different sources of health care financing, a family may face obstacles to obtaining effective health care.

Economic Access

Creating access for those who are economically disadvantaged requires that providers consider many factors. In addition to providing a family with a prescription, for instance, a provider must also make sure there is a way to fill that prescription. It is not enough to prescribe a special diet without ensuring that the individual will have the necessary knowledge and resources to follow that diet.

Coverage by third-party payers also affects economic access. As more small businesses find their health care benefit costs escalating, they may begin to eliminate these benefits. Individuals and families whose incomes are marginal may be unable to purchase insurance because of the high cost of individual policies. Although giving people an incentive to use services wisely is the stated goal of raising deductibles and copayments, the result for some families may be the delay or avoidance of timely care.

Some individuals are unable to obtain health insurance because of preexisting illnesses. These are often the people who are most in need of health care services. Another group concerned about being denied insurance coverage are those with the potential for serious health problems. As genetic testing for potential health problems has become more widespread and the information gleaned from it more exact, insurance companies have been using the results of these tests as a basis for denying coverage to healthy individuals. As more tests become available, this issue will be a growing cause for concern, especially as it relates to access to health care.

Geographic Access

Geographic access to health care is a special concern for those in rural areas. As changes have occurred in the health care system, small rural hospitals have found themselves unable to compete or to manage financially. When a rural hospital closes, residents lose hospital access as well as many diagnostic services. Most health care providers prefer not to work in an area where no hospital is available to provide diagnostic and treatment services; consequently, rural communities are finding it difficult to recruit health care providers.

Geographic access may be a concern for those in urban areas as well. Economically depressed areas of large cities have fewer health care providers, thus forcing the residents of those areas to travel long distances, often using inconvenient public transportation, in order to receive health care. The Healthy People 2000 Report (Public Health Service, 1992) recommended that health care services be made available in locations such as work sites and schools in order to improve access.

Access to health care is also affected by whether all services are available in one location. It is not uncommon for individuals to be required to visit several geographically separate locations in order to receive all needed health care. Some organizations are now offering a single *point-of-service*, meaning one geographic location where providers can take care of all needs. A single point-of-service makes it unnecessary for an individual to go to one location to see a primary provider, to another to see a specialist, to still another for diagnostic tests, and to yet another location for procedures. The single point-of-service makes efficient use of the client's time, lessens the likelihood that the client will fail to follow through with recommended procedures, and simplifies communication between providers.

Sociocultural Access

Sociocultural differences also affect access. When individuals feel uncomfortable in a setting because of their socioeconomic status or because their cultural background and beliefs are not respected, they are reluctant to use the services provided. Making care culturally accessible may mean having translation services, materials in multiple languages, and care providers who understand and are sensitive to cultural differences.

Access to health care is discussed further later in this chapter, in association with key indicators of system effectiveness (Fig. 2-4).

MAINTAINING QUALITY IN THE HEALTH CARE SYSTEM

A wide variety of mechanisms are used to maintain quality within the health care system. Two of the most important are accreditation standards and evaluation processes.

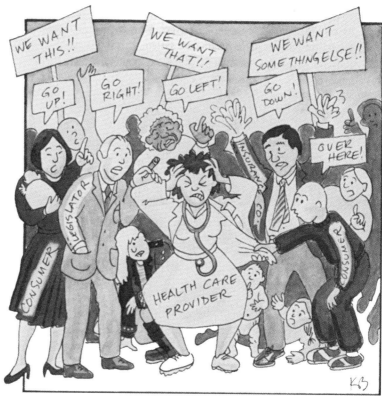

FIGURE 2-4
The impetus for change in health care delivery has been growing.

Accreditation of Health Care Institutions and Agencies

Institutions and agencies providing health care must usually be approved by the governmental jurisdiction in which they are located. Approval may take the form of state licensing, which is usually focused on maintaining minimum standards in order to safeguard public health.

Medicare requires health institutions and agencies that seek payment from its programs to meet specific standards and be Medicare certified. These standards relate to many aspects of care. By designating those to whom payment will be given, Medicare effectively exerts control. Because the costs of private care are so high, most people choose to receive care where it can be reimbursed. When care is not reimbursable, individuals may make other choices.

Health care institutions and agencies may also seek accreditation from nongovernmental bodies that set standards for high quality and provide guidelines to assist in developing policies and procedures. Medicare and Medicaid have granted several of these nongovernmental agencies what is called *deemed status*. This means that the standards of the agency are "deemed" to equal or exceed the Medicare standard. Therefore, a health care agency that has been accredited by the voluntary process is "deemed" to meet the standards set by Medicare and Medicaid, and is not required to pursue an additional accreditation process.

Hospitals, nursing homes, and related organizations may seek accreditation from the Joint Commission on Accreditation of Healthcare Organizations (JCAHO). This is a non-profit, voluntary organization originally established by the American College of Surgeons and the American Society of Internal Medicine to set standards for hospital care. Today's organization has a board of directors with members from a variety of health care and public occupations. The standards of this organization are comprehensive and involve evaluation of the structural aspects of institutions, policies and procedures, and the outcomes of care provided. JCAHO has deemed status for federal programs.

The Community Health Accreditation Program (CHAP) is a separate arm of the National League for Nursing that was established to provide a voluntary accreditation system for community health and home health agencies. This is a peer-reviewed process governed entirely by community health agencies with public representation. This organization has deemed status for Medicare and Medicaid certification.

The National Committee for Quality Assurance (NCQA) reviews and evaluates health maintenance organizations. This is a relatively new, independent nonprofit organization developed by the HMO industry. NCQA has established a set of statistical measures called Health Plan Employer Data and Information Set (HEDIS). These data provide a standard set of information that both employers and consumers can use to compare and evaluate HMOs. Included in the HEDIS data set are nine indicators of quality, seven of which are related to processes and two of which are related to outcomes. Most of these data relate to prevention and not to the effective diagnosis and treatment of illness. The organization's plan is to expand this data set to include more clinical data. Because the data have only been collected for a short time and because all HMOs are not using the same methods for collecting data, the HEDIS statistics have limited value for comparison even though they do provide some important information (Brooks, McGlynn, & Cleary 1996).

Evaluation of Health Care

A variety of evaluation mechanisms are used within the health care system. Some involve evaluating agencies providing care and others involve evaluating client outcomes.

PEER REVIEW AND QUALITY ASSURANCE

The first systematic evaluation of health care services provided to the consumer was established through the Professional Standards Review Organization set up by Medicare and Medicaid. As part of the 1982 revisions of Medicare, the evaluation process was altered to require that hospitals contract with an external medical review organization, called a Utilization and Quality Control Peer Review Organization (abbreviated PRO). These organizations have been established through contracts awarded by the Secretary of Health and Human Services through competitive bidding. Most of the PROs are statewide in scope and are required to have a substantial number of physicians represented in the organization to effectively set standards and review care.

Evaluation may include preadmission, preprocedure, concurrent, or retrospective reviews. The purpose of the reviews is to determine whether care given was necessary and whether it was given in the appropriate manner. For example, the reviews have resulted in an increase in the number of outpatient surgeries (day procedures) performed, and a subsequent decrease in the number of inpatient surgeries. These changes have resulted in significant economic savings. The PRO is also required to evaluate outcomes of care to ensure that the changes made do not jeopardize clients.

OUTCOME MEASUREMENTS

The federal government compiles statistics related to health care outcomes. These include infection rates and morbidity and mortality rates associated with specific hospitals and procedures. In 1995 the federal government began releasing these figures to the public. Health care providers have opposed the release of these numbers without an explanation, fearing that the figures may be misinterpreted. For example, a particular hospital might have the highest maternal–infant mortality in the state, but it might also be the same tertiary care center that serves the greatest number of high-risk pregnant women or women with the most serious complications of pregnancy. Thus the statistic does not reflect a low quality of care but rather the provision of care in the most problematic situations. The government statistics may be helpful in evaluating some aspects of care, however. When a client is considering a particular type of cardiac surgery, for example, specific data regarding the number of those surgeries performed, the percentage of complications, and the associated mortality rates may be useful in comparing one institution with another that also offers the same type of cardiac surgery. One result of outcome studies has been the recommendation that only hospitals that perform a specified number of highly technical surgeries (for example, cardiac surgeries) each year should offer those procedures. Hospitals that perform fewer procedures per year have higher complication and mortality rates.

Evaluating Care. Individual institutions are also establishing ways to measure the outcomes of the care they provide. Outcomes refer to data such as the number of clients admitted with a fractured hip who had uncomplicated recoveries leading to effective rehabilitation and the number of clients who had complications or did not recover. Knowledge of outcomes is essential for planning and, increasingly, for effective marketing. Often data have been collected but are scattered among many different records and are difficult to retrieve. Because data only become valuable for planning when it is organized in a useful framework for analysis, health care agencies have been moving rapidly to the computerization of data and the implementation of standardized protocols for data collection.

The Clinical Pathway. One of the standardized tools used in monitoring outcomes is called the *clinical pathway*. This is also referred to as a critical path, a care map, or an anticipated recovery path. The clinical pathway describes the optimum progression through the system of the individual with a particular health problem. By establishing the desired outcome for Day 2 of the postoperative fractured hip client, it is possible to determine when an individual client is not meeting this desired outcome. The advantage for the individual is that care may be modified immediately to address whatever problem is occurring. The advantage for the system is the ability to aggregate data across all clients and begin to examine what it is working well and what needs to be changed.

POWER IN THE HEALTH CARE SYSTEM

Part of trying to understand any system involves examining some of the unique sources of power and authority within it. If we define power as ''the capability of doing or accomplishing something'' (Ellis & Hartley, 1995, p. 93), then understanding how power is distributed and used in the health care system will help us to function more effectively. Smith (1994) states that as health services and educational preparation for health professions undergo systemic changes, we must give attention to the allocation of power within these services and education systems. Sources of power unique to the health care system are the authority to decide who may enter and leave the system, who may practice within it, and how funding will be controlled.

Regulatory Power

The primary regulatory agencies in health care are governmental bodies. These agencies administer licensing laws that govern who is allowed to practice. There are also agencies that approve or accredit institutions that educate personnel for health care and licensing, or approve those that provide services. Through regulation these agencies have a profound effect on how institutions operate.

Nongovernmental agencies such as the Joint Commission for the Accreditation of Health Care Services (JCAHO) have a great deal of power. For example, although nursing experts taught for years that individualized nursing care plans were important for clients, such plans were often not written. When individualized plans of care were required by JCAHO standards, however, hospitals began putting time, energy, and money into systems for documenting plans of care. Although the JCAHO standards do not mandate any specific format for a plan of care, they do require a method of determining from the record what a particular plan is and how it is being carried out, and proof that the outcomes of a plan are being evaluated.

Financial Power

Because they represent the financial interests of large groups of people and control payments for services, third-party payers have the power to demand changes in the health care system. When they were first established, these agencies did not see their role in health care as anything beyond a financial relationship. As health care costs rose, these agencies began to look for ways of controlling costs to maintain their competitive place in the insurance market. They have set increasingly rigid criteria for payment for services. The standard rates set for payment for procedures have tended to place some restraints on charges (although actual fees often are slightly ahead of payment schedules). By determining whom they will pay for services, insurance companies reduce the choices available to those who carry insurance—and subscribers usually must select from the choices available if they wish to be reimbursed. Third-party payers therefore exert a more powerful influence over institutions and care providers than do individual subscribers.

Physician Power

Physicians historically have had almost unlimited power within the health care system. They determined who entered the system and when, they decided if and when other services and personnel would be used, and they determined when clients would leave the system. As other agencies and professionals in the health care system have obtained some power and independence, the overall power of the physician has diminished. As a group, physicians have opposed changes that would disperse power in the system, arguing that they are the most educated and knowledgeable of all health care providers and that their professional judgment should be accepted. Those favoring increased distribution of power have argued that more competition, more choice for consumers, and input from a greater variety of health care providers will make the system more balanced and more responsive to individual consumers. Despite changes, physicians are still very powerful within the health care system. For example, although the consumer may pay the costs of health care through a third-party payer, the physician is the "customer," who chooses services and whom the facility tries to please by providing those services, supplies, and schedules preferred by the physician.

However, constraints are increasingly being placed on physicians. Payers are reviewing plans for care and refusing reimbursement when care does not follow their established guidelines. Many hospitals routinely review costs associated with care ordered by physicians, and sometimes restrict the physician's ability to order certain high-cost drugs and procedures because payers provide only a flat daily fee that does not extend to cover high-cost items. Care pathways may demand that physicians provide standardized care that leads to quick discharge. These constraints on practice have been disturbing to many physicians. Most health care reform proposals include limitations on the power of physicians in the system.

Consumer Power

The sources of power previously discussed present problems for the client because the client is excluded from them. Clearly the client is involved in only the most basic aspect of entry into the system: determining that he or she needs care. The client cannot enter any institution without the express approval of a physician. The client has no control over who becomes a primary care provider, and, with the advent of HMOs and PPOs, may have limited choice in selecting providers. Funding is usually controlled by third-party payers, and the client is often powerless to determine who will be paid, how much will be paid, and when payments will be made.

Consumers do have rights in the health care system. These are stated in different ways by different institutions and groups, but all revolve around the recognition of the health care consumer as an adult with the ability and right to be self-determining. As a general rule, consumers are not aware of their rights, and even when they are aware they may be reluctant to take of advantage of them. Consumers are in a particularly vulnerable position in the health care system. Because they depend on those within the system for life itself, they are often reluctant to complain or request changes for fear of offending those on whom they depend. When consumers try to exert power within the system, they may be met with resistance, and comments such as "Well, you really do not have the background to understand this issue." Consumers are most often effective in exerting power in the system by working in groups and through established committees and agencies.

The reduction of consumer choice in providers and the consumer's lack of influence over the larger system are some of the concerns that are raised by health care reform. Another concern is that individual insurance coverage may not include certain types of expensive or experimental care. This is of particular concern to those who are diagnosed with hard-to-treat types of cancer; often new treatments continue to be designated as experimental when they are the only alternative available. Consumers are becoming vocal in their demands for care they perceive to be of benefit.

Nurse Power

Nurses historically have had limited power in the health care system, a situation that has its roots in many of the traditional aspects of nursing. Most nurses were women, employees of institutions, and economically unable to take risks. In addition, nursing education did not prepare nurses to try to change the system, but rather to function within it.

As changes leading to health care reform are occurring, nurses sometimes feel that their power is decreasing. When economics are a driving force, as they are in health care reform, those who argue in favor of quality of care may feel that they are not heard. The public in general, and politicians in particular, may have little understanding of the scope of nursing practice and its value to the client. The focus in health care reform has sometimes been on obtaining the cheapest care from the cheapest provider rather than on providing optimum care (Fig. 2-5).

Nevertheless, things are changing in nursing. Nursing education programs try increasingly to educate nurses to act as client advocates and agents of change. Nursing organiza-

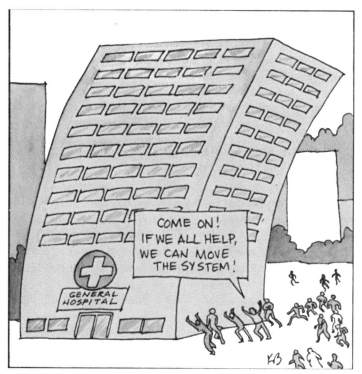

FIGURE 2-5
To have the necessary power to influence the health care system, nurses must develop effective group action.

tions are working to provide nurses with a voice at higher decision-making levels in health care. Collective bargaining and shared governance have provided nurses with mechanisms for demanding recognition of the importance of their role and for being participants in decision-making processes.

Change may not occur as rapidly as desired, and nurses are often frustrated because of their inability to influence the system. Many new graduates are especially distressed to learn that, as individuals, they cannot affect the system. Somehow they expect that if they speak with a voice of reason and act in the best interest of their clients, others will respond positively. By understanding the political realities and the ways in which decisions are made, and by working together to speak with a united voice, nurses may increase their power within the system.

CONTINUING CONCERNS IN THE HEALTH CARE SYSTEM

There are ongoing concerns in the health care system relating to the actual use of health care services by the public, and to the structure of the system itself.

Effective Use of Health Care Resources

Key indicators are specific, measurable aspects of health care that show the effectiveness of the system as a whole and indicate whether access to services is available. Family planning resources, prenatal care, child health statistics, adult health statistics, and dental health information serve as key indicators of effective use of health care resources. In the last 10 years, these key indicators have shown a lack of improvement in access in most areas and, in some areas, even diminishing access (Center for Health Economics Research, 1993).

One example of how a key indicator provides information is a study of contraceptive use by sexually active women. Between 1982 and 1988 contraceptive use by sexually active women in general increased. Public spending for contraceptive services fell by 40% during the 1980s. Teenagers and poor women were less likely to participate in family planning visits in 1988 than in 1982. This demonstrates that while most women were using more contraceptive services, low-income groups were not using these services. Therefore, the conclusion is that there is an economic barrier to access to contraceptive health care services (Center for Health Economics Research, 1993).

In 1990, despite widespread publicity regarding the effectiveness of prenatal care in improving birth outcomes, less than 65% of black and Hispanic women received early prenatal care. There are approximately one-fourth fewer obstetric care providers in low-income than in higher-income areas. Pregnant teens and pregnant black women are more likely to have low-birth-weight babies, and the white to black infant mortality gap has widened since 1990. These indicators appear to represent an access problem created by distribution of resources and possibly exacerbated by cultural barriers (Center for Health Economics Research, 1993).

Childrens' health is evaluated by examining physician visits, immunization rates, and hospitalizations for preventable problems. Whereas privately insured children had an average of 3.4 physician visits per year, those on Medicaid averaged 6.0 visits per year, and those without insurance averaged 2.8 visits. For those on Medicaid, many visits are to hospitals or clinics rather than to primary care providers. There is a concern that this use of emergency services is an inappropriate use of resources for those on Medicaid. Low-income areas have low immunization rates and have 44% fewer physicians who care for children. This health outcome is related to geographical access (Center for Health Economics Research, 1993).

For adults, concern about access focuses on such health services as cancer screening (Pap smears, mammography, and rectal examinations) and availability of ambulatory care. Whereas only 5% of cervical cancer in nonpoor women is diagnosed late, 14% of cervical cancer in poor women is diagnosed late. Elderly adults in poor neighborhoods are more likely to be hospitalized for asthma, congestive heart failure, and pneumonia—conditions that could be treated with effective ambulatory care (Center for Health Economics Research, 1993).

Dental problems respond very well to health promotion and disease prevention strategies. The fluoridation of the community water supply, fluoride toothpaste, dental sealants, and regular oral care all make a significant difference in dental health. However, dental visits for the purpose of education and establishing appropriate dental care habits vary by income—only 53% of those who are poor receive these services, whereas 83% of the nonpoor visit dentists. This has resulted in economic differences in overall dental health. The discrepancy in patterns of dental care is even more pronounced for poor adults compared to nonpoor adults (Center for Health Economics Research, 1993).

Changing the System

We refer to the health care system in the United States as if it were an organized entity, with each part relating to the others in a systematic way. In reality the current situation is more like a nonsystem of many diverse people and organizations, each moving in their own direction. There has been no central authority in the U.S. health care system, no setting of priorities, and no general planning for resource utilization. There are private components and governmental components, nonprofit sectors and profit-making sectors, with individuals and groups all operating independently.

Although this nonsystem has been chaotic, it has produced some of the most significant advances in medicine and health care. Yet, there is a maldistribution of the benefits of those advances; the high infant mortality rate in the United States, for example, which exceeds that of many other major industrialized nations, reflects an imbalance in the distribution of health care (Healthy People 2000, 1992). Some people receive outstanding health care in the most modern of settings. Others receive no health care. Health insurance grows ever more expensive, and many working people are unable to afford coverage for their families. Society is staggering under the increasing costs of governmental programs such as Medicare and Medicaid.

The impetus for change continues to grow. Several states have already instituted efforts to create a more coordinated health care system for their citizens. In recent years, several bills for health care reform were considered by the United States Congress, but none passed. This did not slow the change, but redirected its focus from the governmental sector to the private sector. No one can predict the details of the future system with certainty, but we have tried to point out the major changes currently occurring and the directions in which the new health care system is moving.

Throughout the world there are concerns about health care and its costs. European nations and Canada have long had socialized systems of health care that provided for the needs of all residents. Health outcomes as measured by immunization rates and infant mortality rates have been excellent. In these systems too, however, costs have risen at a rapid rate. Increasing numbers of older citizens have health care needs that are costly to meet. Problems such as unemployment decrease the number of individuals supporting the system. Attempts to control costs have often created long waiting periods for some types of care.

Throughout this chapter we have referred to changes occurring as part of the health care reform process. Some of the specific changes being debated in the political arena are discussed in Chapter 3. In whatever way the system is changed and restructured, nurses will have some continuing concerns.

Nurses are most concerned about client well-being in the midst of a powerful system. As pressures to change increase, nurses continue to speak out for consumers. Who will help consumers cope with their health problems and those of their families? Who will assist them in negotiating the various parts of the health care system? Will the individual identities and unique needs of consumers be addressed or will each person be treated as the mythical "standard client"?

Another important concern of nurses is whether that aspect of health care that we call "nursing," with its focus on the individual, will be maintained. Will the pressures for demonstrating cost-effectiveness result in a loss of caring because it is not always quantifiable? Will the system recognize the critical thinking skills and abilities of nurses as well as their technical skills? Will many educated and skilled nurses be replaced by unlicensed assistive personnel? The future poses many as yet unanswerable questions!

KEY CONCEPTS

- The financing of health care is complex and involves insurance companies, health maintenance organizations, preferred providers, and governmental systems.
- Cost increases have created stress in the health care system and resulted in a variety of approaches to cost containment. A variety of mechanisms for controlling costs and improving patterns of care have been instituted. The federal government has played a major role in the development and implementation of these mechanisms.
- Access to health care must be considered in terms of economic access, geographic access, and sociocultural access.
- Quality of care can be measured and assured by a wide variety of mechanisms. Institutions and agencies providing care receive oversight in the form of governmental approval and accreditation and certifying organizations.
- Power is exerted within the health care system by those who control finances and those who control resources. Historically nurses and consumers have enjoyed little power in the system. Both are working to gain recognition and to more significantly affect the way the system functions.
- There are continuing concerns in health care regarding the effective use of health care resources and changing the health care system.

Critical Thinking Activities

> 1. Identify clients you have encountered from a variety of social, cultural, and economic backgrounds. Given these clients' needs and backgrounds, what type of practitioner would best meet their needs for primary care? What barriers might they meet in trying to gain access to primary care? What might you do to assist these individuals?
> 2. What cost-control measures have you seen in places where you have had clinical practice? Analyze the effects of these cost-control measures on client care.
> 3. Power in the health care system is being actively sought by nurses. How might nurses in the settings with which you are familiar increase their power?
> 4. What changes are occurring in the health care systems in your community? Analyze how these changes may affect nursing practice.

REFERENCES

American Medical Association, Again on the offensive. Am J Nurs 95(8):64–67, 1995

Biordi DL. Accounting for nursing costs by DRG. J Nurs Admin 25(1):6–8, 1995

Brooks RH, McGlynn EA, Cleary PD. Quality of health care: Part 2: Measuring quality of care. N Eng J Med 335(13):966–970, 1996

Case Management Society of America. Standards of Practice for Case Management. Little Rock, AR: Author, 1995

Center for Health Economics Research. Access to Health Care: Key Indicators for Policy. Princeton, NJ: The Robert Wood Johnson Foundation, 1993

DRGs reflect nursing resources. Hospitals 59(19):56, 1985

Eroding care, cuts in RN staff anger AJN readers. Am J Nurs 96(7):69–73, 1996

Halloran E, Halloran DC. Exploring the DRG equation. Am J Nurs 85(10):1093–1095, 1985

How Good Is Your Health Plan? Consumer Reports 61(8)28–42, Aug 1996

McKibbon RC, Bimmer PF, Galliher JM, Hartley SS. Nursing Costs and DRG payments. Am J Nurs 85(12):1353–1355, 1985

Moccia P. Curriculum revolution: Agenda for change (p. 63). New York: National League for Nursing, 1988

Owens C. Managed care organizations. New York: McGraw-Hill, 1995

Public Health Service, Healthy people 2000: National health promotion and disease prevention objectives: Summary Report. Boston: Jones and Bartlett Publ, 1992

Smith GR. Power and health care reform. J Nurs Educ 33(5):194–197, 1994

Yasko JM, Fleck A. Healthcare reform and cost containment in oncology care: Prospective payment (DRGs). Oncol Nurs Forum Apr. 22(3):491–502, 1995

FURTHER READINGS

Angell M, Kassierer JP. Quality and the medical marketplace: Following the elephant. N Eng J Med 335(12):883–885, 1996

Baker CB. School health policy issues in the 1990s. Nurs Health Care 15(4):178–184, 1994

Ballard KA, Gray RF, Knauf RA, Uppal P. Measuring variation in nursing care per DRG. Nursing Management 24(4):33–36, 1993

Blumenthal D. Quality of health care: Part 1: Quality of care–what is it? N Eng J Med 335(12): 891–894, 1996

Buerhaus PI. Managed competition and critical issues facing nurses. Nurs Health Care 15(1):22–27, 1994

Buxton FL Jr. Health care reform hits the laboratory. What (almost) happened in California. Laboratory Medicine 26(2):113–117. 1995

Drayton-Hargrove S, Woods JH. Ethical analysis of health care reform: Implications for diverse communities. Assoc. Black Nrsg Fac Jrnl 6(4):99–103, 1995

Grimaldi P. New PPS rules take effect. Nursing Management 25(11):39–40, 1994

Infante MC. Legally speaking: The legal risks of managed care. RN 59(3):57–59, 1996

Keepnews D, Stanley S. Managed care and nursing's principles. Am Nurs 28(7):5, 1996

Mitchell PH, Krueger JC, Moody LE. The crisis of the health care nonsystem. Nurs Outlook 38(5): 214–217, 1990

Porter-O'Grady T. Building partnerships in health care: Creating whole systems change. Nurs Health Care 15(1):34–38, 1994

Porter-O'Grady T, Wilson CK. The leadership revolution in health care. Gaithersburg, MD: Aspen, 1995

Smith GR. Power and health care reform. J Nurs Educ 33(5):194–197, 1994

Stahl, DA. Subacute care: Creating alternative, Maximizing reimbursement for subacute care.(RUGS III), Nursing Management 26(4):16–17, 1995

The Political Process and the Nursing Profession

The struggle for power is a pervading feature of politics; thus, politics in general as well as the politics of nursing requires the learning of power. (Kalisch & Kalisch, 1982)

Objectives

After completing this chapter, you should be able to

1. Explain the relevance of the political process to nursing.
2. Discuss seven ways you might influence the political process.
3. Outline the current U.S. federal governmental role in health care.
4. Explain common state legislative concerns.
5. Discuss common local political concerns.
6. Discuss the reasons for the existence of the large numbers of nursing organizations.
7. Discuss the major purpose of each specialized organization presented in the chapter.
8. Analyze the ways that nursing organizations seek to affect the health care delivery system and the political processes that control it.
9. Identify how politics is relevant to your participation in organizations.

KEY TERMS

Allocation of resources
Americans With Disabilities Act (ADA)
Appropriations Act
Authorization Act
Conditions of participation
Department of Health and Human Services
Hatch Act
Lobbying

Minimum data set (MDS)
Nurse Practice Act
Occupational Safety and Health Act (OSHA)
Omnibus Budget Reconciliation Act (OBRA)
"Ontario Plan"
Political action committees (PACs)
Resident assessment protocols (RAPs)

Politics is the way in which people in a democratic society try to influence decision-making and the allocation of resources. Because resources (money, time, and personnel) are limited, it is necessary to make choices regarding their use. There is no perfect process for making optimum choices, because whenever one valuable option is chosen, some other option must be left out. Politics is a part of every organization and a part of government at every level. In this chapter we present the political process as we discuss some of the current issues in regard to political decisions and describe ways you can play a role in the political arena and in nursing organizations.

RELEVANCE OF THE POLITICAL PROCESS FOR NURSES

Nurses have always been involved in politics. Florence Nightingale used her contacts with powerful men in government to obtain supplies and the personnel she needed to care for wounded soldiers in the Crimea (Woodham-Smith, 1983). Hannah Ropes was able to fight incompetence and obtain decent care for wounded Civil War soldiers because she understood who the influential people in Washington were and who would be receptive to her efforts on the soldiers' behalf.

Modern times are no different. With all the many different voices competing to be heard in the decision-making circles of any nation, the person who understands power and how the system works is better prepared to achieve desired ends.

Health care is costly, and public dollars can be and are spent in many ways to provide health care. What part of the federal budget should be allocated to health care? What part of the state budget? The local governmental budget? Of the money allocated, what part should be used for preventive health programs? What part for research? What part for care and treatment? What part for education? These questions are answered by legislation and administrative decisions made by governmental agencies. How can the individual citizen affect these decisions?

Nursing organizations are confronted with similar questions. What is the role of the organization? Should resources be spent only on benefits for members? On activities related to general health care? In the political arena? How can nurses affect decision-making? What is my role as an individual nurse within the organization?

If you have opinions regarding an appropriate government role in health care, then politics is for you. If you disagree with current priorities, then politics is for you. If you have ever been blocked in your attempt to provide health care to a client and family because funds or programs were not available, then the political process is relevant to you.

Your practice as a nurse is controlled by a wide variety of governmental decisions. One of the most basic is the Nurse Practice Act of your state. In that document, nursing is defined legally, and the scope of nursing practice is outlined. This document affects what you do each day that you practice. All of the philosophical discussions about the role of the nurse must return to the reality of the nurse's role as legally defined in the state's practice act. Do you care what that role is now or what changes are made in it? Does it make any difference to you what education is required by that law, or if that law requires continuing education? Answering "yes" to any of these questions underlines the relevance of the political process for you.

Many decisions are made within the various nurses' organizations. These organizations speak for nurses in a variety of settings. Are you happy with the way they are spending funds paid in dues? Do you agree with all of the public statements they make? Do you support their mechanisms for decision-making? Are you happy with the image of nurses and nursing the public receives from these organizations? Do you care what these organizations do with their resources? The political process is an important part of their functioning, too.

INFLUENCING THE POLITICAL PROCESS

You as an individual can have an effect on such things as what health care legislation is submitted, the content of the legislation, and what legislation is passed. However, this does not happen without effort and action. Historically, women have been less active in politics than men. This has been the result of a variety of societal factors. Gradually women are assuming a more active role in politics: more are running for and being elected to office, more work with policy-making bodies, and more vote. Because the majority of nurses are women, this changing social climate is important to nursing. Nurses, in particular, have demonstrated increasing political awareness, and some statistics suggest that one in 17 women voters is a nurse and one in 44 voters overall is a nurse.

Each person must determine his or her own level of personal involvement, but there is, in the broad realm of the political process, a way for everyone to find a suitable role. Some of these ways are outlined here, and in Display 3-1.

Becoming Informed

To become informed about legislation and health care, you will need to learn about the sources of information that are available. Your daily newspaper can be an excellent source regarding significant legislation being proposed, when an issue is controversial or of widespread interest. When you rely on the newspaper for information, however, you will sometimes only learn of legislation after it has already been passed.

DISPLAY 3-1
Influencing the Political Process

- Become informed through a variety of sources.
- Vote for candidates or ballot issues that reflect your concerns.
- Vote for officers within professional or political organizations.
- Express your opinions through letters or in public forums.
- Communicate directly with legislators and public officials.
- Work for and/or contribute to nonlobbying nursing organizations or political action committees.
- Work for and/or contribute to candidates who represent your views.
- Testify before decision-making bodies.

Television and radio news reports are usually quite brief and give only an overview of a particular piece of legislation being introduced. This overview may be helpful in alerting you to something that you will want to study more intensively. Some television programs, such as those on public television, do discuss issues in depth. In an attempt to meet the Federal Communications Commission rules regarding equal time, these programs usually make an attempt to present both sides of any issue.

Professional journals usually devote some space to current legislative issues. This is done routinely in the *American Journal of Nursing* and in the *American Nurse*. When major issues are being debated, other nursing periodicals will frequently contain articles of interest. The journals of other health care professions may also carry information regarding current issues.

Nursing organizations and other health-related organizations sometimes hold open meetings to present and discuss legislative issues. Often knowledgeable speakers are present who can help you to understand what is being proposed and the various potential effects of a proposal. Nursing organizations can be excellent sources of information because they often are in touch with legislators and legislative staff.

Newsletters and journals of organizations that have a political focus provide information on what they see as current issues. These organizations include consumer groups such as Common Cause, political groups such as Young Democrats and Young Republicans, and nonpartisan groups such as the League of Women Voters.

Copies of legislation are usually available through your congressional representatives (for federal matters) and your state representatives (for state matters). Along with copies of the legislation, a legislator may send other informational material. Government agencies affected by proposed legislation may also provide information about its potential effects, although they are not allowed to try to influence legislation.

Each source of information is valuable to you, but should be weighed in terms of its known biases. Even the most objective-sounding report can be biased—not only in terms of what is reported, but also in terms of what is not reported. Identifying the groups that support and the groups that oppose a particular viewpoint might help you to recognize bias. Determine whether a group and its members would tend to gain or lose personally by the passage of proposed legislation. Are special interest groups voicing an opinion? When biases are evident, it is advisable to obtain information from groups with divergent viewpoints. Decisions need to be based on firm factual data.

Being informed as a member of an organization is usually an easier task. You can read the publications of the organization. You can attend meetings. You can talk with others in the organization about activities, priorities, and plans.

Once you are informed about the current issues in legislation or within an organization, you are better prepared to form personal opinions about them and to try to influence the outcome of the political process. There are many ways you can affect that process.

Voting

Your individual vote on a ballot issue is significant. It is a common practice to belittle the importance of the individual vote in any election. Recent major elections in this country, however, have demonstrated how important every vote can be. One of the unfortunate

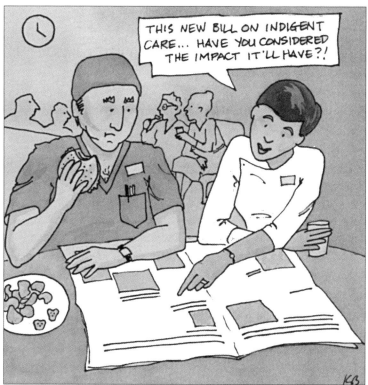

FIGURE 3-1
Sharing your opinions is one avenue of political involvement.

statistics in the United States is that only a very small percentage of eligible people in the United States are registered voters. Nurses, as a group, represent a high percentage of all people who vote. When legislators hear statistics such as "1 in 17 women voters is a nurse," or "1 in every 44 voters is a nurse," they pay attention to the opinions of nurses. Although you cannot vote directly on legislative issues, you can vote for candidates whose positions you support and who share your values. Absentee ballots are always available for those who cannot be present at their polling place on the day of an election. These ballots must be requested well in advance of the election, however (Fig. 3-1).

Voting for officers within organizations may be ignored by a large majority of members. They look at the ballot, cannot identify those running for office and, therefore, do not vote. Most organizations do make an attempt to introduce members to the various candidates. If you do not know the candidates, you can seek information about them: read their prepared statements of position, and learn about their previous activities. The direction and priorities of an organization are usually determined by those elected to office. If you are contributing your dues dollars, you will want to have a voice regarding those who are entrusted with making the decisions.

Shaping Public Opinion

Public opinion does influence the actions of legislators and regulatory bodies. As a registered nurse, you can help to shape public opinion; your judgment about matters that affect health care can help others make their own decisions. Share the knowledge you have gained through your personal experience and research. Do not be afraid to state your own position, although you must be prepared to support your position with evidence if you want to be considered a thoughtful health care professional. Certainly, you will not want to make every social occasion an opportunity to share political positions, but you should take advantage of opportunities that arise to present your concerns to others.

Another means of shaping public opinion is writing a letter to the editor of a newspaper or news magazine. These letters are often read by hundreds, even thousands, of people. The following suggestions will maximize your chances of appearing in print:

- Carefully follow the instructions provided by the publication for letters to the editor. These will generally refer to length, signature, address, and telephone number.
- Your letter is more likely to generate interest and support if you clearly present your opinion with well reasoned arguments.
- Personal experiences that illustrate health care concerns are also useful; however, you must be careful that health care examples do not violate the confidentiality of clients.

Additional information is provided in Figure 3-2.

Within an organization you may use some of these same avenues to influence opinion and action. You can discuss issues with other members, attend meetings, and voice your opinion. Remember that a viewpoint supported by strong reasoned judgment and rationale will be better received than a simple statement of opinion.

Communicating With Legislators and Officials

Legislators are affected by the views of their constituents. Letters received by a legislator usually are reviewed by the legislator's staff; views are tabulated, and letters with significant opinions or information are directed to the legislator for individual consideration. Form letters and postcards receive the least attention from a legislator. Some groups encourage members to sign form letters or postcards, but personal letters always have the greatest impact. A carefully written personal letter that reflects thoughtful and informed opinions on an issue that a person is competent to evaluate will receive the most attention.

As a registered nurse you have expertise in an area of health care that can provide a valuable viewpoint. Identify yourself as a registered nurse in your letter and outline why you are concerned about the issue in question. Legislators often appreciate personal anecdotes from your practice (with identities concealed, of course) that underscore your point.

Concern regarding the rules and regulations of a specific department of government can be addressed to the officials of that department. It is possible for officials to become insulated from the effects of their decision making. Communication from concerned citizens can be as important to them as it is to legislators. Letters to officials should reflect the same care and professional viewpoint as letters to legislators in order to be most effective.

HOW TO WRITE YOUR CONGRESSMAN

How to learn their names . . .

Call your public library, local newspaper, or chapter of the League of Women Voters to learn the names and addresses of your U.S. senators, your representative to congress, your state senator(s), and your state representative(s), (called assemblyman in California, New Jersey, New York, and Wisconsin; delegate in Virginia and West Virginia).

How to obtain a copy of a bill

For a Senate bill, write or visit (no telephone requests filled) the Senate Documents Office, Washington, DC 20510; for a House bill, write or visit the Doorkeeper of the House, U.S. Capitol, Washington, DC 20515.

Ask for the bill by number and enclose a self-addressed and gummed label for fastest service. There is no charge.

Requests are normally filled the day received, unless the bill is out of print, and sent via first class mail. There is a limit of six items per day per person, and of three copies of one bill per person (or of one copy per bill if the bill is 60 pages or longer).

Request a copy of a state bill from the appropriate state legislator.

Copies of a hearing record can be requested from the committee conducting the hearing although they usually are not ready for distribution until several weeks after the hearing.

An alternate to the above procedures, for federal bills and hearing records, is to request a copy from your appropriate senator or representative.

Fundamentals:

1. Address your letter properly: "Hon. _____, House Office Building, Washington, DC, 20515" or "Senator _____, Senate Office Building, Washington, DC 20510".
2. Identify the bill or issue. Try to give the bill number or describe it by popular title.
3. Watch your timing. Inform your congressman while there is still time to take effective action.

(Reprinted by permission of the N.A.A.C.O.G.)

Write to the right persons:

Concentrate on your own delegation. The representative of your district and the senators of your state cast your votes in the Congress and want to know your views.

Be brief:

Be reasonably brief. Your views and arguments stand a better chance of being read if they are stated as concisely as the subject matter will permit. It is not necessary that letters be typed—only that they be legible—and the form, phraseology, and grammar are not important.

Do:

1. Write your own views—not someone else's. A personal letter is far better than a form letter or signature on a petition. Form letters often receive form replies.
2. Give your reasons for taking a stand. The effects of a bill on a certain constituency will be far more helpful.
3. Be constructive. If a bill deals with a problem, but you believe the bill is the wrong approach, outline the correct approach. If you have expert knowledge, share it with your congressman.
4. Say 'well done' when it is deserved. Congressmen appreciate this from people who believe they have done the right thing.

Do not:

1. Don't make threats or promises.
2. Don't berate your congressman. If you disagree with him, give reasons for your disagreement.
3. Don't become a 'pen pal'. Quality is more important than quantity.
4. Don't demand a commitment before the facts are in. A bill rarely becomes law in the same form as introduced, it is possible for a writer to change his or her position once a bill reaches a floor.

The above material, excerpted from *Congressional Record, Nov. 2, 1977,* by Morris K. Udall, was prepared by the Washington office of The American College of Obstetricians and Gynecologists.

FIGURE 3-2

How to write your congressman.

Telephone calls cannot usually be made directly to a legislator but can be made to the legislator's office. Staff keep a record of all calls, and the positions of callers are noted. In some states a toll-free number is maintained for calls to state legislators during the legislative session.

Many governmental agencies have e-mail addresses that allow you to send messages electronically. As the "information highway" becomes more widely accessible, using this form of communication will become easier. Although you may have e-mail access at your place of work, your employer may not allow you to use it for political activity. If you are employed by a government entity, such as a public health department, the law prohibits you from using governmental resources such as e-mail for political activity.

Telegrams are delivered by telephone within 5 hours of being sent. A mailgram is a less expensive type of telegram that is delivered in the regular mail on the next business day after it is sent. These are especially useful ways of communicating to legislators right before an important vote or committee deliberation.

Visiting congressional or state representatives may also be an effective means of expressing your concerns. One of the best ways to arrange to speak with congressional representatives and senators is to contact their local offices. Through these offices you may receive assistance in arranging your visit. They may also help you to arrange other interesting and valuable activities such as attending committee hearings, taking tours, and visiting Congress in session. Appointments should always be made well in advance, as representatives and senators often have busy schedules. If your time is limited, you may have to modify your expectations and meet with a staff member who will relay your concerns. Plan carefully for your visit. It is often helpful to write out concerns and questions. Be sure to leave time for answers to the questions that you pose. Even when you disagree with the position taken by your legislator, be polite and present your concerns calmly. Rudeness will result in the legislator's unwillingness to listen to what you have to say.

These same activities may be useful in working within an organization. Those elected to office do not know the views of members unless communication occurs. For communication to be effective, you must know when and where boards meet, how to get information to board members, and the names of those responsible for specific aspects of the organization's operations.

Group Action

The political process within the nursing profession takes many forms. On one level it is the involvement of nurses in legislative and ballot issues. Nurses can be involved as individuals, but they are far more effective when they work in groups. Because nursing is the largest single health care occupation, nurses have many votes. For this reason, legislators pay attention to positions held by groups of nurses. Furthermore, although nurses do not have high incomes, their combined financial contributions can significantly help a candidate or issue.

NONLOBBYING NURSING ORGANIZATIONAL EFFORT

Most traditional nursing organizations are nonprofit groups and therefore are limited in their political activity. The major role of nonprofit groups in politics involves testifying to facts and concerns within the health care arena. The American Nurses Association (ANA) has an office in Washington, DC, and tries to keep the nursing profession informed about legislative matters of importance in health care. The ANA also provides experts in the nursing profession who testify about proposed legislation. The ANA organized the Nurses Strategic Action Team (N-STAT) to provide nurses with a means to mobilize quickly to influence legislative policy. This organization promotes grassroots involvement in legislative issues, meets with members of Congress, and organizes letter writing and telephone campaigns. It involves some 8000 nurses. You can imagine that receiving letters from 8,000 individuals about a single topic might get the attention of a legislator.

Other nursing organizations, such as the National League for Nursing (NLN) and the Association of Colleges of Nursing, also testify on pertinent issues before the federal government. The Tri-Council is a coalition of the ANA, the NLN, the American Association of Colleges of Nursing, and the National Organization of Nurse Executives, and functions at the national level. This organization provides expert testimony for committees and commissions that are considering health-related legislation. By coordinating efforts, the member organizations are able to present a more united front and a stronger voice for nursing.

Most state and district nurses' associations have legislative committees that monitor legislative and regulatory actions in their areas. They may provide educational events for nurses in regard to current issues, and testify at hearings regarding health-related issues. They may also seek to mobilize letter writing or telephone campaigns.

POLITICAL ACTION COMMITTEES

To take a more active role in seeking the passage of desired legislation, the defeat of undesired measures, and the election of particular candidates, groups form organizations called political action committees (often referred to as PACs). These organizations are registered as political action groups and are free to try to affect the political process. However, they are not considered nonprofit organizations; because they are used for political purposes, donations to these committees are not tax deductible (Fig. 3-3).

The ANA Political Action Committee (ANA-PAC) is a political action organization formed by the ANA. ANA-PAC actually lobbies for the passage or defeat of bills and supports candidates for public office. Since the 1976 federal elections, ANA-PAC has raised funds to support candidates for the Senate and the House of Representatives based on their expressed and demonstrated stands on key health issues such as health care reform proposals, funding for nursing and biomedical research, extension and funding of nursing education, and third-party reimbursement for nurses. Not all candidates endorsed by ANA-PAC were supported financially because of the limited funds available. Candidates' successes are attributable to many factors, but the effect of nursing support has been demonstrated. Many state nursing associations also have political action organizations. These groups serve the same function on the state level as the ANA-PAC does on the national level. Many candidates actively seek the endorsement of nursing organizations that are perceived as influential with voters.

The Nurses' Coalition for Legislative Action is an organization of 28 specialty nursing organizations that works to support the positions of its member organizations at the federal

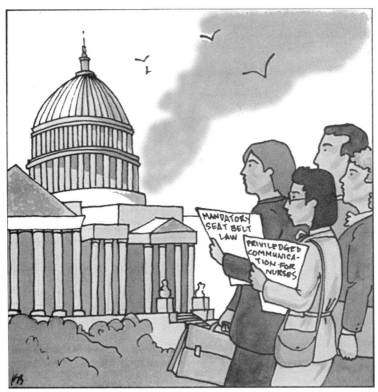

FIGURE 3-3
Nurses may lobby to get desired legislation passed by visiting legislators, by presenting
information and arguments about the bill, and by writing letters.

level. Nurses in specialty organizations have joined this organization as a way of bringing
a larger voice to the support of issues that affect nursing specialty practice.

Although these nursing political action groups have not grown rapidly in size, their
growth has been steady. In addition, nurses are gaining more sophistication in their approach
to the political process. Both of these factors have resulted in nurses gaining increased
power. There is still a long way to go before nurses will have the same kind of power that
is wielded by those in labor, education, and medicine, but change is occurring.

OTHER POLITICALLY IMPORTANT GROUPS

Many organizations in addition to those specifically related to nursing are concerned about
health and social issues. Some are official lobbying groups and others provide information
resources. Groups such as Common Cause (a consumer lobbying group) and the League of
Women Voters, and even church organizations, often act to affect the political process. You
may support these groups by simply donating money for their needs or by being actively
involved in their work.

Testifying for Decision-Making Bodies

Many decisions affecting nursing, and health care in general, are made by committees and commissions at various levels of government. These decision-making bodies frequently hold hearings to gather information before decisions are made. As a nurse, your testimony may have particular value when certain areas of health care are considered. A nurse may testify as either an official representative of an organization or as an independent individual.

You may learn of opportunities to testify through announcements in the newspaper and through professional publications. In general, you must register in advance to testify. In some instances, there is registration at the door before a meeting begins, but for more formal situations, you will have to notify the committee in advance that you wish to testify.

If you have an opportunity to testify, be sure to make your position clear so that the decision-makers know whether you speak for yourself or for a larger group. Prepare your testimony ahead of time, but try to avoid simply reading a statement. A less formal presentation is usually more interesting for the listener. Be prepared with sources for any facts or figures you present, and explain any technical terms you use. Find out whether there will be a time limit for each testimony. If you are given a time limit, make sure that you present your most important arguments and facts first. Most committees will accept written testimony if you cannot be there in person, but the personal presentation is usually more effective.

Individual Support for Legislation and Candidates

You may choose to personally support a specific piece of legislation by contributing money for publicity and campaigning, or by working on a committee that is striving for the passage of a proposal. Funds are needed for printing and distributing literature, newspaper ads, and television and radio announcements. Workers may be needed for secretarial tasks, to contact people in a door-to-door campaign, and to speak on behalf of the issue.

Supporting a candidate for public office is accomplished in the same way. In our political system the reality is that those who have actively supported a candidate during an election campaign are listened to more closely when decisions are being made. Working for a candidate is one way to make your view known. It is also an excellent way to gain first-hand knowledge of the political process (Fig 3-4).

Working In Policy Making Agencies

Nurses have been appointed to major administrative positions in state and federal health agencies and to the staffs of several senators and representatives. The Robert Wood Johnson Foundation has provided one-year fellowships for nurses to study policy in Washington, DC. Nurses who complete these fellowships have the skills and abilities to be effective in influencing health care policy. Nurses have a promising future in the health policy arena.

Seeking Election to an Office

Those elected or appointed to an office, whether it is in a local nursing organization or the U.S. Congress, have considerable power to affect outcomes. Leaders in nursing organiza-

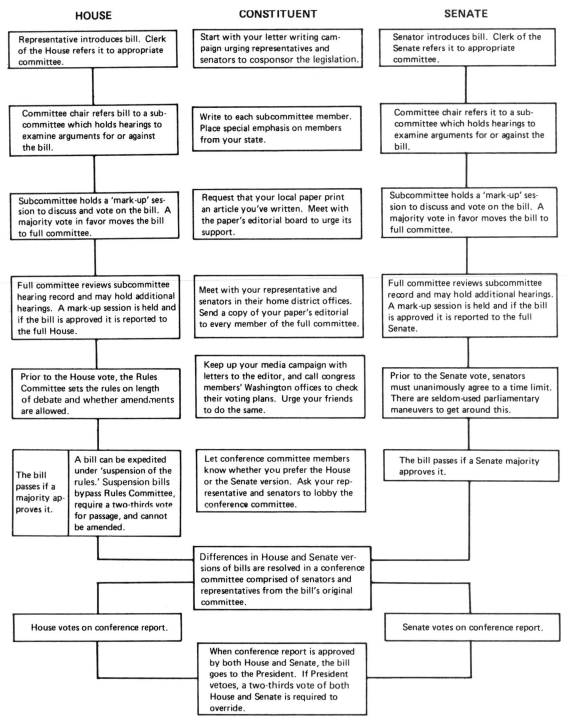

HOUSE

Representative introduces bill. Clerk of the House refers it to appropriate committee.

Committee chair refers bill to a subcommittee which holds hearings to examine arguments for or against the bill.

Subcommittee holds a 'mark-up' session to discuss and vote on the bill. A majority vote in favor moves the bill to full committee.

Full committee reviews subcommittee hearing record and may hold additional hearings. A mark-up session is held and if the bill is approved it is reported to the full House.

Prior to the House vote, the Rules Committee sets the rules on length of debate and whether amendments are allowed.

The bill passes if a majority approves it.

A bill can be expedited under 'suspension of the rules.' Suspension bills bypass Rules Committee, require a two-thirds vote for passage, and cannot be amended.

House votes on conference report.

CONSTITUENT

Start with your letter writing campaign urging representatives and senators to cosponsor the legislation.

Write to each subcommittee member. Place special emphasis on members from your state.

Request that your local paper print an article you've written. Meet with the paper's editorial board to urge its support.

Meet with your representative and senators in their home district offices. Send a copy of your paper's editorial to every member of the full committee.

Keep up your media campaign with letters to the editor, and call congress members' Washington offices to check their voting plans. Urge your friends to do the same.

Let conference committee members know whether you prefer the House or the Senate version. Ask your representative and senators to lobby the conference committee.

Differences in House and Senate versions of bills are resolved in a conference committee comprised of senators and representatives from the bill's original committee.

When conference report is approved by both House and Senate, the bill goes to the President. If President vetoes, a two-thirds vote of both House and Senate is required to override.

SENATE

Senator introduces bill. Clerk of the Senate refers it to appropriate committee.

Committee chair refers it to a subcommittee which holds hearings to examine arguments for or against the bill.

Subcommittee holds a 'mark-up' session to discuss and vote on the bill. A majority vote in favor moves the bill to full committee.

Full committee reviews subcommittee record and may hold additional hearings. A mark-up session is held and if the bill is approved it is reported to the full Senate.

Prior to the Senate vote, senators must unanimously agree to a time limit. There are seldom-used parliamentary maneuvers to get around this.

The bill passes if a Senate majority approves it.

Senate votes on conference report.

FIGURE 3-4

How a bill becomes a law.

tions help to shape the direction and efforts of those organizations. Legislators have power to affect significant regulations and spending plans. Nurses in several states have been effective in shaping health policy by seeking and being elected to office as members of their state legislatures. Eddie Bernice Johnson, elected as a Congresswoman from Texas in 1994, was the first nurse to hold an elective federal office. In the 1996 elections four nurses were candidates for congressional seats, and of these, three were elected to office.

Limitations on Your Political Activity

If you are an employee of any governmental agency, such as a public health department or the Veterans Administration, your political activity is subject to restrictions that do not apply to the general public. Restrictions that apply to the federal government are defined in the Hatch Act. Prohibited activities are mainly those that have to do with supporting a particular political party by being an officer or party spokesperson. The Hatch Act also prohibits any political activity on the part of a government employee, on behalf of a party or in support of legislation, that could be construed as representing his or her government agency.

The Hatch Act does not interfere with a private citizen's right to support parties and candidates financially, to join political parties, to work for or against measures that will appear on a ballot, or to participate in nonpartisan (ie, not connected with a political party) elections as a candidate. Each state has its own version of the Hatch Act. If you are employed by a governmental agency of any kind, you should investigate the limitations that your employment may place on your political activity.

THE FEDERAL GOVERNMENT'S ROLE IN HEALTH CARE

Federal legislation has affected nursing and health care in very important ways. If you understand key concepts regarding the federal government's involvement in health care and how federal legislation has affected health care delivery, you will be more effective in the political arena.

Federal Agencies Related to Health Care

The federal government operates in the health care field in complex ways. Literally dozens of federal agencies are involved with health care in some way. The Department of Health and Human Services (DHHS) is a cabinet-level administrative unit of the federal government with four major service divisions (Display 3-2).

The Public Health Service (which includes the Centers for Disease Control and Prevention and the National Institutes of Health [NIH]), the Food and Drug Administration, the Health Resources Administration, and the Health Care Financing Administration (which administers Social Security, Medicare, and Medicaid) are all part of the DHHS.

The Federal Budget Process

Because funding is a driving force in all decision-making, you will find it useful to understand something of the federal budget process. The availability of government funding for

DISPLAY 3-2
Major Service Divisions of the Department of Health and Human Services

OFFICE OF HUMAN DEVELOPMENT SERVICES
Administration on Aging
Administration for Child, Youth, and Families
Administration for Native Americans
Administration for Public Service

PUBLIC HEALTH SERVICE
Centers for Disease Control and Prevention
Food and Drug Administration
Health Resources Administration
Health Services Administration
National Institutes of Health
Alcohol, Drug Abuse, and Mental Health Administration

SOCIAL SECURITY ADMINISTRATION
Systems
Governmental Affairs
Family Assistance
Hearings and Appeals
Operational Policy and Procedure Assessment

HEALTH CARE FINANCING ADMINISTRATION
Health Standards and Quality Bureau
Bureau of Quality Control
Bureau of Program Operations
Bureau of Program Policy
Bureau of Support Services
Office of Child Support Enforcement

each federal program depends on two separate legislative actions. The first action is the authorization act. This is a bill, passed by both the House of Representatives (where any revenue bill must originate) and the Senate, that describes a program and outlines the rules under which funds for the program can be expended. It also sets a ceiling on the amount of money that can be provided. It is under these authorization acts (often referred to by the "title" of the section of the authorizing act) that funds are dispensed for all the health-related activities described in this chapter.

The second necessary legislative action is the appropriations act. The appropriations process establishes the Federal budget and the specific amounts of money appropriated for actual spending for each previously authorized program. Both the House and the Senate pass a budget appropriations act. Then a joint House and Senate committee meets to achieve a compromise that both will accept. The final result is called the "Omnibus Budget Reconciliation Act" (OBRA), which includes the compromises the budget committee has worked out between the House and Senate versions of the budget. Each budget act—for example, OBRA 1995—is identified by the year in the title. The amount appropriated for any program cannot exceed the amount originally authorized, but it can be, and frequently is, less. This is sometimes confusing because two monetary amounts, the authorized amount and the budgeted (or appropriated) amount, may be reported in connection with the same act.

The budget act may also place restrictions on the people and organizations who receive federal funds. It is under this authority that the federal government sets standards for nursing homes that receive reimbursement through Medicaid and Medicare. The rules and regulations for nursing homes, called the "conditions of participation," included in OBRA '87 (the budget reconciliation act for 1987) were very extensive. These rules and regulations did not take effect until October 1, 1990. This allowed the affected organizations to begin the process of change to meet the new requirements.

Historically, a third factor has affected the amount of money available for a specific federal program: the participation of the executive branch of government in decisions regarding how and when available funds will be spent. If money that has been authorized and appropriated has not been spent by the end of a budget period, it is lost. This money must then be reauthorized and reappropriated. The executive branch has used this mechanism to withdraw support for programs it opposes.

Federal Support for Nursing Education

Beginning in 1964 the Federal government provided funding to support nursing education through what was initially the Nurse Training Act and later called the Nurse Education Act. Initially the funding was very generous and included money for buildings, classroom renovation, equipment, faculty development, and student scholarships and traineeships. As the shortage of nurses abated and priorities changed in Washington, DC, the amount of funding gradually declined.

Every two years, when the biennial budget is passed, nurses try to rally congressional support for additional funding for nursing education, but so far they have not been successful. Funds currently appropriated through the Nurse Education Act are limited and primarily used to support education for advanced nursing practice and graduate degrees. Other federal funds are used to support research in nursing. The future of any federal support for nursing education is uncertain (White, 1995).

Occupational Safety and Health

The Occupational Safety and Health Act (OSHA) mandates actions and prescribes safety equipment to improve the health and safety of the working environment. OSHA regulations have required health care employers to provide the equipment, supplies, immunizations, and education to enable the implementation of CDC recommendations for universal precautions. After the CDC established new and broader guidelines (referred to as Standard Precautions), OSHA was expected to make those guidelines mandatory through regulation. However, the antiregulatory stance of the 1994-1996 Congress was reflected in the failure of OSHA to upgrade infection control requirements.

OSHA has recently undertaken a study of back injuries in nursing homes. The potential cost of preventing such injuries is so great, however, that in 1996 businesses lobbied Congress to forbid OSHA to even collect data on the problem. The bill to limit OSHA in this way was not successful.

Many people think that the rules and regulations created by OSHA are too cumbersome. Nevertheless, concern for the safety of the working person is of considerable importance to nurses. Occupational injuries create major health problems for the adult population. They are costly not only in terms of health and personal loss but also in terms of lost productivity. Nurses also are affected by the provisions of OSHA in their own work environments. They, too, are subject to injury and accident on the job. The safety concerns of nurses in the workplace are discussed in Chapter 11.

Nurses in occupational health nursing are also involved in OSHA through educating workers about job safety. In some situations safety precautions are time consuming and uncomfortable, and workers may be tempted to ignore them. Nurses may be able to help workers understand the importance of following health and safety regulations. Occupational health nurses also assist management in planning to make the environment safe and in establishing appropriate procedures for treating injuries.

A current safety concern of health care workers is violence in the workplace. Nurses in psychiatric settings have long recognized the hazards they face in working with aggressive, violent, and sometimes out-of-control clients. Emergency rooms are sites where the violence of society spills over into the health care setting. Even obstetric units may encounter violence by family members. Nurses are asking that healthcare workplaces be mandated to provide safety from violence. (See Chapter 11 for a further discussion of violence in the workplace.)

Nursing Home Regulations

OBRA '87, the federal budget bill passed for 1987, contained regulations that for the first time mandated a national standard for quality of care in long-term care facilities receiving any federal money through Medicare or Medicaid. This legislation also required an admission assessment of every individual admitted to long-term care according to a standardized minimum data set (MDS). Based on critical data (termed ''triggers''), resident assessment protocols (RAPs) and plans of care must be established. They are also required to limit the use of both chemical and physical restraints and to establish programs that maintain residents at the highest levels of functioning. Training for nursing assistants was mandated, and the requirements for supervision by licensed nurses were increased. Although the provisions of this act were set to take effect in October 1990, there were delays because of legal challenges to the requirements and because of the extra time that was needed to establish monitoring mechanisms. Therefore, some of the provisions of OBRA '87 took effect as late as 1994. Despite earlier concerns, it is now clear that these regulations have positively affected the care environment in nursing homes. The use of restraints has decreased, resident rights are more effectively supported, and basic care needs are being identified and met.

Family Health Concerns

The Maternal--Child Health Act, Title V, was created to improve health in the nation through benefits such as nutritional support for children and pregnant women, health supervision, and well child care. Part of the money appropriated was earmarked for nursing research projects and nursing research training. Since its inception, the Maternal--Child Health Act has never been fully funded. This means that even those who are eligible for services under the provisions of the act may not receive them because of budget limitations.

The Americans with Disabilities Act of 1990 brought to fruition an effort begun 20 years earlier to guarantee equal access and opportunity to those with disabilities. A disability is defined in the act as ''a physical or mental impairment that substantially limits activities of daily living'' (ADA, 1990). In 1973 the Rehabilitation Act began the effort by providing the disabled with physical and vocational access to organizations and institutions that received federal funds. The Americans with Disabilities Act moved beyond that and now requires accessible workplaces, nondiscriminatory practices, and access to public services such as transportation and the telephone. It also provides legal avenues for redress when the provisions of the act are not carried out. Nurses play a key role in educating the disabled about their rights under the law and acting as advocates in the community (Watson, 1990).

The Women's Health Equity Act addressed the unmet health needs of the women of the United States. Although women make up 52% of the population, only 13% of NIH research dollars were directed toward women's health issues in 1990 (Sharp, 1990). For example, although heart disease was, and still is, the major cause of death in women, no women were included in any of the major heart disease studies. This bill brought together concerns about adequate breast cancer research, women's infertility and contraceptive needs, and the inclusion of women as subjects in research studies (ANA testifies . . . , 1994).

The Family and Medical Leave Act of 1993 issued a mandate to businesses with more than 50 employees to provide unpaid leave for those wishing to take time off without pay to care for an ill family member (Wimberly, 1993). There was opposition to this act from those who believe that this will place an unfair burden on businesses. However, family leave is well established in European countries. In Europe, leave with pay is available in some circumstances.

Future Federal Legislation

Many issues will come before Congress in the next two years. One concern is the effect on health care of millions of poor people as changes in eligibility for public assistance are implemented. People who are not on public assistance are not eligible for Medicaid; therefore, as individuals and families are removed from Medicaid, they will most likely enter the ranks of the uninsured, further burdening the system with the need to provide uncompensated emergency care. How these problems will be addressed has not yet been determined.

Dissatisfaction with the restructuring of health care systems has led to widespread provider and consumer discontent. The resulting pressure caused Congress to pass a bill in 1996 mandating that all insurers allow 48 hour stays for mother and baby post delivery. Other areas of dissatisfaction are generating demands for legislation to address other specific health concerns. A current proposal is the Patient Safety Act that would require agencies to inform patients of their staffing ratios, and would include "whistle blower" protections for staff reporting poor care.

STATE-LEVEL LEGISLATIVE CONCERNS

Many issues that vitally affect the health care arena are decided at the state level. Because the health care issues in each state are different, only some general areas of concern are outlined here.

State Agencies and Health Care

State institutions range from those that care for the mentally retarded and the mentally ill to penal systems and institutions of higher education. Health care is a consideration in all of these settings. When budgets are planned, topics as diverse as immunization and contraception may be part of the debate. Nurses often can advocate for those who are unable to speak for themselves in regard to their own health care needs. Sometimes nurses who work in these settings are unable to deliver quality care because of severe budgetary deficiencies. All nurses can support efforts to provide quality health care in such settings.

Nurse Practice Acts

Nurse practice acts are being discussed and revised in many states. This process is long and difficult, and requires intense political effort on the part of nurses to avoid creating problems for the profession. One current concern related to placing the act before a state legislature for action is the pressure to lessen the standards or allow unlicensed assistive personnel to perform more nursing tasks. The Pew Report (Pew, 1995) suggested that laws regarding scopes of practice for health professionals have been too specific and that the health care system would be enhanced by greater flexibility. Ontario, Canada, for example, has a new health professions licensing act that limits the use of titles (such as registered nurse) but otherwise places few limits on health care activities. The act provides a list of 27 tasks that are restricted to specific health professions. These tasks include such activities as performing surgery (which is limited to physicians), prescribing drugs (which is limited to physicians and dentists), and piercing the skin to inject drugs (which is limited to physicians, dentists, and nurses). Except for the specifically named acts that are restricted, anyone with the proper training may perform any other activity. One concern about this law is that it reduces health care to performing tasks and does not recognize that the decision making and judgment behind the tasks are critical to safe and effective outcomes. Many state legislatures are examining the ''Ontario Plan'' with interest to determine the outcomes of this approach to licensing.

LOCAL POLITICAL CONCERNS

The budgetary process always seems to be at the root of most political and legislative concerns. Because only a limited amount of money is available, budgets are always developed through a series of compromises. In order to gain one objective, it is sometimes necessary to recognize that there will be no funds for achieving another. In most communities, budgets for public health departments, school nurses, and so forth are developed over a period of several months. Hearings are often held, at which members of the public may ask questions and address issues. Nurses have often found that involvement at this planning stage is most rewarding. Determining priorities for health care is essential, and nurses often can speak with authority on these matters. Nurses actually employed in a public department undergoing review may be limited in making their views known because of regulations governing their action in the political sphere. For this reason it is significant that nurses outside of government institutions recognize the importance of community health. It is not only the practice of the public health nurse that is affected by the priorities of the agency. For example, a nurse who is employed in a hospital may wish to refer a discharged patient to a public health nurse for follow-up, only to find that, owing to changes in the ordering of priorities, home visits for the identified purpose are no longer being made.

In many communities decisions about the allocation of federal money are made at the local level. The most recent Congress has had a goal of creating large block grants where priorities would be decided locally. Support for alternative health care centers, blood pressure screening, and senior citizen centers may depend on whether those who are knowledgeable about the benefits of these services are willing to voice their advocacy in local decision-making bodies.

HEALTH CARE REFORM

The United States is the only major industrialized country other than South Africa that does not provide some type of government-sponsored health care for all citizens. Through Medicare and Medicaid, and the widespread effects of the military, public health, and Indian health systems, the federal government is already deeply involved in the provision of health care. President Clinton's proposal for a national system of managed competition was defeated, pushing most of the impetus for reform to the states.

As each state debates this issues, common questions recur.

- Do people have a right to health care?
- If there is such a right, what level of health care can people expect to receive? Routine preventive services? Surgery and hospitalization for all conditions? Or treatment only for serious life-threatening conditions?
- Should catastrophic illnesses, transplantation, and experimental treatments be included?
- What about fertility-enhancing services? Should abortion services be available?
- How can health care be transformed into an effective, coordinated system?
- How will changes in the health care system be financed?

These are difficult philosophical and ethical questions, and there are no simple answers.

Factors Leading to Health Care Reform

After the recent demise of federal health reform efforts, many people thought that health care would remain essentially the same. This thinking did not take into account the reality of the rapid rate of increase in health care costs, the feelings of individuals about their rights with respect to health care, or people's fears about losing coverage. Health care providers, insurance companies, and managed care organizations have created a monumental change in the entire system.

More and more people are being drawn into managed care organizations for health care coverage because of their lower-cost premiums. Managed care companies are negotiating very restrictive contracts that put providers at risk for managing individuals who require high-cost care. In an effort to become more competitive, health care agencies are restructuring, downsizing, merging, and changing the basic framework in which they do business. Mergers of hospitals, systems, and providers have resulted in a few large entities dominating the health care marketplace in most metropolitan areas. Individual health care professionals have found their jobs changing or even disappearing. Managed care plans favor primary care physicians and are limiting the use of specialty physicians. For the first time, physicians' incomes are dropping.

People who receive health insurance through an employer have fewer choices as more employers are offering their workers only one or two options in health care coverage. The number of employers who do not provide any health insurance coverage, even for full time workers, is increasing. In the past, individuals whose employer did not provide coverage often purchased private health insurance. This option is becoming prohibitively expensive. Although legislation has been passed that requires insurers to continue providing individuals with a company policy for a period of time after they leave employment, the cost of the policy is often a deterrent to continuing. Many who choose not to purchase expensive insurance express the concern that they are gambling with their family's future, but often they do not feel they have a choice.

People who are unemployed or underemployed often do not have health insurance. These same people are often not eligible for health care through public assistance. Therefore, these people do not receive preventive health care or prompt attention to health problems as they arise. When they have major health care needs, people without insurance seek care in emergency rooms—one of the most costly forms of health care. Regulations require that emergency rooms provide care to those with critical problems; therefore, people are treated and may be admitted for surgery and major care regardless of their ability to pay. Costs mount and bills often simply remain unpaid. Hospitals historically have absorbed these costs by passing them on to those who do pay their bills. As insurance companies and the government become more stringent about reimbursement, this method of absorbing costs is becoming increasingly difficult, and some hospitals will be in serious financial trouble if an answer to this problem is not found.

The number of people with chronic illnesses continues to grow as the population ages and those with chronic illness live longer lives. In the past, many of these individuals found themselves completely excluded from health insurance coverage because of their "preexisting condition." New legislation has required that health insurance benefits be portable; this means that if an individual has insurance through one employer and then changes jobs, the second employer's insurance must provide coverage. Some states have passed legislation requiring that insurers provide an option for the person with a preexisting illness. Some insurers have responded to this by trying to retreat to states where this option is not required.

Nursing's Agenda for Health Care Reform

The ANA, the NLN, and almost 60 other nursing organizations cooperated in presenting Nursing's Agenda for Health Care Reform (American Nurses Association, 1991) to legislators, health care agencies, and the public. Nursing's agenda was based on the belief that any health care system must provide quality health care, must have access for all citizens, and must be cost effective. One aspect of this was a federally defined standard package of essential health care benefits. The goal of this package was to provide primary care and prevention that would be financed by a mix of public and private sources. Nursing suggested improving access to health care, which is often affected by geographical, economic, and cultural factors, by delivering it in schools, workplaces, and the home. Nursing also suggested controlling costs through managed care, and implementing the plan in steps.

One key concern of nurses has been direct reimbursement of nursing care. This has been of special concern to primary health care nurses. The availability of funding for nursing care will, to a great extent, determine whether the public will be able to use such services.

Physicians (through the American Medical Association) have consistently supported provisions for direct payment only to physicians or for care ordered by physicians. Other organizations of direct care providers (social workers, nurses, psychologists, and so forth) are seeking greater breadth in reimbursement. Third-party payment funds a large percentage of the health care in the United States; if this avenue of funding is closed to nurses and other direct care providers, then their ability to provide services is severely curtailed. Physicians believe that controlling access to third-party payment will control health care costs. Limiting access would also preserve the physician's unique position of power in the health care setting.

Although planning for health care reform at the federal level was dropped as a result of political opposition, many of the issues that nursing supported are being discussed, and proposals contained in nursing's agenda are being adopted at state and local levels. Nurses continue to support plans that provide comprehensive access to health care and provide mechanisms for nurses to work to the full extent of their abilities.

The Role of the States in Health Care Reform

Many states are moving ahead toward health care reform at the state level. States instituting health care reform have asked for waivers from the federal rules governing Medicaid in order to incorporate all Medicaid funds into their planning.

Hawaii has the oldest universal health care plan in the United States. Perhaps because it is less populous than other states and small in size, its citizens were able to build a consensus regarding a coordinated health system for the state. Some individuals are covered through employers. For those without this coverage, health care coverage is available through a state system. One of the difficulties Hawaii has experienced has been the distribution of health providers to smaller communities throughout the islands.

Oregon has been one of the most innovative states. Oregon has attempted to institute universal health care for certain basic services. In order to determine what services should be covered in the basic guarantee, a series of meetings to discuss priorities were held all across the state. The result was a prioritized list of services. Prioritization was based on the importance of the service to saving life, the number of people served, and whether treatment would significantly alter health outcomes. This rationing of services was defended based on the rationale that without it, some individuals would have access to every possible service, whereas others would have no services at all. Although this sounds rational, the results have upset some people. For example, a liver transplant would be funded for a child with biliary atresia, but not for an adult with liver failure. Bone marrow transplants are funded in certain instances where the success rate is high and not in cases (such as breast cancer) where success is very unlikely. All preventive services such as immunizations, pap smears, and mammograms are included in the funding. Of course, those with private health plans have access to any services they choose. The prioritization affects only insurance funded through taxes.

Minnesota has been another leader in trying to assure that basic health care is available to all residents of the state through a program called MinnesotaCare. A plan has been developed there that provides a basic safety net of health care coverage for everyone. Nurses have been influential in the process of determining the structure and coverage of care there (Maynard, 1995). Other states are also instituting reforms, some more extensive than others.

Malpractice Reform

All of the plans address concerns regarding malpractice suits and the cost to the system of litigation. Most include some type of dispute mechanism as an alternative to court proceedings. Plans vary with respect to the presence of caps on awards, limits on attorney's fees, the approach to punitive damages, and the statute of limitations.

NURSING ORGANIZATIONS

A student once said that it seems that every time nurses identify a problem, their first action is to form a new organization. Although this may be something of an exaggeration, it contains some bit of truth. When you first learn about the great number of nursing and nursing-related organizations, it may all seem confusing and their purposes and functions may seem duplicative (Fig. 3-5).

The existence of a large number of diverse organizations for nurses is, in many ways, a reflection of nursing itself. The profession offers a wide variety of employment opportunities to its members with distinct and varied contributions and interests in health care. When nurses become committed to a particular specialty group, they have a tendency to

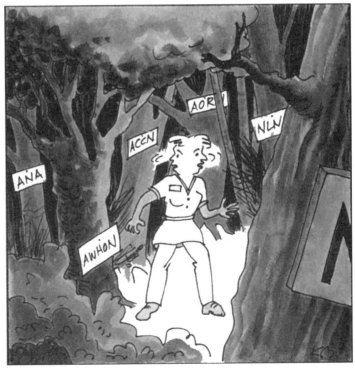

FIGURE 3-5
The large number of nursing organizations may seem overwhelming

want to advance the purposes and interests of the people working in that area. For example, operating room nurses have more in common with other operating room nurses, in terms of interests and concerns, than they have with nurses involved in hospice care. Likewise, nurses involved in hospice care would probably prefer to share concerns with one another than to discuss them with critical care nurses. With more than 2.2 million nurses in the United States, it is understandable that there are many different areas of nursing interest and therefore many different nursing organizations.

The formation of a large number of nursing organizations has resulted in concern regarding the overlapping of function and interrelationships among some of the organizations. Unfortunately, there has often been a spirit of competition rather than one of cooperation among these groups in the past. Because nurses traditionally have not had high incomes, joining more than one organization has not been a desirable option for economic as well as philosophical reasons.

Nursing organizations have recently made a concerted effort to promote cooperation. Nurses are better informed about the various organizations and receive better salaries than in the past. However, these facts have not resulted in significantly greater participation by professional nurses in their organizations. Some people specifically do not join because of philosophical differences, but many nurses seem to be apathetic and do not recognize the importance of nurses acting together. Some, because they are combining a job with family and home responsibilities, feel they do not have the time or energy to become involved. Nurses need to recognize the potential for power that they possess as a group. As the nation moves toward health care reform, this has never been a more critical issue. (Appendix B provides an overview of the many nursing and nursing-related organizations).

American Nurses Association

The ANA, the professional association for registered nurses, had its origins in a meeting of nursing leaders at the World's Fair in Chicago in 1890. Through their suggestions and efforts the alumnae organizations of ten schools of nursing sent delegates in 1896 to form a committee to organize a professional association. The resulting organization was called the National Associated Alumnae of the United States and Canada. The name was changed in 1899 to the Nurses' Associated Alumnae of the United States and Canada. In 1901, Canada was dropped from the title because the state laws of New York (where the organization was incorporated) did not allow for representatives from more than one country. The name American Nurses Association was adopted in the United States in 1911 and Canadian nurses formed their own organization.

The ANA has been identified as the organization for registered nurses. As such, it has always had as its primary interest the concerns of the nurses it represents. Throughout history, the organization has been active in issues relating to licensure (see Chapter 7), collective bargaining (see Chapter 12), nursing education (see Chapter 6), and a host of other concerns facing nurses and nursing.

MEMBERSHIP

The ANA membership comprises the 50 state nurses' associations and the 3 territorial constituent units. State nurses' associations (SNAs) comprise the district nurses' associations

(DNAs). The individual nurse belongs to the ANA through the SNA. Prior to 1982, when the federation model was adopted, individual nurses were members of the ANA. The change to membership through the SNAs was made because it was thought that SNAs would be able to recruit more members and have greater control. However, there has not been an increase in membership. Each state is free to establish its own membership plans; however, membership is limited to registered nurses. The only exception to this rule is the admission to membership of some new graduates who have not yet passed the licensing examination.

It is regrettable that fewer than half of the registered nurses in the United States participate in the ANA. Those who do participate are often the leaders in the nursing profession. One reason for the low level of membership is the high cost of membership. Annual dues to the national association and the state and district associations are paid together, and in most parts of the country they are more than $300 combined. Another reason nurses have for not joining is a lack of time to participate in activities. Many nurses have the dual responsibilities of job and home and feel that they have no time left for involvement in a professional organization. Other nurses do not see how the benefits available through membership in the association are personally valuable. Some explain that they are just not interested in the issues and concerns of the organization. Finally, some nurses do not join because they do not agree with the position of the ANA on major issues; this has been especially true with regard to the role of the SNAs in collective bargaining and with regard to some of the ANA's positions on nursing education.

Those who are active in the ANA believe that its work is severely hampered by the low level of membership. The funds of the organization are limited by the number of members. Because some specific programs, such as the collective bargaining programs, are costly to the state association, there has been a strong move to require nurses to belong to the association if it serves as a bargaining agent. In some states the state association has set a specific percentage of an agency's staff that must be members before they will become the bargaining agent for the nurses in that agency.

A current controversy involves differing views regarding the purpose of the professional organization. Many nurses believe that the organization should be primarily concerned with what it can do for the individual nurse. Others believe that a truly professional approach focuses on what the individual nurse can contribute to the profession through the organization. Some think that the organization should be an advocate in the realm of economic security. Another point of controversy is the organization's stand on political issues.

In 1995, the California Nurses Association experienced a great deal of internal turmoil because of a perceived lack of support from the ANA regarding the massive changes being created by health care reform (Costello, 1995). As a result the CNA delegate assembly voted to withdraw from the American Nurses Association and to establish itself as an independent "international" organization. This enabled the CNA to keep all of the dues within the state for its own purposes, but it also deprived CNA members of a voice and opportunities at the national level. Some nurses who did not support the separation of the CNA from the ANA joined ANA affiliate organizations in bordering states during the dispute. The ANA tried to resolve the problems, but was unsuccessful; instead, it subsequently established another organization called ANA-California. ANA is encouraging nurses in California who are interested in being part of the national organization and its efforts to join this new organization.

ACTIVITIES AND SERVICES

The ANA has been referred to many times throughout this book. As a professional association it has been involved in all the issues that nursing has confronted. There has not been universal support within the nursing community for all of the activities that the ANA has championed or for the stands that it has taken. In any group as large as nursing, it is perhaps inevitable that there should be a wide range of viewpoints.

Advancement of the Profession. The ANA supports work on such policies as the ANA Social Policy Statement (American Nurses Association, 1980). These activities are ongoing efforts to support the advancement of nursing as a profession. The ANA also supports research on topics related to the profession itself, such as historical patterns of licensure (Snyder & LaBar, 1984).

One of the most significant services the ANA offers to its members is certification through the American Nurses Credentialing Center. Recognition for expertise in a particular area is usually granted based on demonstration of knowledge through testing and clinical practice, although the criteria for certification vary among specialties.

Legislative Activity. The ANA is extensively involved in legislative activity. The organization often represents the profession in testimony before Congress on numerous issues affecting nursing. The need to be geographically closer to legislators in order to have greater participation in legislative efforts was the major reason for the relocation of the ANA offices to Washington, DC in 1992. The organization provides testimony for or against legislation that will affect the profession, either directly or indirectly: legislative topics include funds for nursing education, collective bargaining issues, concerns for higher education, and human rights issues. It also testifies on health-related issues affecting the general public, such as the quality of care in nursing homes and health care reform. A newsletter, *Capitol Update*, is published monthly and provides information to the reader regarding issues currently being addressed in the Capitol.

Collective Bargaining. An activity that has a major impact on the economic welfare of nurses is the organization's support of collective bargaining. This is also one of the most controversial services of the ANA. The SNAs are the official bargaining representatives in most instances (see Chapter 12). The ANA works with the states and territories to help them in this role and to develop strategies and techniques for collective bargaining. The ANA serves as the primary bargaining agent for nurses employed by federal institutions such as the Veterans Administration facilities. Initially, the major concerns of the economic and general welfare sections of the ANA focused on adequate remuneration for nurses. Today, with nurses' salaries significantly higher than in earlier years, the emphasis is shifting to practice concerns.

Other Resources and Services. In addition to its activities, the ANA provides direct services to members. These include access to a group professional liability insurance plan and group insurance for health, disability, and accident coverage. From time to time the ANA also provides access to group travel arrangements and purchasing discounts.

Through its educational services, the ANA produces and distributes a wide variety of nursing educational materials, such as films, as well as a biennial report entitled ''Facts About Nursing.'' This report provides basic statistical information that is used by many organizations and individuals. Reports of committees and commissions and special studies supported by the ANA are also published.

The *American Nurse* is the official publication of the ANA; official announcements of ANA business are published in this paper. The paper also contains current news of relevance to nursing and health care, editorials, letters, and classified advertisements. The *American Journal of Nursing* is the official journal of the organization. It is published monthly and contains some current news, but its major focus is professional articles. It is published by Lippincott-Raven Publishers and retains autonomy over its own content.

The ANA also publishes many pamphlets and informational resources that are of value to nurses. A complete list of publications is available from the organization.

Organizations Related to the ANA

Because it is an official professional association, the ANA is related to other organizations in unique ways. These organizations operate autonomously from the ANA, but are closely tied to it.

INTERNATIONAL COUNCIL OF NURSES

The International Council of Nurses (ICN) is the international organization for professional nursing, with membership comprised of national nursing organizations. The ANA, as a constituent member of the ICN, sends delegates to its convention and participates in its activities. The ICN is interested in health care in general, and nursing care in particular, throughout the world. It works with the United Nations when appropriate, and with other international health-related groups, such as the International Red Cross.

The ICN concerns itself with such issues as the social and economic welfare of nurses, the role of the nurse in health care, and the roles of the various national nursing organizations throughout the world, and their relationships to their governing bodies. The primary governing body of the organization is the Council of National Representatives, which meets biennially.

The ICN has representatives from 104 national nurses' organizations. The organization is governed by the Council of National Representatives, which consists of all the presidents of the member organizations. Activities of the organization are carried out by its Board of Directors, the officers, volunteer nurse members of constituent organizations, and employed staff, including an executive director. The ICN maintains headquarters in Geneva, Switzerland.

Every 4 years a quadrennial congress is held. This meeting is open to all nurses and to delegates from the national organizations. Concerns addressed at recent congresses focused on such issues as career ladders, educational standards, research, human rights, and nursing's roles in the planning of a national health policy.

AMERICAN NURSES FOUNDATION

In 1955, the ANA established the American Nurses' Foundation (ANF) as a tax-exempt, nonprofit corporation for the purpose of supporting research related to nursing. It is independently financed and self-governing. The Board of Trustees is composed of members of the Board of Directors of the ANA, other nurse members, and non-nurse members from other health-related fields and from the public. To accomplish its varied objectives, the ANF solicits gifts and contributions from individuals and organizations. These gifts are tax deductible.

The ANF maintains a three-pronged approach to supporting research. The first objective is to conduct policy analyses to provide nursing leaders and public policy-makers with the information they will need for decision-making. The second objective is related to developing a group of ''nurse scholars'' who engage in study of such areas as journalism and public policy. Support is directed toward independent study, research, and doctoral and postdoctoral work for these nurse scholars. The third objective is to facilitate the research and educational activities of ANA. This includes providing consultation and funding for groups within the ANA that wish to initiate projects.

AMERICAN ACADEMY OF NURSING

The American Academy of Nursing (AAN) was established by the ANA in 1973 as an honorary association within the ANA. The original members were chosen by the Board of Directors of the ANA. The AAN is now an independent organization, and new members are selected by those currently in the AAN. Those elected to the AAN are called fellows and may use the title Fellow of the American Academy of Nursing (FAAN). The purpose of this organization is to recognize nurses who have made significant contributions to the profession of nursing.

National Student Nurses Association

The National Student Nurses' Association (NSNA) is a professional organization for students in schools of nursing and was started in 1952. Although it works with the ANA, it is a fully independent organization, run and financed by nursing students. It sponsors its own annual convention.

Although the NSNA is an autonomous organization, it has close ties with the ANA. Members of the NSNA serve on selected committees within the ANA, speak to the House of Delegates at the ANA convention to provide a student viewpoint, and work together with the ANA in regard to current issues.

Each state has a state nursing student association that operates in the same relationship to the state professional organization as the NSNA does to the national organization. State conventions and workshops are held in many states. State issues are addressed by the state association in the same way that national issues are addressed by the NSNA. Local nursing student organizations may or may not exist in individual schools of nursing. These local organizations may be closely tied to the state and national groups, or they may be independent. It is possible for an individual student to join the state and national student nurses' organizations even if no local counterpart exists.

A major project of the NSNA is ''Breakthrough into Nursing,'' which is designed to recruit and maintain the enrollment of minorities in schools of nursing. The project has enlisted nursing students to speak to minority teenagers to interest them in nursing early in their scholastic careers, and to act as preceptors and tutors to increase the retention of minority students when they enroll in schools of nursing.

N.S.N.A. STUDENT BILL OF RIGHTS

The following Student Bill of Rights and Responsibilities was adopted by the NSNA House of Delegates in April 1975.

1. Students should be encouraged to develop the capacity for critical judgment and engage in a sustained and independent search for truth.

2. The freedom to teach and the freedom to learn are inseparable facets of academic freedom: students should exercise their freedom with responsibility.

3. Each institution has a duty to develop policies and procedures which provide and safeguard the students' freedom to learn.

4. Under no circumstances should a student be barred from admission to a particular institution on the basis of race, creed, sex, or marital status.

5. Students should be free to take reasoned exception to the data or views offered in any course of study and to reserve judgment about matters of opinion, but they are responsible for learning the content of any course of study for which they are enrolled.

6. Students should have protection through orderly procedures against prejudices or capricious academic evaluation, but they are responsible for maintaining standards of academic performance established for each course in which they are enrolled.

7. Information about student views, beliefs, and political associations which instructors acquire in the course of their work should be considered confidential and not released without the knowledge or consent of the student.

8. The student should have the right to have a responsible voice in the determination of his/her curriculum.

9. Institutions should have a carefully considered policy as to the information which should be a part of a student's permanent educational record and as to the conditions of its disclosure.

10. Students and student organizations should be free to examine and discuss all questions of interest to them, and to express opinions publicly and privately.

11. Students should be allowed to invite and to hear any person of their own choosing, thereby taking the responsibility of furthering their education.

12. The student body should have clearly defined means to participate in the formulation and application of institutional policy affecting academic and student affairs.

13. The institution has an obligation to clarify those standards of behavior which it considers essential to its educational mission and community life.

14. Disciplinary proceedings should be instituted only for violations of standards of conduct formulated with significant student participation and published in advance through such means as a student handbook or a generally available body of institutional regulations. It is the responsibility of the student to know these regulations. Grievance procedures should be available for every student.

(continues)

N.S.N.A. STUDENT BILL OF RIGHTS

15. As citizens and members of an academic community, students are subject to the obligations which accrue them by virtue of this membership and should enjoy the same freedom of citizenship.
16. Students have the right to belong or refuse to belong to any organization of their choice.
17. Students have the right to personal privacy in their living space to the extent that the welfare of others is respected.
18. Adequate safety precautions should be provided by schools of nursing, for example, to and from student dorms, adequate street lighting, locks, etc.
19. Dress code, if present in school, should be established by student government in conjunction with the school director and faculty, so the highest professional standards possible are maintained, but also taking into consideration points of comfort and practicality for the student.
20. Grading systems should be carefully reviewed periodically with students and faculty for clarification and better student–faculty understanding.

(Reprinted by permission of the National Student Nurses' Association, Inc © 1978)

FIGURE 3-6
NSNA Student Bill of Rights.

The NSNA is frequently asked to testify before congressional committees when issues relevant to nursing education are being considered. In this role the organization becomes the public voice for all nursing students.

In 1975, the NSNA developed a Student Bill of Rights. This document carefully balances the rights of students with the responsibilities of students. It supports the view of students as competent adults who are engaged in an educational program. The rights that are outlined relate to educational programs, to the rules and policies of an institution, and to freedom in personal life and decision-making (Fig. 3-6).

In the past it was not uncommon for schools of nursing to require membership in the student nurse organization at local, state, and national levels. With increasing emphasis on student rights and freedom of choice, this practice is no longer followed and has led to recruitment problems for many of the nursing student organizations. Students are busy, with full lives and limited funds. Some do not understand that the efforts of the organization benefit them in ways not immediately apparent. The activities of the student organization cannot occur without a wide membership base for funding and for credibility. Certainly, the profession of nursing and the situation of the individual nursing student would be adversely affected if the NSNA did not remain a viable and active force.

National League for Nursing

Another major nursing organization is the National League for Nursing (NLN), which was established in 1952 and is often referred to as "The League." The forerunner of the NLN was the National League of Nursing Education that was organized under the title of the American Society of Superintendents of Training Schools for Nurses of the United States and Canada. Established in 1893, it was the first nursing organization in the United States. The name was changed to the National League of Nursing Education in 1912. This organization then fused with six other organizations and committees to form one in 1952. The groups that joined together to form the National League of Nursing Education included the National Organization for Public Health Nursing (established in 1912), the Association of Collegiate Schools of Nursing (established in 1933), the Joint Committee on Practical Nurses and Auxiliary Workers in Nursing Services (established in 1945), the Joint Committee on Careers in Nursing (established in 1948), the National Committee for the Improvement of Nursing Services (established in 1949), and the National Nursing Accrediting Service (established in 1949). The stated mission of the NLN is "to improve education and health outcomes by linking communities and information. The NLN achieves its missions through collaborating, connecting, creating, serving, and learning" (NLN, 1995).

MEMBERSHIP

The NLN offers membership to individuals and agencies, and is unique among nursing organizations in offering membership and participation to consumers, to non-nursing members of health care teams, and to institutions concerned with nursing service and nursing education, as well as to registered nurses. The NLN began a major restructuring beginning in 1995 that was designed to enhance its effectiveness (Bowles, 1996).

ACTIVITIES AND SERVICES

The NLN works in a complementary, rather than competitive, manner with the ANA. Whereas the ANA speaks as the official voice of nurses, the NLN seeks to unite the interests of nursing with those of the community.

Until 1982 the NLN produced the licensing examination for the state boards of nursing. Although it no longer has this responsibility, it does have a large testing service that produces standardized tests to be used in the nursing program admission process, achievement tests for various levels within a program, the NLN mobility exams which are used to provide advanced placement credit, and diagnostic examinations for those preparing for the NCLEX exams.

Accreditation Services. Most students are aware of the accreditation services, especially if they are attending an NLN-accredited school. Accreditation, which is voluntary, is one of the longest-standing services that the NLN has provided. Initially accreditation was performed by the National Nursing Accrediting Service, which merged with other groups to form the NLN. Beginning in 1997, a separate but related organization, the National League for Nursing Accrediting Commission (NLNAC), has been charged with accrediting responsibilities. This change was necessary to meet the requirements of the Department of Education for a structure that clearly separated the accreditation process from any potential for conflict of interest within the organization. There were many changes in the accreditation process in 1995 and 1996, when the National Advisory Committee on Institutional Quality and Integrity (NACIQI), which acts in an advisory capacity to the Secretary of Education,

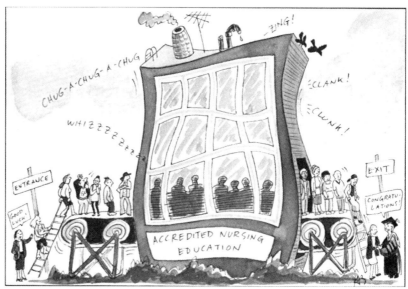

FIGURE 3-7
Accreditation is designed to help ensure that the desired outcomes of education are achieved.

established a new framework for voluntary accreditation with many additional regulatory features (Tanner, 1996).

The goals of accreditation include providing the public with well-prepared nurses, guiding students in the selection of a program, ensuring the public of the quality of a school and its faculty, and stimulating the continued improvement in schools (Fig. 3-7). Recently there has been a significant push toward evaluating the "outcomes" of various educational programs rather than focusing more heavily on the process of education and its structure. The criteria for accreditation developed by each educational council reflected an outcome-oriented approach after June 1991.

Program and Professional Development. The NLN also offers consultation to schools that are seeking to improve their programs or that are initiating new programs, and to health agencies that are seeking to improve services. This consultation usually takes the form of personal visits to the school by paid staff and appointed members, but consultations at NLN headquarters or by telephone are also offered.

The NLN sponsors continuing education workshops and conferences throughout the country, often repeating a workshop in different locations to spare nurses and others the expense of travel. Subjects are determined in consultation with the councils and are geared to current needs and interests. Curriculum, research, accreditation, testing and evaluation, student recruitment and retention, political awareness and health care legislation, and a nurse executive series are regular subjects for continuing education. The NLN has developed and conducted workshops designed to assist the new graduate with the state licensing examination. The constituent leagues, which are grouped by regional assemblies, also offer workshops designed to meet the interests of particular areas of the country.

Division of Research. When any group needs figures on nursing education, it cites data gathered by NLN's Division of Research. The division is a primary provider of statistics on nursing education, and each year surveys all schools of registered and practical nursing for enrollments, admissions, and graduations. It also conducts a yearly survey of newly registered nurses regarding the characteristics of their employment. Every 2 years the nurse–faculty census is taken; every 3 years data are gathered on men and minorities in schools of nursing. These data are published in the annual *Nursing Data Book*. The division also publishes the yearly "blue books," which contain essential information about state-approved schools of registered nursing and practical nursing.

Information and Publications. The career information service answers the thousands of inquiries about nursing education that arrive each year by mail and by telephone. The NLN publishes annual lists of accredited schools of associate degree, baccalaureate, master's, diploma, and practical nursing programs, plus a list of doctoral programs and information on scholarships and loans. (Each of these booklets carries a nominal price.)

Through its journal, *Nursing & Health Care: Perspectives on Community,* and a newsletter, *NLN Update,* members are kept informed about current issues. Sometimes NLN spokespersons offer testimony on legislation or rulings significant to the organization. The NLN publishes a number of texts and references regarding curriculum, ethics, public policy, nursing administration, long-term care, and other topics of interest to nursing. It also produces many educational videos.

National Council of State Boards of Nursing

Although it is not a nursing organization like those previously discussed, our discussion would not be complete without mention of the National Council of State Boards of Nursing, Inc. (NCSBN). This organization was organized in 1978 to replace the Council of State Boards that had been part of the ANA. The purpose of this organization is to provide a forum for the legal regulatory bodies (whatever their particular state titles might be) of all states to act together in the development of the licensing examinations, and in other matters of common concern. There is one delegate to this council from each state agency. The actions of this council are particularly important because its membership represents the legal authority for the control of nursing education and nursing practice.

Although each state agency must operate within its own laws, it does have authority to establish many specific rules and regulations. Working together, the state boards hope to promote uniform standards for the nursing profession. One of the agenda items they have addressed is the development of a Model Nurse Practice Act. Much energy has gone into the development, validation, and establishment of computerized testing for the licensing examination for both registered and practical nursing. Currently the organization is studying the methods used to approve and license advanced practice nurses and the concerns associated with multistate practice.

Organizations Representing Licensed Practical Nurses

Two nursing organizations are concerned primarily with advancing the interests of practical (vocational) nurses. These two organizations are the National Federation of Licensed Practical Nurses (NFLPN) and the National Association for Practical Nurse Education and Service (NAPNES).

The National Federation of Licensed Practical Nurses (NFLPN) is one of the professional organizations for practical nurses. Founded in 1949, its membership is limited to licensed practical and vocational nurses. The NFLPN has assisted the ANA in some of its activities, and actively supports the need for the practical nurse in health care. State and local groups of the NFLPN are active in regard to educational issues affecting the licensed practical nurse, and have supported the associate degree as the appropriate educational preparation for the responsibilities of the licensed practical nurse in the current health care system.

The National Association for Practical Nurse Education and Service was organized as the Association of Practical Nurse Schools in 1941. Its purpose was to address the needs of practical nursing education. The name was changed in 1942 to the National Association for Practical Nurse Education and, in 1959, it added ''and Service'' to that title. The official publication of the organization is *The Journal of Practical Nursing*, which it has been published since 1951. It also publishes a newsletter, *NAPNES Forum*, that keeps members alert to activities of the organization. Membership is open to licensed practical/vocational nurses, practical/vocational nursing students, faculty, directors, and others interested in promoting the purposes of the organization. It was the first organization to provide accreditation for practical nursing programs, although that role now rests with the NLN affiliate.

North American Nursing Diagnosis Association

The North American Nursing Diagnosis Association (NANDA) is open to individuals as well as to group members. The purpose of this group is to work toward uniform terminology and definitions to be used in nursing diagnosis, and to share ideas and information regarding this topic. Members identify and research problems nurses manage, prepare documentation, and submit these to NANDA to be included in the consideration process. The problems are then reviewed by committees. Those that meet the basic criteria for nursing diagnoses are submitted to the membership. Defining characteristics are identified, and conditions that form the etiology or are related to the development of the diagnosis are identified. A national convention held every 2 years is the final forum for the debate and discussion of proposed new nursing diagnoses. The general outline of the taxonomy (classification system) was established by a group of nursing theorists and then accepted by the organization.

Clinically Related Organizations

Some of the earliest specialty organizations were related to specific clinical practice areas of nursing. A major focus of these organizations now is continuing education related to a particular nursing specialty. Most of these groups also have some mechanisms, such as certification, for recognizing achievement in the field. One of the earliest specialty organizations, founded in 1941, was the American Association of Nurse Anesthetists, a group of approximately 24,000 members, of whom 40% are men.

Specialty organizations also include groups that began as auxiliaries to specialty physicians' organizations such as the AWHONN: The Association of Women's Health, Obstetric and Neonatal Nurses. This organization was started for nurses affiliated with physicians who were "fellows" of the American College of Obstetricians and Gynecologists. As more members joined and nurses became more active, groups such as this one became autonomous (see Appendix B for a listing of the major specialty groups.)

The overlapping purpose and actions of the Councils on Practice of the ANA and the corresponding specialty organizations have caused some concern. One attempt to promote a more cooperative effort was the creation of the Nursing Organization Liaison Forum (NOLF), which operates as a forum within the ANA.

One of the newest nursing organizations is the National Alliance of Nurse Practitioners (NANP), organized in 1986. Its purpose is to promote the health care of the nation by promoting the visibility, viability, and unity of nurse practitioners. Its activities focus on advancing the role of the nurse practitioner in the health care delivery system. Issues related to the reimbursement of nurse practitioners are of major concern to this organization.

Groups Related to Ethnic Origin

As the movement for self-determination and preservation of identity arose within ethnic groups in the United States, nurses within various ethnic groups began to unite to achieve a greater voice in health care. Some ethnic groups are nationally organized; others are organized on a more local level. As these groups have become stronger and more organized, their interests have included the recruitment and support of nursing students from the particular ethnic groups they represent. These ethnic groups also encourage their members to become more politically involved in nursing and nursing leadership.

Honorary Organizations

Sigma Theta Tau is an international organization established in collegiate schools of nursing to recognize those who have superior ability and leadership potential, and those who have made important contributions to nursing. Candidates may be asked to join during the senior year of a baccalaureate program, or any time thereafter. Sigma Theta Tau has established a nursing library at its headquarters in Indianapolis that has reference abilities to support advanced scholarship; the organization also provides the first "on-line" nursing journal that can be accessed by computer. Local chapters may maintain funds to support individual research projects, hold research conferences, and recognize those who have made significant contributions to nursing.

Alpha Tau Delta is a professional nursing fraternity. Students who are enrolled in baccalaureate nursing programs and demonstrate scholarship and personality characteristics in line with the organization's professional goals are eligible for membership.

Religiously Oriented Organizations

The National Council of Catholic Nurses and the Nurses' Christian Fellowship (primarily a nondenominational Protestant group) were organized to assist nurses in sharing concerns and integrating their work and their religious beliefs. These two organizations place special emphasis on meeting a patient's spiritual needs and on dealing with ethical issues.

Educationally Oriented Organizations

Since the 1960s, there has been a great deal of change and development in nursing education as it has moved from the hospital into the educational setting. During this time there has been an increasing emphasis on educational methods, curriculum development, and research.

Within several major geographical regions of the United States, educational organizations extending membership to schools of nursing, members of the state boards of nursing, and other interested individuals, were developed to promote interstate and interinstitutional cooperation in seeking pathways to improved nursing education and scholarship. These organizations are the Western Institute of Nursing (WIN), the Council on Collegiate Education for Nursing of the Southern Regional Education Board (CCEN/SREB), the New England Organization for Nursing (NEON), the Midwest Alliance in Nursing (MAIN), and the Mid-Atlantic Regional Nursing Association (MARNA).

The National Organization for the Advancement of Associate Degree Nursing (NOAADN) has four purposes: to speak for associate degree nursing education and practice, to reinforce the value of associate degree nursing education and practice, to maintain endorsement of registered nurse licensure from state to state for the associate degree nurse, and to retain the registered nurse licensure examination for graduates of associate degree nursing programs. Membership is open to individuals, states, agencies, and organizations.

The American Association of Colleges of Nursing (AACN) was formed to assist collegiate schools of nursing in working cooperatively to improve higher education for professional nursing. Membership is restricted to deans and directors of programs that offer a baccalaureate degree in nursing, with an upper-division nursing major, and that are part of a regionally accredited college or university. In 1996, this organization instituted planning to become an accrediting organization for baccalaureate and higher degree programs in nursing. When plans are completed, both the NLNAC and the AACN will be offering accreditation for these programs.

Hospital schools of nursing have formed the National Association of Hospital Schools of Nursing, the aim of which is to support quality education in hospital-based programs. As the number of hospital-based schools of nursing has declined, this organization has decreased in size (Fig. 3-8).

Political Action Organizations

Specific rules and regulations govern the conduct of individuals and groups in the political realm. A nonprofit professional organization may provide expert testimony in regard to an issue, but is prohibited from actively lobbying on the behalf of legislation or candidates. As nurses have become more politically active, one of the routes they have chosen for affecting the political process has been the formation of specific political groups. The financing of these groups must not be related to any nonprofit organization, and membership must be voluntary. Political action groups are free to undertake lobbying efforts as well as to work on behalf of candidates.

As discussed previously, since 1974, the ANA has sponsored a political action committee. Formerly known as N-CAP, the group is now called ANA-PAC. Many individual states also have political action organizations for nurses.

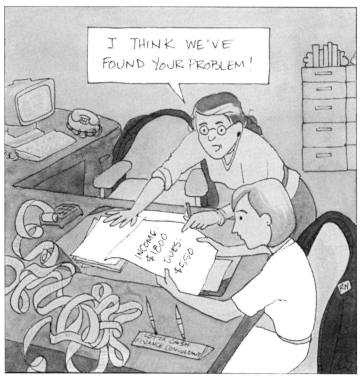

FIGURE 3-8
Deciding which organizations to join is an economic as well as a philosophical decision.

Miscellaneous Organizations

The Gay Nurses' Alliance was an outgrowth of the movement of homosexual individuals to be accepted without having to disguise their sexual orientation. This group has primarily focused on the issue of gay rights. They also provide a forum for individuals to address the difficulties they may face in the nursing profession.

The American Assembly for Men in Nursing was formed by those who believed that, as a minority in the profession, men needed to speak about issues with a united voice. The membership has expanded to include women who are concerned about gender issues in nursing. The organization has addressed the issue of discrimination toward men in nursing and seeks to present nursing as a profession in which both men and women can contribute and excel.

Nurses House, Inc. provides assistance for nurses in need. It originated from a bequest in 1922 from Emily Bourne, who donated $300,000 to establish a country place where nurses might find needed rest. As the need for this residence decreased, supporters of this endeavor sold the estate and invested the proceeds. Income from the investment and funds donated by nurses (and friends of nurses) are used to provide guidance and counseling for nurses with emotional and chemical dependency problems, encouragement to homebound nurses, and temporary financial assistance to nurses who are ill, convalescing, or unemployed. Nurses House seeks members and donations to assist in continuing these activities.

KEY CONCEPTS

- Because scarce resources are allocated through the political process, nurses will find that understanding this process is essential to influence the health care system.
- Every individual nurse has many opportunities to affect the political process. This may be done simply through keeping informed, through voting, or through trying to shape public opinion. Communicating with legislators and officials can be done as an individual of as part of a group. Testifying presents issues of importance, and individual support may be given to those running for office. You may even make the decision to run for a public office.
- The federal government is active in health care through many existing agencies within the Department of Health and Human Services and within other branches of government. The federal budget process affects the health care services that are available through the many legislative acts affecting health care.
- Many factors are coming together in support of health care reform. Nursing organizations are supporting efforts to reform health care access, quality, and cost control. The major reform proposals take different approaches to funding, managing reimbursement, malpractice reform, the role of the states, determining who should be covered, and determining what benefits should be included in new health care plans.
- A political process is part of any large organization and nursing organizations are no exception. Understanding the political process will help you to be a more effective participant in a large organization.
- The wide variety of organizations that exist in nursing are often confusing to the new nursing graduate and to the public. These organizations represent nurses and special interest groups in nursing.
- A major nursing organization is the American Nurses Association, whose membership is open to registered nurses only. It is recognized as the voice of professional nursing. It is also active in issues related to the economic welfare of nurses.
- The National Student Nurses Association addresses the interests and needs of nursing students. This is a fully autonomous organization open to nursing students only.
- Another major nursing organization is the National League for Nursing which, historically, has championed better nursing education. Membership is open to individuals and agencies interested in nursing. The NLN is responsible for the accreditation of nursing programs throughout the United States.
- Two nursing organizations exist expressly to serve the needs of licensed practical (vocational) nurses. These groups are the National Federation of Licensed Practical Nurses and the National Association for Practical Nurse Education and Service.
- Organizations also exist that represent specialty groups in nursing. Members are usually drawn together by their common interests and concerns. The organizations provide continuing education and, in some instances, certification.
- Some organizations, such as Sigma Theta Tau, are honorary in their focus. These groups strive to bring recognition to nurses and nursing.

- A wide variety of other organizations meet the special needs of their membership. This may relate to social interests, ethnic background, or other common denominators.

Critical Thinking Activities

1. Identify a political issue about which you feel strongly. Write a letter to a governmental official that provides sound rationale in support of your position.
2. Identify an aspect of health care reform that concerns you. Analyze the various proposals currently before Congress or your state legislature in regard to that specific concern. Rank the proposals in order of your preference, providing rationale for your decision-making.
3. In a small group, divide the various proposals for health care reform among all the participants. Hold a discussion in which you analyze the proposals.
4. Identify a current health care issue in your state or province. Investigate that issue and form a position that you can support with data.
5. Contact your state nurses' association and find out if your state has a political action organization. If it does, contact that organization and ask what the current issues are in the state. Investigate those issues.
6. As a new graduate, assume you have $400 per year to spend on membership in a nursing organization. Which organization would you join? Provide a clear rationale based on both economic and professional reasons for your choice.
7. In trying to decide which organization to join, how would you go about learning the focus of several groups that have attracted your interest? What process could you use to ensure that you are joining the group that best serves your needs?
8. If you could develop a method for reducing the number of nursing organizations, what criteria would you suggest be used to support the continuation of existing groups? Provide the rationale for each criterion you suggest.
9. Do you believe that there are too many nursing organizations? Give the rationale for your answer.

REFERENCES

American Nurses Association. Nursing's Agenda for Health Care Reform. Washington, DC: American Nurses Publishing Co., 1991

American Nurses Association. Nursing: A Social Policy Statement. Kansas City, MO: American Nurses Association, 1980

ANA testifies on women's health issues. Capitol Update 12(5):5, 1994

Bowles C. The NLN makes a new road: An interview with NLN CEO Patricia Moccia. NHC Perspectives on Community 17(2):82–87, 1996

Costello K. ANA weak on protecting nursing practice. Calif Nurse 91(8):4, 16, 1995

Division of Nursing, U.S. Dept. of Public Health, Funding and Application Data for Grant Programs Administered by the Division of Nursing, National League for Nursing 1964–1990

Kurzen CR. Contemporary Practical/Vocational Nursing. Philadelphia: JB Lippincott, 1989

Lasswell H. Politics: Who gets what, when, how. New York; Meridian Books, 1986, p. 3.

Maynard CA. Stakeholders in the political process: Nurses' role in MinnesotaCare. Nurs Policy Forum 1(5):18–25, 1995

Sharp N. Women's Health Equity Act of 1990. Nurs Management 21(12):21–22, 1990

Snyder ME, LaBar C. Issues in Professional Practice: I. Nursing: Legal Authority for Practice. Kansas City, MO: American Nurses Association, 1984

Tanner CA, Accreditation under siege. J Nurs Educ 35(6):243-244, 1996

Watson PG. The Americans with Disabilities Act: More rights for people with disabilities. Rehabil Nurs 15(6):325–328, 1990

White KM. Federal observer: The future of health professions education: How will the Nurse Education Act fare? Nurs Policy Forum 1(5):8–9, 1995

Wimberly JW Jr. The family medical leave act of 1993. AAOHN J 41(11):551–557, 1993

Woodham-Smith C. Florence Nightingale. New York: Atheneum, 1983 (reprint of 1951 edition)

FURTHER READING

The American Nurse. Kansas City, MO: American Nurses Association, monthly newspaper

Capitol Commentary. A monthly publication regarding federal health actions and activities published by the ANA.

Cassetta RA. ANA governmental affairs: Working for you in Washington. Am Nurse 26(4):16, 1994

Cassetta RA. RNs fight for recognition of women's health issues. Am Nurse 26(2):1, 16, 1994

Cella KJ. Legislation: NAFTA NIOSH & OSHA. Imprint 43(2):31–32, 1996

Chaffee M. Insider's viewpoint: The nurse in Washington internship (NIWI). Nurs Policy Forum 2(1): 12–15, 18–19, 1996

Chinn P. Looking into the crystal ball: Positioning ourselves for the year 2000. Nurs Outlook 39:251–256, 1991

deVries C, Vanderbilt M. The Grassroots Lobbying Handbook: Empowering Nurses Through Legislative and Political Action. Washington, DC: American Nurses Publishing Co., 1991

deVries C, Vanderbilt M. Key players on bill hear ANA input on reform. Am Nurse 26(4):1, 20, 1994

Fry ST. Ethical implications of health care reform. Am Nurse 26(3):5, 1994

Griffith HM. Needed–A strong nursing position on preventive service. Image 25(4):272–284, 1993

Hall-Long BA. Nursing's past, present, and future political experiences. NHC Perspectives on Community 16(1): 24–28, 1995

Headline News. American Journal of Nursing, A regular column in each month

Helms LB, Anderson MA, Hanson K. "Doin' politics": Linking policy and politics in nursing. Nurs Admin Quart 20(3): 32–41, 1996

Huston CJ. Nursing and political action in the 20th century: From separation to fusion. Revolution 5(3):50–53, 1995

Keepnews D. Issues: ANA challenges Pew Health Profession's findings. Imprint 43(3):24–25, 1996

Keepnews D, Marullo G. Policy imperatives for nursing in an era of health care reform. Nurs Admin Quart 20(3):19–31, 1996

Ketter J. ANA, Dept of Labor discuss workplace issues. Am Nurse 26(6):1, 3, 1994

Rodwell CM. An analysis of the concept of empowerment. J Adv Nurs 23(2):305–313, 1996

Scott K. RN career security is ANA goal for reform. Am Nurse 25(9):1, 6, 1993

Sharp N. Legislative effects: It's politics, not policy. Nurs Management 26(12):18–19, 1995

Simpson M, Hanley B. Nurse policy analyst: Advanced practice role. Nurs Health Care 12(1):10–15, 1991

Welch JK. Political action can save jobs for American nurses. Revolution 5(4):71–73, 1995

See also the official publication of your state nurses' association.

Understanding the Development of Nursing as a Profession

You have learned about the health care delivery system and how it operates and is financed. You have also had the opportunity to consider the employment settings in which nurses seek positions, and you have gained an exposure to the importance of the political process to nursing. To continue in your understanding of the role you are about to assume, learning about the history and development of the profession will help you to appreciate the heritage of the discipline and the events that resulted in nursing offering the opportunities and challenges it provides today. Nursing is considered a relatively young profession by many people. Others believe that it has yet to achieve professional status. The educational processes by which we prepare nurses continue to experience change and modification. Are you interested in how this might affect you and your career in nursing? In this unit we present a history of nursing that describes its growth from an apprentice-type training to a profession that encompasses doctoral degrees. You will learn about some of the individuals who made significant contributions to the profession. We also discuss and describe the various educational routes by which you can prepare for a role as a nurse and conclude with a discussion of the future of nursing education.

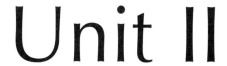

Unit II

Exploring Nursing's Origins

History can open the door to storehouses of information that can be used to assist with the development of reasoned conclusions about specific phenomena. Critical thinking cannot help but be fostered and strengthened by the study of history. (Donahue, 1993)

Objectives

After completing this chapter, you should be able to:

1. Describe the health care practices of early civilizations.

2. Analyze how each of the three historical images of the nurse has influenced the development of nursing as a profession.

3. Explain the significance of the "Dark Ages of Nursing" to the development of the nursing profession.

4. Discuss the contribution of Florence Nightingale to nursing and its development.

5. Explain the impact of the Civil War on the development of nursing in the United States.

6. Describe the early development of nursing schools in the United States.

7. Delineate the characteristics of early nursing programs.

8. Identify the first organizations created by and for nurses and discuss the purpose of each.

9. Discuss the history of hospitals and long-term care facilities in the United States.

10. Identify the factors that influenced the development of health care facilities and explain why each was important.

KEY TERMS

Almshouse
Ancient cultures
Civil War
"Dark Ages of Nursing"
Flexner Report
Florence Nightingale
Folk image of nursing

Hospitals
Long-term care facilities
Nursing organizations
Pesthouse
Religious image of nursing
Servant image of nursing
"Uncommon women"

It is impossible to specify a particular date or time period at which nursing, as we know it now, came into being. The same can be said of medicine. Our best speculations regarding their origins must necessarily be tied to our knowledge of cultures that existed in the past, and to the contributions these cultures left for posterity. As you might anticipate, these cultures were many and varied. They reflected the events and developments (or lack of the same) that characterized each given period in history. In this chapter we will review some of the various cultures and historical events that have contributed to nursing's history.

HEALTH CARE IN ANCIENT CULTURES

The life of primitive societies was necessarily a nomadic one. Well-defined groups, built around the nucleus of family relationships, wandered in search of food, warmth, and an environment that supported life. Solidarity among these scattered groups, organized for the convenient management of human affairs, existed for purposes of mutual protection. Anthropologists believe that primitive groups originated in Africa and migrated across the world. Ice ages in the northern latitudes drove these groups back to the warmer climates found around the Mediterranean Sea, in India, and in China, where civilizations developed. Historians suggest that the movement of early tribes radiated from the interior of Europe and Asia toward the warm shores of the Mediterranean Sea, India and China (Jamieson & Sewell, 1944). The regions around the Mediterranean Sea were thought to occupy the center of the earth with all areas to the east known as ''eastern'' and all those to the west known as ''western'' (Donahue, 1996, p. 28). The sophistication of health care practices varied considerably from one culture to another.

Egypt

The ancient Egyptians, who settled in the long, narrow valley that lay along the banks of the Nile River while other cultures were settling along the Indus, Euphrates, and Tigris rivers, developed a community considered to be much more advanced than others. By the year 5000 B.C., stone implements had been developed to facilitate work, followed by the wheel and cart, and animals were domesticated to help with heavy burdens. A system of irrigation increased the productivity of the fertile soil.

In Egyptian culture, treating disease was considered the responsibility of priests. The Egyptians, like the people of all early cultures, looked on natural phenomena as the work of the gods. Health and security meant keeping the gods happy.

The oldest medical records so far discovered and deciphered are those from Egypt, dating back as far as 3000 B.C. Early records were carved in stone or written on papyrus. The Egyptians developed an elaborate pharmacopoeia that classified more than 700 drugs, and a system of community planning that helped to avoid public health problems, especially those related to disease transmitted through water sources. Egypt is credited with being one of the healthiest of the ancient countries, perhaps because of the progress it made in the fields of hygiene and sanitation. The Egyptians developed strict rules around such things as cleanliness, food, drink, exercise, and sexual relations. They also established a ''house of death,'' which was located at a site away from civilization. Mummies that have survived to the present day clearly show that the Egyptians were skilled in wrapping and embalming their dead. It is also believed that they were accomplished in dentistry, often filling teeth with gold. The oldest known medical books come from Egypt. These books outline surgical techniques and methods of birth control, describe disease processes, and suggest remedies. Out of this culture came the first physician known to history, Imhotep (2900–2800 B.C.). He was recognized as a surgeon, an architect, a temple priest, a scribe, and a magician. Although women in ancient Egypt received more respect than women in other Eastern countries, it is not clear whether nurses existed as such. Women most likely worked in the temples, along with priest–physicians, holding the rank of priestess or serving as midwives or ''wet nurses.''

Cultures of the Fertile Crescent

Several cultures made their homes in a crescent-shaped strip of land that extended from the Persian Gulf on the east to the Mediterranean Sea on the west. This area, known as the Fertile Crescent, enjoyed a warm, hospitable climate and rich soil, and benefited from the water provided by three great rivers–the Tigris, the Euphrates, and the River Jordan. The Fertile Crescent is often referred to as the ''cradle of civilization.'' Because the cultures that settled there were often warlike and took possession of land by con-quering the empire in power, the boundaries of these early societies sometimes over-lapped.

PALESTINE

The Hebrews made their home in the area called Palestine, at the western end of the Fertile Crescent and adjacent to Egypt. This region included what is now Israel, as well as some of the surrounding area. The society of the Hebrews was primarily an agricultural one, and the country was ruled by kings. The Hebrews are credited with more democratic sharing of knowledge than any of the other ancient civilizations. Under the leadership of Moses, the adopted son of the Egyptian Pharaoh's daughter, the Hebrews developed the Mosaic Code, which included an organized method of disease prevention. The code emphasized the iso-lation of people with communicable diseases, differentiated clean from unclean, and covered every detail of personal, family, and public hygiene. With regard to their treatment of women, Nutting and Dock (1935) write:

All the stern and ungraciously sounding texts relating to the 'uncleanliness' of women, which when considered only in the abstract seem so needlessly humiliating, are in reality witnesses of the extreme care and solicitude of the Jews for the health of their women, and of the sanctity and beauty of their family life. These regulations secured to women the personal isolation and privacy, quiet, and con-sideration necessary on hygienic grounds, and especially made the time of childbirth a period of isolation and quiet, of cleanliness of body and clothing, and of rest for mind and body (pp. 62–63).

Bible scriptures such as Leviticus 7:16–19 and 19:5–8, which forbade the eating of meat past the third day after an animal was slaughtered, were no doubt written because of the effects of the warm climate and lack of refrigeration. Similarly, Mosaic and Talmudic regulations regarding the slaughtering of animals, which included requirements for exami-nation and inspection to check for diseases of the internal organs, were in keeping with the advanced sanitary ordinances of Hebrew society.

Hebrew culture recognized one god who had power over life and death. From this belief evolved the role of the priest as supervisor of medical practices relating to cleansing and purification. Priest–physicians took on the function of health inspectors. The writings of the early Jewish rabbis taught that visiting the sick was a duty, even if the sick were Gentile. Houses for the sick during this early period were called "Beth Holem."

BABYLONIA

The life-style of the Babylonians was entirely different from that of the Egyptians or the Hebrews. Babylonia was located in the southern part of present-day Iraq, although its borders differed from those of the modern country. Each city was an autonomous community governed by a divine ruler and a priest–king. Women never enjoyed much esteem in Babylonian society; polygamy was acceptable, and woman's role was a domestic one.

The Babylonians are credited with being skilled mathematicians and astrologers. Many of the beliefs of the Babylonians were based on their study of nature, their belief in the potency of numbers, and their observations of the movement of stars and planets. The division of the year into months, weeks, days, hours, and minutes is said to have originated with the Babylonians.

The Babylonians believed illness to be the punishment for sin and for displeasing the gods. A cure was brought about by purifying the body, usually by incantations and the use of herbs. Temples, in which the purification occurred, became centers of medical care (Fig 4-1). Preventive medicine consisted of doing what it was believed the gods desired. Babylonia is the source of the second oldest surviving medical records (Nutting & Dock, 1935). In Babylonian culture, surgery was more advanced than internal medicine, which concerned itself primarily with banishing demons and avoiding evil spirits.

In 1900 B.C., Hammurabi, King of Babylonia, developed the famous Code of Hammurabi. The principal source of our knowledge of this code is a stone monument found in 1901 and preserved today in the Louvre in Paris. This code, which may represent the first sliding scale for fee payment, divided the public into three classes. Those classified as "gentlemen" were expected to pay their surgeons in silver coins rather than in goods or services. A surgeon who bungled an operation on a "gentleman" risked paying a heavy price; the surgeon might have his hands cut off if the surgery was not successful. This puts the malpractice rates absorbed by physicians today in a different light.

ASSYRIA

The history of the Assyrians began around 2300 B.C. This nation was centered in the northern part of present-day Iraq, and extended into what is now Syria and southern Iraq as it conquered other nations. After ceaseless warfare, the Assyrians took possession of the land of Babylonia. The Assyrians are characterized as a hardened, war-like group whose laws were severe, and who made frequent use of the death penalty. They believed in good and evil spirits, in magic, and in many gods. They also believed that ill health was a punishment for sin and that a person's body could be occupied by evil spirits. The practice of medicine developed around these religious beliefs.

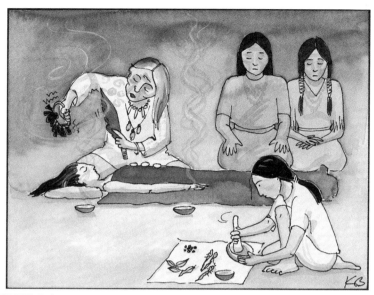

FIGURE 4-1
Internal medicine concerned itself with banishing demons by incantations and the use of herbs.

Persia

Persia, one of the most extensive empires of the Near East, was located in what is now modern-day Iran and, at one time, extended throughout the Fertile Crescent. The Persians' quest for territory and power resulted in their conquest of much of that area. They believed in Zoroaster, a prophet who wrote the sacred books of Persia. His writings introduced the world to the concept of two creators—one good, and one evil—and to the sacred elements of fire, earth, and water. The writings of Zoroaster also introduced the concept of immortality as a mental state. The Persians adopted the cultural practices of the lands they conquered, including many of the medical and surgical practices of Egypt. They established early schools to prepare priest–physicians, from which evolved three types of physicians—those who healed by the knife, those who healed with herbs, and those who healed through exorcism.

Greece

Greek civilization developed on a peninsula that extended out into the Mediterranean Sea from the southeastern part of Europe. The ancient Greeks are remembered in part for their worship of gods and goddesses and also for their emphasis on healthy bodies, which led them to found the Olympic games. In Greek mythology, Asklepios (sometimes spelled Aesclepius or Asclepius), son of Apollo, was taught the healing arts by Cheiron, a wise centaur. Asklepios is usually represented as carrying a staff, to show that he traveled from place to place, around which is entwined a serpent, representing wisdom and immortality. Some people believe that when the army medical services fashioned the caduceus, the symbol of the medical profession, the staff and serpent that were incorporated into the symbol came from this legend.

Exquisite temples, located on beautiful sites, were built as shrines to Asklepios; these temples became social and intellectual centers as well as places to obtain cures. The curative process usually began with animal sacrifice and continued through various purifying rituals. In addition to these shrines, two other institutions, the xenodochium and the iatrion, offered care to the sick in ancient Greece. The xenodochium first offered care to travelers and later to people who were sick and injured. This may have been the forerunner of the city or county hospital as we know it today. The iatrion was a facility offering ambulatory care and would have corresponded to our outpatient clinics.

It is rather surprising that from this society, so heavily steeped in mythology, animal sacrifice, and faith in the power of the gods, came the Father of Modern Medicine. Hippocrates was born about 400 B.C. on the island of Cos. He stressed natural causes for disease, treated the whole patient with a patient-centered approach to care, and introduced the scientific method of solving patient problems. His teaching emphasized the necessity of accurate observations and careful record keeping. Hippocrates did not attribute ill health to an infliction by the gods but rather believed that health depended on an equilibrium existing among the mind, the body, and the environment. From his philosophy evolved the humoral theory of disease, which has lasted for centuries.

Many other early physicians came from Greece, although some eventually practiced their skills in Rome after Greece was conquered by the Roman Empire. Galen, Aesclepiades, and Pedanim Dioscorides were all Greek physicians who worked in Rome.

Rome

The medical advances of the ancient Romans fell short of those of the Greeks. Medical practices were often borrowed from the countries the Romans conquered, and the physicians from those countries were made slaves who provided medical services to the Romans. At one time the Roman Empire was quite extensive, stretching across the entire northern border of Africa and Egypt. The Romans clung to gods, superstition, and herbs when faced with disease, but their hygiene and sanitation were fairly well advanced. Their genius found its best expression in the area of public hygiene rather than in medicine per se. Many homes were equipped with baths, and cleanliness was valued. The Romans also constructed public baths.

Roman society was divided into two classes: the patricians, who were an affluent and privileged group, and the plebeians, who represented the poor or lower class and were denied citizenship. Patrician women in Roman society had more privileges than women of similar economic status in other ancient cultures. Women were quite independent and were allowed to own property, appear in public, and campaign publicly for causes they believed should be advanced. They could even entertain guests and sit with them at the table.

India

Located in the southern part of the Far East, India was essentially isolated by mountains from other parts of the ancient world. People who migrated from central Asia in ancient times traveled through the mountain passes. Excavations indicate that the first civilizations in India (3000–1500 B.C.) were highly developed, with systems of sanitation, bathrooms and public baths, and other amenities. The Vedic age began in 1500 B.C. and was characterized by worship of the eternal spirit Brahma. Brahmanism (also known as Hinduism) was to become a major religion in India, out of which developed the stratification of Indian society into four different castes and the concept of sacrifice to satisfy gods. Sources of information about health practices come from the Vedas, a sacred book of Brahmanism dating back as far as 1600 B.C. and considered by some to be the oldest known written material. Medicine, as described in the books of *Ayur Veda* (or the Veda of Longevity), emphasized hygiene and prevention of sickness and included discussions of major and minor surgery, children's diseases (including inoculation against smallpox), materia medica, and diseases of the nervous and urinary systems (Nutting & Dock, 1935; Jamieson & Sewall, 1944). Their practice of surgery may have been the most highly developed of any ancient culture.

Siddhartha Gautama, who lived about 500 B.C., was a Hindu ascetic who, at age 29, left his wife and child to find salvation and to develop a more intimate relationship with the spiritual. He attained a state called "enlightenment," declaring himself Buddha and offering a new religious philosophy known as Buddhism. Buddhism emerged as the major religion of early India, although some would consider it more of a moral discipline than a religion. Buddha aspired to bring peace and contentment (Nirvana) to all, which he believed could be achieved by freeing the self of all desires and worldly things. During the Buddhist period, under the rule of King Asoka, India developed an advanced understanding of disease prevention, hygiene and sanitation, medicine, and surgery. The importance of prenatal care to both mother and infant seemed well understood and practiced. Buddhism disregarded the caste system of the earlier religion, and made education and the right to peace possible for everyone. Public hospitals were constructed during this time, and some vital statistics were collected. These hospitals were staffed with nurses whose qualifications were similar to those expected of today's practical nurses. The main difference was that, in almost all cases, Indian nurses were men. In rare instances, old women were permitted to assume this role. Donahue (1996, p. 48) states that three main qualities of character were required of these attendants—high standards, skill, and trustworthiness.

China

Ancient China was located far to the northeast of India, across the range of the Himalaya Mountains and, like India, was cut off from the Mediterranean world. The Chinese are thought to have come from central Asia around 3000 B.C. (Jamieson & Sewall, 1944). Chinese civilization developed along the banks of the Yellow River. The ancient Chinese followed the teachings of Confucius, who sought to relieve the country's oppression by reviving ancient customs as a basis for a government ideal. Patriarchal rule dominated, and emphasis was placed on the value of the family as a unit. Ancestor worship attained great importance. Great emphasis was place on the value of knowledge in solving life's problems, and rules of etiquette were important. Women were considered vastly inferior to men; a woman's value was determined by the number of sons she could produce. A daughter was always severed from connection with her family when she married; her obligations and loyalties were automatically transferred to the family of her husband. Although young married women were treated almost as slaves, old women were received with love and given a position of high esteem in families.

The early Chinese established the philosophy of the yang and the yin. The yang represented the active, positive, masculine force of the universe, and the yin represented the passive, negative, feminine force. The Chinese believed that these two forces operated in contrasting and complementary ways. Health practices based on this philosophy focused on prevention and good health was believed to result from a balance between the yang and the yin.

China's medical knowledge extends far back in history. Dissection was performed in China before 2000 B.C. The development of elaborate materia medica was of major significance; many of the drugs used by the Chinese in ancient times, such as ephedrine, are used in modern medicine. The Chinese developed acupuncture skills that are still being practiced today. They also studied the circulation and placed great stress on the behavior of the pulse. Principles of examination emphasized the following guideposts: ''look, listen, ask, feel.'' Baths were used for the reduction of fever and bloodletting was used as a method of helping an evil spirit escape from the body.

The Americas

Early civilization in the Americas may have begun 10,000 or even 20,000 years ago (Donahue, 1996, p 64). It is thought that early inhabitants probably came from Central Asia, gaining access across a land bridge over the Bering Strait into Alaska. Like other early tribes, they were nomadic, wandering in search of food and shelter. Several groups, including the Mayas, Incas, Aztecs, and Toltecs, developed a high degree of civilization.

The sun god was particularly important to these cultures. Rites, ceremonies, herbal treatments, charms, and, in some instances, human sacrifice, contributed to healing practices. Health was a balance among man, nature, and the supernatural. Medicine, pharmacy, nursing, religion, and magic often were not viewed as separate entities. Medicine men (known first as shamans and later as priests) were responsible for curing ills of both the body and the mind, and disease was believed to result from displeasing the gods.

Little is known about the role of the nurse in these early civilizations, although the status enjoyed by Indian women was good and American Indians made significant contributions to modern-day medicine and medical practice. The Aztecs in particular had hospices for the care of the ill, used minerals as drugs, soporifics to decrease pain, and assisted women with childbirth (Donahue, 1996).

HISTORICAL PERSPECTIVES OF NURSING

Writings about early health care make little or no mention of nursing or nurses. Health practices varied depending on the level of development of a society. Ritualistic ceremonies and worship of gods were common and the role of healer was assumed by various individuals within the culture. Each primitive society had its own curative agents, taboos, and practices, some more advanced than others. A sound theory of disease was absent from most early cultures.

Although ancient cultures developed medicine as a science and a profession, they showed little evidence of establishing a foundation for nursing, with the possible exception of the male attendants in early Buddhist hospitals in India, and of midwives, who had an established role in several cultures. It was not until the early Christian period that nursing as we think of it began to develop.

Muriel Uprichard identifies three heritages from the past that inhibited the progress of nursing. They are ''the folk image of the nurse brought forward from primitive times, the religious image of the nurse inherited from the medieval period, and the servant image of the nurse created by the Protestant-capitalist ethic of the 16th to 19th century'' (Uprichard, 1973, p 24). Whether or not they impeded progress, these concepts of the nurse have certainly had an impact.

The Folk Image of the Nurse

Since the time of the first mother, women have carried the major responsibility for nourishing and nurturing children, and caring for elderly and aging members of the family. It is difficult to pinpoint a particular time or place for the beginning of nursing as we know it. It is reasonable to assume that early tribes and civilizations had needs for health care. It is also reasonable to assume that within those tribes and civilizations there were people who demonstrated adeptness and a special interest in meeting the needs of those who were sick, injured, or bearing children. These ''nurses'' received their education largely through trial and error, by advancing those methods that appeared to be successful and by sharing information. Superstition and magic played a significant role in treatment; folklore abounded, and a close relationship existed between religion and the healing arts.

Nursing skills primarily evolved from intuition. For example, during the process of planning a diet for the family, the wise woman would have noticed that eating certain foods resulted in episodes of diarrhea and vomiting, whereas eating other herbs, roots, and leaves had a soothing effect on the body. Families developed recipes that were handed down from generation to generation; effective treatments and cures were recorded and shared.

The Religious Image of the Nurse

The first continuity in the history of nursing began with Christianity. Christ's teachings admonished people to love and care for their neighbors. With the establishment of churches in the Christian era, groups were organized as orders whose primary concern was to care for the sick, the poor, orphans, widows, the aged, slaves, and prisoners, all in the name of charity and Christian love. Christ's precepts placed women and men on a parity, and the early church made both men and women deacons, with equal rank. Unmarried women had unprecedented opportunities for service. Although these opportunities represented positive changes, they also fostered certain limitations as well. Because nursing developed an image closely tied to religion and religious orders, strict discipline was expected. Absolute attendance to the orders of persons of higher rank (eg, priests or physicians) was demanded. Nursing was characterized by this type of thinking for many years.

THE DEACONESSES

One group of women of particular significance to the history of nursing were the deaconesses of the Eastern Christian Church. These women, who were required to be unmarried or widowed, were often the widows or daughters of Roman officials, and thus had breeding, culture, wealth, and position. These dedicated young women practiced ''works of mercy'' that included feeding the hungry, clothing the naked, visiting the imprisoned, sheltering the homeless, caring for the sick, and burying the dead. The deaconesses were the earliest counterparts to the community health nurses of today. When they entered homes to distribute food and medicine they carried a basket (which would later become the contemporary visiting nurse's bag). No discussion of nursing history would be complete without mentioning Phoebe, who is often referred to as the first deaconess and the first visiting nurse. She carried Paul's letters and cared for him and many others. In the Epistle to the Romans, dated about A.D. 58, reference is made to Phoebe and to her work.

THE WIDOWS AND THE VIRGINS

Two other groups—the Order of Widows and the Order of Virgins— shared many common characteristics with the deaconesses and carried out similar responsibilities. Members of the Order of Widows were not required to have been married. It seems that the title of widow was used to designate respect for age. Those who were married, however, took vows never to remarry if widowed. The Order of Virgins emphasized virginity as essential to purity of life, and virgins were ranked equal to the clergy. Because these women often visited the sick in their homes, they are sometimes recognized as the earliest organized group of public health nurses. The movement peaked in Constantinople in about A.D. 400, when a staff of 40 deaconesses lived and worked under the direction of Olympia, a powerful and deeply religious deaconess. The influence of the deaconess order diminished in the fifth and sixth centuries, when church decrees removed clerical duties and rank from the deaconess.

Although the position of deaconess originated in the Eastern Christian Church, it spread west to Gaul and Ireland. In Rome, women who served in comparable positions were known as matrons. Active during the fourth and fifth centuries, these Roman matrons held independent positions and had great wealth, which they contributed to charity and to nursing. Among these Christian converts were three women who contributed significantly to nursing. The stories of these women are told in Display 4-1.

THE ROLE OF THE MONASTIC ORDERS

The monastic orders also developed during this period, including the order of Benedictines, which still exists. The monasteries played a large role in the preservation of culture and learning as well as in offering refuge to the persecuted, care to the sick, and education to the uneducated. By joining a monastic order, young men and women were able to follow the career of their choice while living a Christian life. The learning of the classical period would have been lost when the Roman empire fell were it not for the monks and monasteries.

One of the earliest organizations for men in nursing, the Parabolani brotherhood, was established at this time. Responding to needs created by the Black Plague, this group re-

DISPLAY 4-1
Roman Matrons

FABIOLA

Fabiola, a charming and beautiful young woman, was born into an influential and wealthy Roman family. Growing up in a lavish home, she enjoyed a happy social life. However, her marriage to a worthless gentleman resulted in divorce. She married a second time, and was no happier in her second marriage. Under the influence of Marcella, she converted to Christianity and, after the death of her second husband, began her career of charity. Fabiola's new beliefs made marriage after divorce a sin. She publicly acknowledged this, committed her life to charitable work, and in 390 A.D. built the first public hospital in Rome described as a *nosocomium*. Here she cared for the sick and poor whom she gathered from the streets and highways, personally washing and treating wounds and sores that repulsed others. Later in her life she is said to have built a hospice for strangers at Ostia, a seaport of Rome. St. Jerome tells of some of her work and her attributes in his writings. She died about 399, and scores of Romans are said to have attended her funeral to show their respect for her.

MARCELLA

A Roman woman of means, Marcella made her luxurious home into a monastery for women. Here other matrons such as Fabiola and Paula became involved in Christian study. Much inspiration came to them through a great friend and teacher, St. Jerome. Marcella devoted her life to instruction, charitable work, and prayer and became recognized as an authority on interpretation of biblical passages. She assisted St. Jerome in his translation of the Hebrew prophets. During the sack of Rome, her home was invaded by warriors who expected to find valuables stored there. When they found little more than a bare building, they whipped Marcella, hoping she would reveal the hiding places of riches. After the assault she is said to have fled to St. Paul's church, which was nearby. There she died as a result of her injuries.

St. PAULA

Learned, wealthy, and broken-hearted by the death of her husband, Saint Paula was also a scholar of Marcella. She is said to have assisted St. Jerome (whose lifetime exceeded that of all the women with whom he associated), in the translation of the writings of the prophets. St. Paula traveled to Palestine and devoted a fortune to the establishment of hospitals and inns for pilgrims traveling to Jerusalem. In Bethlehem she organized a monastery, built hospitals for the sick, and developed hospices for pilgrims, where tired travelers and the ill received care. Some credit her with being the first to teach nursing as an art rather than a service. She had a daughter, Eustochium, who joined her mother in the adoption of Christianity, and with her expressed its ideals through charitable work.

portedly organized a hospital and traveled throughout Rome caring for the sick. At the same time, monastic nurses such as the famous St. Brigid, St. Scholastica (a twin sister of St. Benedict), and St. Hilda, founded schools, tended to the sick, and gave to the poor.

During this period (approximately A.D. 50 to 800), the first hospitals were established. Many of these hospitals, located outside the monastery walls, are still standing. There were more than 700 hospitals in England by the middle of the 16th century. The Hotel Dieu in Lyons was established in 542 and the Hotel Dieu in Paris around 650. The Hotel Dieu in Paris was staffed by the first order specifically devoted to nursing, the Augustinian Sisters. The Santo Spirito Hospital in Rome, the largest medieval hospital, was established by papal order in 717.

The Crusades, which swept northern Europe, lasted for almost 200 years (1096–1291). The deaconess movement, suppressed by the Western Church, became all but extinct. Military nursing orders evolved as a result of the Crusades. The Knights Hospitallers of St. John was one such order. It was organized to staff two hospitals that were located in Jerusalem and had as its grand master a monk named Gerard. He drew up codes and introduced the black robe with a white Maltese cross that became the uniform for the brethren (Kalisch & Kalisch, 1995). The same cross was later used on a badge designed for the Nightingale School; this badge was the forerunner of the nursing pin as we know it today. The symbolism of the pin will be discussed later in this chapter. The Knights, organized as a nursing order, soon became famous for their hospitality and care and their numbers, possessions, and wealth increased. At times they were required to defend the hospital and its patients. In Germany, a women's order called ''consorores'' was founded specifically to perform hospital work. Although they took vows, the women were not granted the same status as the Knights, and they lived outside the monastic precincts.

Two other monastic orders were founded during this period as well; the Knights Templars in 1118 and the Knights of the Teutonic Order in 1190. The Hospitallers and the Templars played significant roles during the Crusades. Secular orders of nurses also came into existence at this time. Operating much like the monastic orders, members of these groups could terminate their vocations at any time and were not bound to the vows of monastic life. Examples of the secular orders include the Order of Antonines (1095); the Beguines of Flanders, Belgium (1184); the Misericordia (1244); and the Alexian Brothers, founded during the bubonic plague epidemic of 1348. The only nursing education offered to these dedicated people was in the form of an apprenticeship; a newcomer to the organization would be assigned to a more experienced person for instruction.

The inquiring student is encouraged to seek greater depth of knowledge about the various nursing orders, their purposes and goals, and the lives of those who devoted their energies to the care of the sick and the poor by consulting the nursing references given at the end of this chapter.

MUSLIM CULTURE

Little has been written in nursing history books regarding health care practices and the role of nursing in early Muslim cultures. Recently, attention has been drawn to an 11th century Muslim ''Nightingale'' named Rufaida Al-Asalmiya, who was a nurse during the time of the Prophet Mohammad. Rufaido Al-Asalmiya lived in Al-Media (Yethreb), a region of what is now Saudi Arabia, where her father was a healer. While assisting her father, Rufaido developed many nursing skills. With the permission of the Prophet Mohammad, she began to train women and young girls in the art of nursing. She is also said to have developed the first code of nursing conduct and ethics, long before it was introduced in the western world. When the holy war began, she is reported to have provided care to the Muslim army in battle, enjoining her Muslim nurses to assist her. She continued this care after the battle ended, setting up tents near the mosque of Nabvi where she provided care and health education. A building at the Aga Khan University School of Nursing has been named in her honor (Jan, 1996).

The Servant Image of the Nurse

The Middle Ages were followed by the Renaissance and the Reformation (occurring from the 14th through the 16th centuries). During the Renaissance, also known as the Age of Discovery, a new impetus was given to education, and, to some extent, to medical education. For example, Ambroise Pare (1510–1590), a French surgeon, revived the method of tying blood vessels to stop hemorrhaging, believing that procedures based on acute observation were better than those based on ancient doctrines. Andreas Vesalium (1514–1564) published a treatise of surgery and anatomy that refuted the teachings of Galen, who up to that point had been the undisputed authority on medicine. Nursing education, however, was all but nonexistent during this period.

The Reformation, a religious movement inspired by the work of Martin Luther, began in Germany in 1517. It resulted in a revolt against the supremacy of the pope and the formation of Protestant churches across Europe. Monasteries were closed, religious orders were dissolved, and the work of women in these orders became almost extinct.

The Reformation brought about a change in the role of women. The Protestant Church, which stood for freedom of religion and thought, did not grant much freedom to women. During the Reformation, women were no longer revered by their churches and encouraged toward charitable activities, but were deemed subordinate to men. Their role was defined within the confines of the home; their duties were those of bearing children and caring for the home. Work in hospitals no longer appealed to women of high birth. Hospital care was relegated to "uncommon" women, a group comprising prisoners, prostitutes, and drunks (Fig. 4-2).

Women faced with earning their own living were forced to work as domestic servants, and although nursing was considered a domestic service, it was not a desirable one. The nurse was considered the most menial of servants. Pay was poor, the hours were long, and the work was strenuous. Nursing care was not subject to inspection and was not governed by standards. The same bed linen might be used for several patients, even though suppurating wounds were common. Thus began what may be called the "Dark Ages" of nursing.

The image of nurses and nursing during this time was described by Charles Dickens (1936) through the characters of Sairey Gamp and Betsy Prig in his book *Martin Chuzzlewit*:

She was a fat old woman, this Mrs. Gamp, with a husky voice and a moist eye, which she had a remarkable power of turning up, and only showing the white of it. Having very little neck, it cost her some trouble to look over herself, if one may say so, at those to whom she talked. She wore a very rusty black gown, rather the worse for snuff, and a shawl and bonnet to correspond . . . . The face of

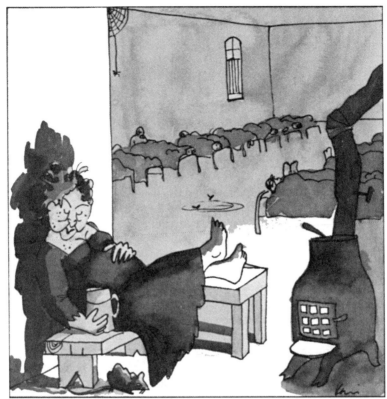

FIGURE 4-2
From the Middle Ages to the 19th century, nursing was often left to "uncommon women."

Mrs. Gamp—the nose in particular—was somewhat red and swollen, and it was difficult to enjoy her society without becoming conscious of a smell of spirits. Like most persons who have attained to great eminence in their profession, she took to hers very kindly; insomuch, that setting aside her natural predilections as a woman, she went to a lying-in or a lying-out with equal zest and relish (p. 318).

Mrs. Prig was of the Gamp build, but not so fat; and her voice was deeper and more like a man's. She had also a beard (p. 417).

The 16th and 17th centuries found Europe devastated by famine, plague, filth, and horror. In England, for example, King Henry VIII had effectively eliminated organized monastic relief provided to orphans and other displaced persons. Throughout Europe vagrancy and begging abounded, and those caught begging were often severely punished by being branded, beaten, or chained in galleys where they served as oarsmen. Knowledge of hygiene was insufficient; the poor suffered the most. Social reform was inevitable. Several nursing groups were organized. These groups gave money, time, and service to the sick and the poor, visiting them in their homes and ministering to their needs. Such groups included the Order of the Visitation of Mary, St. Vincent de Paul, and in 1633, the Sisters of Charity. The last group became an outstanding secular nursing order. They developed an educational program for the intelligent young women they recruited that included experience in a hospital as well as visiting in the home. Receiving help, counsel, and encouragement from St. Vincent de Paul, the Sisters of Charity expanded their services to include caring for abandoned children. In 1640, St. Vincent established the Hospital for Foundlings in Paris. Later, in 1809, the Sisters of Charity established a nursing order in the United States, under the direction of Elizabeth Bayley Seton. Other branches of this order were to follow, variously called the "Gray Sisters," the "Daughters of Charity," or the "Sisters of St. Vincent de Paul," to name a few.

The Beginning of Change

Those countries in Europe that remained Roman Catholic escaped some of the disorganization caused by the Reformation. During the 1500s the Spanish and the Portuguese began traveling to the Americas. In 1521, Cortes conquered the capital of the Aztec civilization in Mexico and renamed it Mexico City. Early colonists to the area included members of Catholic religious orders, who became the doctors, nurses, and teachers of the new land. In 1524, the first hospital on the American continent, the Hospital of Immaculate Conception (Hospital de Nuestra Senora O Limpia Concepcion), was built in Mexico City. Mission colleges were founded. The first medical school in America was founded in 1578 at the University of Mexico, the second at the University of Lima prior to 1600.

Farther north, Jacques Cartier sailed up the St. Lawrence River in 1535 and established French settlements in Nova Scotia. He was followed by Franciscan Friars, Jesuits, Dominicans, and other settlers and explorers. In 1639, three Augustinian nuns arrived in Quebec to staff the Hotel Dieu which opened that year. The Ursuline Sisters, an order of teaching nuns who accompanied the Augustinians from France, are credited with attempting to organize the first training for nurses on this continent. They taught the Indian women of the area to care for their sick during a smallpox epidemic. Jeanne Mance, who had been educated at an Ursuline convent, came to Montreal from France in 1642. She is considered to be the founder of the Hotel Dieu of Montreal as well as the co-founder of Montreal itself. She returned to France in 1657 to recruit financial support and staff, and returned with three French hospital nuns from the Society of St. Joseph de la Fleche to staff the Hotel Dieu (Donahue, 1996).

In Europe, outstanding men of medicine made vital and valuable contributions to medical knowledge. Among lay persons influencing social change during this time was a young minister in Kaiserwerth, Germany, Theodore Fliedner (1800–1864). With the assistance of his first wife, Friederike, Fliedner revived the deaconess movement by establishing a training institute for deaconesses at Kaiserwerth in 1836. During a fund-raising tour through Holland and England, Pastor Fliedner met Elizabeth Fry of England, who had brought about reform at Newgate Prison in London. Greatly impressed with Mrs. Fry's accomplishments, the Fliedners followed her example and first worked with women prisoners in Kaiserwerth. Later they opened a small hospital for the sick, and Gertrude Reichardt, the daughter of a physician, was recruited as their first deaconess. The endeavors at Kaiserwerth included care of the sick, visitations and parochial work, and teaching. A course in nursing was developed that included lectures by physicians.

Friederike, who played a large part in helping to bring Theodore's visionary plans to fruition, was herself deeply dedicated to the deaconess movement. While away from home promoting deaconess activities, she learned that one of her children had died. A second child died shortly after her return, and she herself died in 1842 after the birth of a premature infant. Pastor Fliedner was also assisted in his work by his second wife, Caroline Bertheau, who had some nursing experience before her marriage. In 1849 Pastor Fliedner traveled to the United States, where he helped to establish the first Motherhouse of Kaiserwerth Deaconesses in Pittsburgh, Pennsylvania. With the help of four deaconesses, the Motherhouse of Kaiserwerth Deaconesses assumed responsibility for the Pittsburgh Infirmary, which was the first Protestant hospital in the United States. The hospital is now called Passavant Hospital.

In England, at about the same time, Elizabeth Fry (1780–1845) organized the Institute of Nursing Sisters, a secular group often called the Fry Sisters. Two other groups followed shortly; the Sisters of Mercy, a Roman Catholic group formed by Catherine McAuley (1787–1841), and another Catholic group called the Irish Sisters of Charity, formed by Mary Aikenhead (1787–1858).

THE NIGHTINGALE INFLUENCE

The three images discussed in the previous sections—the folk image, the servant image, and the religious image—all influenced the development of nursing. In the latter half of the 18th century, however, one woman dramatically changed the form and direction of nursing and succeeded in establishing it as a respected field of endeavor. This outstanding woman was Florence Nightingale.

Born on May 12, 1820, the second daughter of a wealthy family, she was named after the city in which she was born—Florence, Italy. Because of her family's high social and economic standing, she was cultured, well traveled, and educated. By the age of 17 she had mastered several languages and mathematics and was extremely well read. Through the influential people she met, she was expected to select a desirable mate, marry, and assume her place in society.

Florence Nightingale had other ideas, however. She wanted to become a nurse, but this aspiration was unthinkable to her family because of the hospital conditions of the day. She continued to travel with her family and their friends and, in the course of these travels, met Sidney Herbert and his wife, who were becoming interested in hospital reform. She began collecting information on public health and hospitals and soon became recognized as an important authority on the subject.

Through friends she learned about Pastor Fliedner's institute at Kaiserwerth. Because it was a religious institution under the auspices of the church, her parents would permit her to go there, although she could not go to English hospitals. In 1851 she spent 3 months studying at Kaiserwerth.

In 1853, she began working with a committee that supervised an ''Establishment for Gentlewomen During Illness.'' She eventually was appointed superintendent of the establishment. As her knowledge of hospitals and nursing reform grew, she was consulted by both reformers and physicians who were beginning to see the need for ''trained'' nurses. Despite her growing reputation as a respected expert, her family continued to object to her activities.

When the Crimean War broke out later that same year, war correspondents wrote about the abominable manner in which the sick and wounded soldiers were cared for by the British Army. Florence Nightingale, by then a recognized authority on hospital care, wrote to her friend Sir Sidney Herbert, who was then Secretary of War, and offered to take a group of 38 nurses to the Crimea. (At the same time, he had written a letter requesting her assistance in resolving this national crisis. Their letters crossed in the mail.) Her achievements in the Crimea were so outstanding, despite the toll they took on her own health, that she was later recognized in 1907 by the Queen of England, who awarded her the Order of Merit.

In 1856, she returned to England, her health broken. Much has been written of her ''illness,'' and many have suggested that it was, to a large degree, a neurosis. She retreated to her bedroom, and for the next 43 years conducted her business from her secluded apartment.

Throughout her lifetime, Florence Nightingale wrote extensively about hospitals, sanitation, health and health statistics, and especially about nursing and nursing education. She crusaded for and brought about great reform in nursing education.

In 1860, she devoted her efforts to the creation of a school of nursing at St. Thomas' Hospital in London, financed by the Nightingale Fund. The basic principles on which Miss Nightingale established her school included the following:

- Nurses would be trained in teaching hospitals associated with medical schools and organized for that purpose.
- Nurses would be carefully selected and would reside in nurses' houses designed to encourage discipline and form character.
- The school matron would have final authority over the curriculum, living arrangements, and all other aspects of the school.
- The curriculum would include both theoretical material and practical experience.
- Teachers would be paid for their instruction.
- Records would be kept on the students, who would be required to attend lectures, take quizzes, write papers, and keep diaries.

In many other ways Florence Nightingale advanced nursing as a profession. She believed that nurses should spend their time caring for patients, not cleaning; that nurses must continue learning throughout their lifetime and not become ''stagnant''; that nurses should be intelligent and should use that intelligence to improve conditions for the patient; and that nursing leaders should have social standing. She had a vision of what nursing could and should be.

Florence Nightingale died in her sleep at the age of 90. The week during which she was born is now honored as National Hospital Week. The enthusiastic student is encouraged to learn more about this fascinating woman in Cecil Woodham-Smith's book *Florence Nightingale.*

EARLY SCHOOLS IN THE UNITED STATES

After the establishment of the Nightingale School in England, nursing programs flourished, and the Nightingale system spread to other countries. In the United States, the growth of nursing education received an additional push because of the Civil War.

The Influence of the Civil War

The Civil War broke out in the United States in 1861. Although social reform was on the rise, the nursing profession was still in an embryonic, unorganized stage. There was neither an army nurse corps, nor an organized medical corps. There were no ambulance services or MASH units. Responding to the nursing needs created by the war, in which it is estimated that 618,000 men died (Donahue, 1996, p. 247) many women volunteered to help. After a brief training course, they performed nursing duties. Many religious orders also volunteered and provided service. A steamer, captured from the Confederates, was converted into a floating hospital and anchored near Vicksburg. Considered the first Navy hospital ship, the *Red Rover* was staffed through the volunteer efforts of the Catholic Sisters of Mercy, who became the first "Navy" nurses. An account of some of the contributions of nurses during the Civil War and afterward is found in Table 4-1.

The serious need for trained nurses, created by the Civil War, was undoubtedly a significant factor in the development of nursing in the United States. The conditions exposed during the Civil War coupled with the popularity of Florence Nightingale in England provided the impetus necessary to heighten the interest in nursing education in the United States.

TABLE 4-1. Nurses of the Civil War and Their Contributions*

Nurse	Contribution
Sojourner Truth (1797–1883)	Born into slavery and named Isabella, this African American was sold three times by the time she was 13, the last time for $300. She married an older slave and bore him 5 children, some of whom were also sold into slavery. In 1843 she changed her name to Sojourner Truth. She nursed Union soldiers, worked for improvement in sanitary facilities and sought contributions of food and clothing for black volunteer regiments. She supported her travel from sales of her *Narrative of Sojourner Truth: A Northern Slave* (1850) dictated to Olive Gilbert because she was illiterate. She continued her work as a nurse/counselor for the Freedmen's Relief Association after the war (Whitman, 1985, p. 814–816).
Dorothea Lynde Dix (1802–1881)	A Boston school teacher already known for her humanitarian efforts on behalf of the mentally ill, was commissioned as Superintendent of Women Nurses for All Military Hospitals during the Civil War when she was past 60 years of age. Her authority was often challenged by the physicians.
Mary Ann Ball Bickerdyke (1817–1901)	Called "Mother" Bickerdyke by the troops, this Illinois woman challenged the work of lazy corrupt medical officers. She served under fire in nineteen battles. Her efforts were recognized by the government in the launching of the hospital ship, the *SS Mary A. Bickerdyke* in 1943.

(continued)

TABLE 4-1. *(continued)*

Nurse	Contribution
Walt Whitman (1819–1892)	A well respected poet who worked as a volunteer in hospital wards after searching for a brother who had been wounded. Dressed wounds, wrote letters, read to soldiers, brought gifts and food. Later wrote about the war and suffering of soldiers.
Harriet Ross Tubman (1820–1913)	An abolitionist sometimes called "Conductor of the Underground Railroad," this black nurse was commended for caring for the sick and wounded without regard for color.
Mary Livermore (1820–1905)	Another untrained nurse of the Civil War, she later became a suffragist and advocated education for all women. Addressing the sixth annual convention of the Nurses' Associated Alumnae, she described the activities of the Civil War nurses.
Clara Barton (1821–1912)	Served as a volunteer with the Sixth Massachusetts Regiment. Independently operated a large-scale relief operation. Was instrumental in founding the American Red Cross in 1882. Called "little lone lady in black silk" (Donahue 1996, p. 255)
Kate Cummings (1828–1909)	A volunteer in the southern army, her diaries chronicled the work of the "matrons" who served in the Confederate hospitals.
Louisa May Alcott (1832–1888)	Served as a volunteer nurse during the Civil War. From these experiences she wrote a small book entitled *Hospital Sketches* which described the work of the volunteer nurses of the Civil War. The nurse character of the book was Miss Tribulation Periwinkle.
Jane Stuart Woolsey (1830–1891)	One of three sisters from a cultivated and elite northeastern family with colonial ancestry, Jane served the Union Army as supervisor of the nursing and cooking department. She provided much narrative to describe the conditions of the day, authoring a book entitled *Hospital Days*. Later she served as the directress of the Presbyterian Hospital in New York.
Abby Howland Woolsey (1828–1893)	A sister of Jane, she too served as a volunteer nurse for the Union Army and fought diligently for the abolition of slavery. Helped found the Bellevue Hospital Training School for Nurses and wrote one of the first books on the organization of nursing schools–*A Century of Nursing with Hints Toward the Organization of a Training School (1876)* (Whitman, 1985, pp. 904–906).
Georgeanna Muirson Woolsey (1833–1906)	Another Woolsey sister involved in war efforts, she benefited from a month-long nursing training experience in New York when selected by the Woman's Central Association of Relief as one of a group of a hundred for leadership potential. She wrote of her war experiences in a book entitled *Three Weeks at Gettysburg*. She later helped found the Connecticut Training School for Nursing in New Haven, enjoying the support of her husband, Dr. Francis Bacon (Whitman, 1985, pp. 903–906).
Susie King Taylor (1848–1901)	Born into slavery, as a young girl she secretly learned to read and write. While serving as a volunteer nurse for the Union Army, she also worked as a teacher.

* Much of the information contained in the above table was gathered from the work of Kalisch and Kalisch, 1995, except as otherwise noted.

The Establishment of Early Schools

As with many other significant events that have evolved from a variety of influences, it is difficult to pinpoint the first nursing program in the United States. As early as 1798, a pioneer physician, Dr. Valentine Seaman, is said to have initiated the first system of instruction for nurses at New York Hospital (Donahue, 1996, p. 235). A society was formed in 1839 under Quaker influence, called the Nurse Society of Philadelphia, and a combined Home and School were opened. Historical records also show that prior to 1850, some intermittent preparation had been provided to individuals who cared for the sick and a plan of instruction had been developed for women who would supply maternity service in the home under the guidance of Dr. Joseph Warrington, who was obstetric physician to the Philadelphia Dispensary for the Medical Relief of the Poor.

In 1850, a commission of the Massachusetts Legislature recommended that institutions be formed to educate nurses. A plan for educating nurses was included in the formation of the New England Female Medical College, and a few nurses were educated through this institution. Other hospitals operated training programs, although the studies lasted only 6 months. The Woman's Hospital of Philadelphia, which operated under the direction of two female physicians, opened a training school in 1861, but it made little progress until endowed in 1872. Despite these efforts, the nursing services provided by the majority of hospitals operating during the 1860s were disorganized and inadequate. In many cases, nursing services were rendered by women who had been arrested for drunkenness or disorderly conduct and were serving out 10-day sentences. The better hospitals benefited from the work of Catholic sisters or Protestant deaconesses, although most of them were also untrained.

In 1869, responding to the impetus given nursing during the Civil War, the American Medical Association established a committee to study the issue of training for nurses. The committee, chaired by Dr. Samuel D. Gross (1805–1884), was charged with identifying the best possible method to organize and manage institutions for training nurses. Their report concluded that every large hospital should have a nursing school, emphasized that the union between religious exercises and nursing would be conducive to the welfare of the sick, and recommended that schools be placed under the guardianship of county medical societies (Donahue, 1996, pp. 265).

The efforts of several influential and socially prominent women of the time were significant in establishing structured training for nurses. An editorial written by Sarah J. Hale, editor of *The Godey's Lady's Book and Magazine*, entitled "Lady Nurses," advocated the elevation of nursing to the level of a profession and recommended providing an education "especially adapted for ladies who desire to qualify themselves for the profession of nurse" (Hale, 1871, pp. 188-189).

The New England Hospital for Women and Children is often credited with being the first hospital to establish a formal 1-year program to train nurses in 1872. It operated under the guidance of a female physician, Susan Dimock, who had received her medical education in Europe and had some knowledge of the work of Florence Nightingale. Five probationers started the program on September 1. It was from this school that Melinda Ann (Linda) Richards graduated in 1873 to become American's first trained nurse. This school was the alma mater for the first black nurse graduate, Mary Eliza Mahoney, in 1879.

By 1873, three additional schools had opened: the Bellevue Training School in New York City, the Connecticut Training School, and the Boston Training School. Typically, these schools did not admit males. In 1888 the Mills School of Nursing at Bellevue Hospital opened to train male nurses for patient care. Separate schools to educate black nurses also opened; among them Spelman Seminary in Atlanta in 1886, Hampton Institute in Virginia and Providence Hospital in Chicago in 1891, and Tuskegee Institute in Alabama in 1892 (Kalisch & Kalisch, 1995). Table 4-2 identifies some of the early schools.

Characteristics of the Early Schools

The life of the nursing student at the turn of the century was not an easy one. The strong militaristic and religious influences over nursing were embodied in the expectations held for nursing students. "Monastic and military traditions heavily influenced not only the actual workings of the schools of nursing but also the public's conception of them. The nurse in training was expected to yield to her superiors obedience characteristic of a good soldier and actions governed by the dedication to duty derived from religious devotion." (Kalisch & Kalisch, 1995, p. 111)

Typically, nursing students were about 21 years of age, single, and female. The first weeks or months of their education were spent as probationers, or "probies," and their duties were those that helped with the operation of the hospital but did little to educate them as nurses. For example, much time was spent washing, scrubbing, polishing, folding, stacking, and the like. Rules of conduct were rigid and unforgiving and early superintendents saw it as their responsibility to "discipline" pupils, ensuring that they possessed good morals, were honest, conscientious, obedient, respectful, loyal, passive, and devoted to duty. Nursing students were expected to be unselfish, thinking not of themselves but of the happiness and well-being of others (Fig. 4-3).

Initially, nursing education was largely an apprenticeship and resulted in students providing much of the work force of hospitals. The work day was long and arduous, often starting at 5:30 in the morning and ending with nursing prayers very late at night, and consisted primarily of work on the hospital wards. Instruction was provided by the superintendent or her assistants. There was no standardization of curriculum and no accreditation. The few lectures that were part of the program were usually given by physicians and scheduled at 8 or 9 p.m. after a long day of work. A seven-day work week was the standard and the help needed on the hospital units took precedence over the education of the young women. Lectures would be canceled if their services were needed.

As schools developed, facilities to house nursing students became necessary. Although some of the early programs provided sleeping quarters in the hospital, nursing students were usually housed in a building next to the hospital, often referred to as the "nurses' dorm." The nurses' residence was often controlled by a "housemother," or, in religious affiliations, by a Deaconess or Sister who served the same purpose. Housemothers assured that codes of behavior were adhered to and that curfews were enforced. Violations usually resulted in expulsion from the program or the loss of a part of the uniform such as the bib section of an apron. This signified to all that some infraction had occurred. Young women who were attracted to nursing because of the imagined glamour of wearing a long crisp white apron and ministering to sick (though handsome) young men, often became discouraged with the severe duties and routine. The attrition rate was high in the early schools.

TABLE 4–2. Early North American Training Schools for Nurses*

Date	Name and Place	Comments
1798	New York Hospital - New York	Dr. Valentine Seaman initiated a system of instruction for nurses. His lectures covered the topics of anatomy, physiology, maternal nursing, and care of children.
1839	Philadelphia Dispensary - Philadelphia	Dr. Joseph Warrington provided obstetrical training to a group of women who would work with the families who would otherwise not receive care. The Nurse Society of Philadelphia grew out of this training.
1861	Bellevue Hospital - New York	Dr. Elizabeth Blackwell converted Bellevue Hospital into a training center for nurses. About 100 women were trained to provide care during the Civil war in an intensive 4-week course.
1861–1862	Women's Hospital of Philadelphia - Philadelphia	Opened a training school but it progressed slowly until 1872 when it became endowed - the first endowed school of nursing in America. Organized and conducted by two female physicians.
1862	New England Hospital for Women and Children - Boston	Dr. Marie Zakrzewska, a colleague of Dr. Blackwell's offered a 6 month program to nurses.
1872	New England Training School - Boston	An expansion of the New England Hospital Program has been identified as the first formal school for nurses, under direction of Dr. Susan Dimock. The first graduate was Linda Ann Richards. Mary Mahoney, the first black nurse also graduated here.
1873 - May	Bellevue Training School - New York	First of a trio of schools modeled after the Nightingale model - Lavinia Dock was one of the early graduates.
1873 - October	Connecticut Training School - New Haven	Second of the trio of schools started in 1873–introduced first textbook, *New Haven Manual of Nursing,* which was written by a committee of nurses and physicians.
1873 - November	Boston Training School - Boston - attached to Massachusetts General	Third of the trio–Linda Richards became superintendent of nurses in November 1894. Idea for school initiated by the Woman's Educational Association. Medical staff did not support initiation of the school.
1874	St. Catharine's General and Marine Hospital - Ontario, Canada later called the Mack Training school.	Patterned after the Nightingale schools, this program included instruction in the art of nursing, chemistry, sanitary science, physiology, and anatomy.
1877	Training School of the New York Hospital - New York	Offered an 18-month course to prepare graduates for nursing.
1878	Boston City Hospital Training School - Boston	Required graduates to complete a 2-year program of study.
1884	Toronto General Hospital - Toronto, Canada	Mary Agnes Snively became superintendent of this school, which had early beginnings in 1877.
1884–1885	Farrand Training School for Nurses - Harper Hospital, Detroit	Considered one of the better schools, students had 2 annual series of lectures, approximately 20 hours total.
1886	Spelman Seminary - Atlanta, GA	The first separate school to educate black nurses who were often denied admission to other schools.
1888	Mills School of Nursing at Bellevue Hospital - New York	First school established for male nurses. Prepared them to give general patient care.
1889	Johns Hopkins School of Nursing - Baltimore	Program opened under direction of Isabel Hampton Robb. Mary Adelaide Nutting graduated 1891.
1890	Montreal General - Montreal, Canada	Although wanting a nursing program as early as 1835, hospital conditions would not allow. Nora Gertrude Livingstone established school in 1890.

*Information for this table was gathered primarily form Donahue, 1995 and Kalisch & Kalisch, 1995.

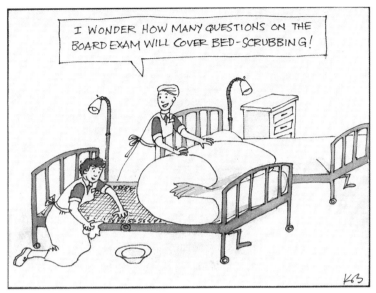

FIGURE 4-3
The duties assigned to probationers may have helped operate the hospital but did little to educate the nurse.

Although there were some changes in the curriculum—work hours were decreased, the length of study was increased, and the theory component was organized into specific areas of care such as medical, surgical, and obstetrical nursing—hospital-based programs remained largely unchanged through the 1940s and 1950s. The following is a quote from a special publication developed on the occasion of the closing of a diploma school:

In 1921, a nurse was discharged for "cigarette habit." Skirts of nurses' uniforms were getting shorter but there was periodic measurement to be sure some were not too short.

The year 1924 would see Deaconess' first student protest. Student nurses were required to wear their hair long in those days. A number of them though made arrangements with a barber in the Victoria Hotel to stay open late one evening and they all went down and had their hair bobbed in the latest style. They were deprived of their caps for several weeks and ordered to wear switches and what-nots, their punishment comparatively slight, since "banks and other business regularly dismissed employees for social offense." (Deaconess Hospital School of Nursing 1980, p. 10.)

Students provided the majority of care given and were seen as such a commodity to the hospital that even very small hospitals established nursing programs. This proliferation of schools became a serious concern as early as 1905. Early pioneers and advocates for nursing championed for programs with a sound educational foundation, and for reasonable working hours. During the time Isabel Hampton was "Principal" of the Johns Hopkins

TABLE 4–3. Early Nursing Textbooks*		
Date	Author	Title/Topic
1878	A committee of physicians and nurses	*Hand-book for Family and General Use*
1885	Clara Weeks Shaw	*A Textbook of Nursing for the Use of Training Schools, Families and Private Students*
1890	Lavinia Dock	*The Textbook on Materia Medica for Nurses*
1893	Diana Kimber	The first anatomy book for nurses, *Anatomy and Physiology*
1889 (about)	Isabel Hampton	*Nursing: Its Principles and Practices for Hospital and Private Use*
1894 (about)	Isabel Hampton Robb	*Nursing Ethics*

Training School (a position she accepted in 1889 and continued until her marriage to Dr. Robb in 1894), she arranged for a regular period of two hours of free time during a day that was limited to twelve hours. She would have liked to limit it to eight. Time was allowed for recreation and for meals (Jamieson & Sewell, 1944, p. 432).

Early Textbooks and Journals

There were few textbooks prior to 1900, a factor that complicated the learning process. Many of the lectures presented by physicians were given from notes they had taken while medical students. The first nursing textbook was reportedly the *Hand-book of Nursing for Family and General Use,* written by a committee composed of physicians and nurses associated with the Connecticut Training School at New Haven Hospital. Other books followed over the next two years. Table 4-3 describes some of the early textbooks.

Nursing journals also appeared toward the end of the 19th century. Five different journals for nurses were published before 1901. The first appeared in 1886 and was entitled the *Nightingale.* In 1889, under the direction of Mary E.P. Davis, a company was formed with 550 cash subscriptions and a new journal called the *American Journal of Nursing* made its debut in October 1890 (Fig. 4-4). The journal continues to be published today (Kalisch & Kalisch, 1995, pp. 115–116).

THE BEGINNING OF NURSING ORGANIZATIONS

By the end of the 19th century, conditions had reached a point at which changes were most effectively accomplished through organizations. Nursing pioneers saw this as an opportunity to bring about changes in nursing practice and nursing education.

Nursing Organizations in England

In England, the establishment of an organization for nursing was driven by the energies of Mrs. Bedford Fenwick (Ethel Gordon Manson), a prominent leader who, in 1887, campaigned for nurse registration. She believed that standards were necessary to improve nursing. Although her ideas for nurse registration were not well accepted, she founded the British

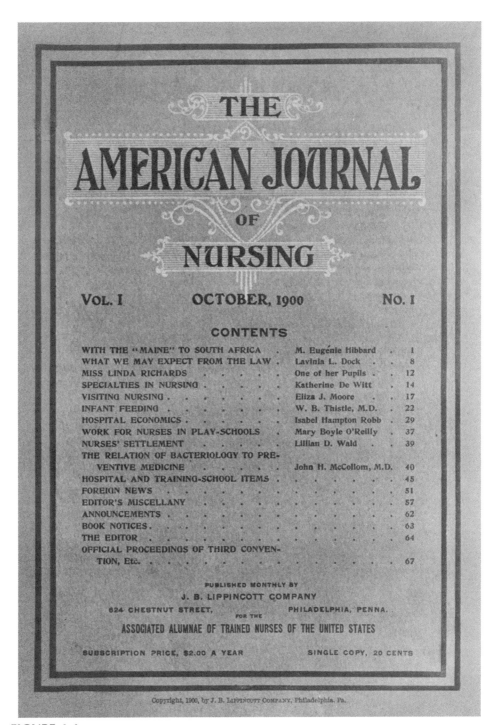

FIGURE 4-4
Cover of the first issue of the American Journal of Nursing.

Nurses' Association in 1888. It grew rapidly to 1000 members by the end of the first year. It later became the Royal British Nurses' Association.

The American Society of Superintendents of Training Schools for Nurses

In 1893, the World's Fair and Columbian Exposition was held in Chicago to celebrate the 400th anniversary of Columbus' arrival in the United States. The Fair provided the meeting place for many professions and artisans. The first nurses' meeting was held in the Hall of Columbus from June 15–17, 1893, as a part of the International Congress of Charities, Corrections, and Philanthropy. The nursing meeting was chaired by Isabel Hampton and was attended by both American and Canadian nurses. Attendees included such individuals as Lavinia Dock–suffragist, nurse activist, historian, and educator–who spoke on the relation of training schools to hospitals. An address sent by Florence Nightingale was presented to the group. The papers presented were later compiled in a publication, *Nursing the Sick, 1893*. The day following the meeting, Isabel Hampton arranged a meeting of a small group of leaders to discuss the possibility of a nursing organization. This meeting resulted in the formation in 1896 of the American Society of Superintendents of Training Schools for Nurses, so named because the majority of the attendees were directors of nursing schools and the membership was restricted to those nurses associated with nurse training. Concern for the standards of nursing education was primary, and a committee to study nursing education was quickly appointed. In 1907, the Canadian members formed their own organization called the Canadian Society of Superintendents of Training Schools. The American organization changed its name in 1912 to the National League for Nursing Education (Donahue, 1996, p. 326).

In 1952, the National League for Nursing Education became the National League for Nursing when six organizations merged into one. The organizations involved in the merger were the National Organization for Public Health Nursing (est. 1912), the Association of Collegiate Schools of Nursing (est. 1933), the Joint Committee on Practical Nurses and Auxiliary Workers in Nursing Services (est. 1945), the Joint Committee on Careers in Nursing (est.) the National Committee for the Improvement of Nursing Services (est. 1949), and the National Nursing Accrediting Service (est. 1949).

Nurses' Associated Alumnae of the United States and Canada

As the number of nurses increased throughout the United States and as hospitals formed individual alumnae groups, the need arose for an organization of trained nurses. At the third meeting of the American Society of Superintendents of Training Schools in 1896, a committee prepared a constitution and bylaws for such an organization with the delegates representing the various alumnae associations. The constitution was accepted a year later and the Nurses' Associated Alumnae of the United States and Canada was formed. The first president was Isabel Hampton Robb. The purposes of the group were:

1. To establish and maintain a code of ethics;
2. To elevate the standards of nursing education;
3. To promote the usefulness and honor, the financial and other interest of the nursing profession (American Nurses' Association, 1941, p. 2).

When it was discovered that New York law would not permit foreign membership in an incorporated association, the words "and Canada" were dropped from the title in 1901 and Canadian participation was prohibited. In 1911, the name of the organization in the United States became the American Nurses Association.

In 1908 the Provisional Organization of the Canadian National Association of Trained Nurses was formed, which was renamed the Canadian Nurses Association in 1924. This group also had as a primary concern the education of nursing students, the improvement of nursing care, the amelioration of conditions for nurses, and state registration of nurses to protect the public.

The International Council of Nurses

The International Council of Nurses, the oldest of all international nursing organizations, was formed in 1899. Founded by Mrs. Bedford Fenwick, it held its first meeting in Buffalo, New York, at the World Exposition in 1901. Mrs. Fenwick was the first president of the organization. The membership was originally composed of self-governing national nurses' associations rather than individual members, although until 1904 individual members could belong because few countries had organized nursing associations. Its purpose was to encourage communication between nurses of all nations and to provide opportunity for nurses from all parts of the world to meet and discuss concerns about the profession and about patient care. At the present time, the International Council of Nurses meets once every 4 years.

It is not within the scope of this chapter to discuss the origin of all the many nursing organizations in the United States. A quick review of Appendix B will give you insight into the tremendous number of specialty and special interest groups that now exist in nursing. The information provided in this Appendix will help you to research individual organizations that may be of interest to you. As you review Appendix B, you will understand why some critics suggest that nursing has too many organizations working in too many different directions.

THE DEVELOPMENT OF HOSPITALS IN THE UNITED STATES

The history of hospitals in the United States can be traced back to the mid-1700s when most cities built *almshouses,* also called poorhouses at the time. Almshouses provided food and shelter for the homeless poor, and served as homes for the aged, the disabled, the mentally ill, and the orphaned. *Pesthouses* were also built at this time to isolate people with contagious diseases, especially those diseases contracted aboard ship. These facilities housed people suffering from cholera, smallpox, typhus, and yellow fever, as well as the more common communicable diseases such as scarlet fever. Pesthouses would open and close as the need indicated.

Neither almshouses nor pesthouses were institutions from which most individuals would want to seek or receive care. They were crowded and unsanitary, with insufficient heat and ventilation. Cross-infection was common and mortality was high. Those with the financial means were cared for in their homes.

The first hospital founded in what was to become the United States was started in Philadelphia in 1751, at the urging of Benjamin Franklin. Franklin believed that the public had a duty to provide care to the poor, friendless, sick, and insane. A bill, passed that year, authorized the establishment of the Pennsylvania Hospital (Kalisch & Kalisch, 1995). The New York Hospital in New York City was established in 1773, primarily to prevent the spread of infectious diseases brought by sailors and immigrants. Massachusetts General Hospital in Boston opened its doors in 1816, and New Haven Hospital in Connecticut in 1826.

These early hospitals cared for people with acute illnesses and injuries, but did not admit the mentally ill. Several governmental hospitals were established for this purpose. The first such facility was established as a department of the Pennsylvania Hospital in 1752. The second was founded in Williamsburg, Virginia, in 1773; the third, known as the Friend's Hospital, was located near Philadelphia in 1817. By 1840, eight hospitals to treat the mentally ill had been established (Kalisch & Kalisch, 1995). The cruel and inhumane treatment of patients in the early mental hospitals is legendary. Dorothea Dix, mentioned in Table 4-1, campaigned vigorously for and brought about much reform in the area of mental health treatment. Although she was never educated as a nurse (she was a schoolteacher), Dix volunteered as a nurse during the Civil War and is included in the Nursing Hall of Fame because of her significant contributions to the profession.

The earliest hospitals left much to be desired. Most were housed in large buildings that had been converted into temporary quarters. Often they were dirty, rank with infection, and poorly ventilated. Linen was used for several patients before it was laundered. Draining, suppurating wounds were common. The stench was overwhelming, and it is said that nurses used snuff to make working conditions more tolerable (Kalisch & Kalisch, 1995). Hospitals constructed during the early 19th century often followed a block plan in their design and the buildings resembled large barns. In the 1850s, Massachusetts General Hospital constructed a facility divided into wards or pavilions, each one a separate building with high ceilings and good ventilation. The buildings were built of wood because it was believed they would need to be replaced after 20 years because of contamination (Kalisch & Kalisch, 1995 p. 22).

Factors Affecting the Development of Hospitals

Six developments can be cited as major forces that each played a unique role in the continued development of hospitals and patient care:

- Advances in medical science
- The development of medical technology
- Changes in medical education
- The growth of the health insurance industry
- Greater government involvement in health care delivery
- The emergence of professional nursing

ADVANCES IN MEDICAL SCIENCE

By the end of the colonial period two medical schools had been established in the United States. Before that time physicians learned their skills through an apprenticeship with a practicing physician. As medicine became more of a science, advances occurred. One of the most significant was the discovery of anesthesia and the rapid advances in surgery that were to follow. The germ theory also did much to advance the practice of medicine because it inspired the development of agents or techniques that would sterilize or serve as antiseptics. The growth of hospitals in the United States was a direct result of advances such as these that made hospitals safer and more desirable. The discovery of sulfa and antibiotics in the mid-1930s and mid-1940s, respectively, heralded even greater changes.

THE DEVELOPMENT OF MEDICAL TECHNOLOGY

The development of specialized medical technology was a natural successor to the advances in medical science. The first hospital laboratory was opened in 1889, and x-rays were used in diagnosis in 1896. The electrocardiogram (ECG) was invented in 1903 and the electro-encephalogram (EEG) in 1929 (Haglund & Dowling, 1993).

CHANGES IN MEDICAL EDUCATION

Advances in medical education also had a significant impact on the development of health care in this country. The Flexner Report (see Chapter 5) was completed in 1910, and it led to changes in the structure and content of curricula in medical schools. It also expanded the role of hospitals to include education and research and resulted in internships and residencies for medical students.

GROWTH OF THE HEALTH INSURANCE INDUSTRY

The growth of the health insurance industry is another factor responsible for the development of hospitals. Although there were some antecedents, most sources indicate that the first hospital insurance plan was initiated at Baylor University Hospital in 1929 to serve the needs of schoolteachers in Dallas, Texas (Raffel & Raffel, 1989). The approach used there was to form the model for Blue Cross plans around the country.

Today figures vary as to what percentage of the population is protected against the costs of medical care by some type of insurance. They range from 85% to 90%. There is great concern for the approximately 35 million individuals who have no protection (Raffel & Raffel, 1989).

GREATER INVOLVEMENT OF THE GOVERNMENT

In early times the government was involved in health care delivery primarily at a local level, building almshouses and facilities for the insane. By 1935, the government was providing grants-in-aid to assist in the establishment of public health and other programs to furnish health assistance to citizens. In 1946, the Hill-Burton Act resulted in the construction of many hospitals and other health facilities. The initiation of Medicare and Medicaid in 1965 made another significant impact on the health care industry because the legislation encouraged capital construction and the development of hospitals through the manner in which the system of reimbursement was structured.

THE EMERGENCE OF PROFESSIONAL NURSING

Another force that significantly influenced the growth of hospitals was the development of professional nursing. Haglund and Dowling (1993, p. 139) cite two ways in which advances in nursing contributed to the growth of hospitals. First, they ''increased the efficiency of treatment, cleanliness, nutritious diets, and formal treatment routines'' that resulted in patient recovery. Second, they resulted in considerate, skilled patient care that made hospitals acceptable to all people, not just the poor. The role of the nurse and nursing influences the health care delivery system more today than ever before.

HISTORY OF THE NURSING HOME

Like our acute care facilities, the nursing home had a rather harsh beginning. In the 19th century, almshouses and poorhouses were constructed by the government to shelter the destitute elderly. These facilities attracted a strange mixture of residents, including those who needed asylum and detention, as well as the poor, the chronically disabled, and the mentally ill. According to the moral perspective that prevailed at the time, poverty and disability were viewed as indications of an undisciplined, improvident, and even profligate life. A person who was housed in a "county poorhouse" often had no financial resources and no family to provide care and assistance, and endured a certain social stigma. In time these almshouses became the community "dumping grounds" for all of society's cast-offs. The early facilities for the country's dependent elderly offered the same grim surroundings as the early hospitals. They were unsanitary, overcrowded, and poorly ventilated. Residents were expected to work to assist with their keep if they were able. Care was provided by individuals who sought employment there as a last resort. Appropriations to manage these facilities were meager because the majority of citizens did not identify with the institutions that housed the poor and the transient, who probably had no previous history of contributing to the community.

As the United States grew as a society, various groups became concerned about the conditions that existed in the poorhouses. Eventually, patients were separated according to condition and the mentally and chronically ill were reassigned in different hospitals. An increasing number of churches and fraternal organizations started homes to care for their elderly members. As a result of the Social Security Act of 1935, private (for-profit or proprietary) nursing homes emerged during that decade. Raffel and Raffel (1989, p 205) state, "The original exclusion of benefits for patients in public institutions (since repealed) apparently stemmed from congressional concern about conditions in county poorhouses and a desire to get them closed."

In the postwar period, the Hill-Burton Act of 1948, which supported hospital construction, was expanded to include voluntary (nonprofit) nursing homes, and some states also developed grant programs. Since 1950, government funding for nursing home care has increased steadily and culminated in the 1965 Medicaid program, which now covers 40% of all nursing home costs (Callopy et al., 1991). Governmental regulation of nursing homes has become increasingly involved and complex.

As changes in funding occurred and as short-term acute care hospitals became increasingly specialized, the role of the nursing home changed. It was affected by the deinstitutionalization movement in the 1950s and 1960s, which saw large numbers of the elderly population discharged from mental hospitals. Nursing homes began to assume the role of providing specialized care for the elderly. By the 1960s, this role was well established, but the nursing home industry was plagued by constant reports of substandard and negligent care and, in some instances, charges of absolute abuse of patients and misuse or embezzlement of their funds. This resulted in even greater scrutiny and regulation by the government.

Today *nursing home* is a broad term that encompasses a wide spectrum of facilities ranging from special units in acute community hospitals to a campus of care retirement centers. The facilities are licensed by each state in which they exist, each state having its own definitions and requirements. Only about 6% have 200 beds or more. Approximately 75% are certified by Medicare as "skilled nursing facilities," a necessary qualification if Medicare funds are to pay for the care. The major reason for admission to a nursing home is functional dependency rather than diagnosis. The use of nursing homes will continue to grow in the future as the population grows older, with an estimated national expenditure of $131 billion anticipated by the year 2000 (Williams & Torrens, 1993).

THE AMERICAN HOSPITAL ASSOCIATION

The American Hospital Association was founded in 1899 as the Association of Hospital Superintendents with a membership of nine. Its purpose was to establish and maintain high standards of hospital service, care of the sick, and control and prevention of disease. Nurses who held positions as hospital administrators played roles in the early development of this organization although these roles might have been somewhat passive. It has been suggested that "this passivity cast a negative influence over nurse training standards" (Kalisch & Kalisch, 1995, p. 132).

KEY CONCEPTS

- Nursing has its roots in all endeavors to care for the sick and injured; therefore, it is difficult to pinpoint a particular period in history when nursing first began.
- Nursing's history has influenced the way the profession is recognized by the public. There were three significant images of the nurse in the past: the folk image, the religious image, and the servant image.
- The "Dark Ages of Nursing" occurred during the Reformation, when only those individuals who could not find other employment cared for the ill.
- Florence Nightingale had a significant impact on the form and direction of nursing and established it as a respected field of endeavor. Many of her precepts are still a part of nursing.
- The Civil War in the United States demonstrated the serious need for trained nurses to care for the sick and wounded.
- Early nursing schools were developed in the United States for the purpose of nursing service as much as for the purpose of educating young women. The programs were rigorous; often a 7-day work week was comprised of 14-hour work days.
- Nursing organizations, the forerunners of today's associations, began to emerge toward the end of the 19th century as the pioneers of early nursing visualized the need for change in nursing education and nursing practice.
- Acute care hospitals have a history reaching back into the ancient past. Advances in medical science, the development of medical technology, changes in medical education, the growth of the health insurance industry, government involvement, and the emergence of professional nursing all affected the development of modern hospitals.
- Long-term care facilities have a history similar to that of acute care hospitals; both often started as facilities to house the poor and indigent. Today's nursing homes provide specialized care to the elderly or disabled and rehabilitation services to others.

Critical Thinking Activities

1. If you had the power to change one single event in the history of nursing what would it be? Why would you make that change? How do you think that would have effected nursing today?
2. Knowing what you do about the history of the image of nursing, how will you, as a nurse of the future, advance the image of nursing? What aspects of the role are most critical? Who are the people who most need to be influenced? What are the aspects of the profession that should be changed?
3. Imagine that you are an instructor in an early nursing program. There are no textbooks. There are no nursing journals from which you can assign reading. How would you go about teaching the students for whom you are responsible?
4. Select one of the nursing leaders of the past that you would like to interview. Why did you choose that person? What would you like to ask that individual? How would you use the information that person shared with you?
5. Research a particular nursing specialty organization. Why did you choose that organization? Compare and contrast the philosophy of the organization with your own.

REFERENCES

Collopy B, Boyle P, Jennings B. New Directions in nursing home ethics (A Hastings Center Report Special Supplement, March-April) Hastings Center Rep 21(2):1-16, 1991

Dickens C. Martin Chuzzlewit. *In* The Works of Charles Dickens, vol II. New York: Books Inc, 1936

Deaconess Hospital School of Nursing. Eighty-One Years of Nursing: 1989-1980. Spokane, WA: Deaconess Hospital, 1980

Donahue MP. Why nursing history. In MM Styles & P Moccia (Eds.) On Nursing: A Literary Celebration (p 147). New York, National League for Nursing Pub. No. 14-2513, 1993

Donahue MP. Nursing: The Finest Art, 2nd ed. St Louis: CV Mosby, 1996

Jan R. Rufaida Al-Asalmiya, the first Muslim nurse. Image: Journal of Nursing Scholarship. 28(3): 267-268, 1996

Haglund CL, Dowling WL. The hospital. In Williams SJ, Torrens PR: Introduction to Health Service, 4th ed. New York: Delmar Publishers, Inc., 1993: 135–176

Hale S. Lady nurses, Godey's Lady's Book and Magazine 82:188, 1871

Jamieson EM, Sewall M. Trends in Nursing History, 2nd ed. Philadelphia: W.B. Saunders Co., 1944

Kalisch PA, Kalisch BJ. The Advance of American Nursing, 3rd ed. Philadelphia: J.B. Lippincott Co., 1995

Nutting MA, Dock LL. A History of Nursing. New York: GP Putnam's Sons, 1935

Raffel MW, Raffel NK, The U.S. Health System: Origins and Functions, 3rd ed. New York: John Wiley & Sons, 1989

Uprichard M. Ferment in nursing. *In* Auld E, Birum LH: The Challenge of Nursing. St Louis: CV Mosby, 1973:24–31

Whitman A. American Reformers. New York: H.W. Wilson Co., 1985

Williams SJ, Torrens PR. Introduction to Health Service, 4th ed. New York: Delmar Publishers, Inc., 1993

FURTHER READING

Aaronson LS. A challenge for nursing: Reviewing a historic competition. Nurs Outlook 37(6):274–279, 1989

Backer BA. Lillian Wald: Connecting caring with activism. Nurs & Health Care 14(3):122–129, 1993

Bunting S, Campbell JC. Feminism and nursing. Adv Nurs Sci 12(4):11–24, 1990

Bullough VL, et al. The Emergence of Modern Nursing. New York: Macmillan, 1969

Calhoun, J. The Nightingale Pledge: A commitment that survives the passage of time. Nurs & Health Care 14(3):130–136, 1993

Christy T. Equal rights for women: Voices from the past. Am J Nurs 2(2):288–293, 1971

Christy T. First fifty years. Am J Nurs 9(9):1778–1784, 1971

Christy T. Portrait of a leader: Lavinia Lloyd Dock. Nurs Outlook 17(6):72–75, 1969

Christy T. Portrait of a leader: M. Adelaide Nutting. Nurs Outlook 17(1):20–24, 1969

Christy T. Portrait of a leader: Isabel Hampton Robb. Nurs Outlook 17(3):26–29, 1969

Christy T. Portrait of a leader: Isabel Maitland Stewart. Nurs Outlook 17(10):44–48, 1969

Dolan JA. Nursing in Society: A Historical Perspective, 14th ed. Philadelphia: WB Saunders, 1978

Griffin GJ, Griffin JK. Jensen's History and Trends of Professional Nursing, 7th ed. St Louis: CV Mosby, 1973

Hanson KS. The emergence of liberal education in nursing education, 1893–1923. J Prof Nurs 5(2):83–91, 1989

Kalisch BJ, Kalisch PA. Heroine out of focus: Media images of Florence Nightingale: I. Popular biographies and stage productions. Nurs Health Care 4(4):181–187, 1983

Kalisch BJ, Kalisch PA. The nurse–detective in American movies. Nurs Health Care 3(3):146–153, 1982

Kalisch BJ, Kalisch PA, Scobey M. Reflections on a television image. Nurs Health Care 5(5):248–255, 1981

Larisey MM. Attic treasures: A look at nursing history. Nurs Forum 25(1):20–24, 1990

Melosh B. Not merely a profession: Nurses and resistance to professionalization. Am Behav Scientist 32(6):668–679, 1989

Parsons M. The profession in a class by itself. Nurs Outlook 34(6):270–275, 1985

Pennock, MR. Makers of Nursing History. Portraits and Pen Sketches of One-hundred and Nine Prominent Women. New York: Lakeside Publishing Co., 1941

Roberts MM. American Nursing: History and Interpretation. New York: Macmillan, 1954

Sleeper R, et al. Issues in Health Care: The Edna A. Fagan Health Care Lecture Series. Publication No. 14-1599. New York: National League for Nursing, 1976

Woodham-Smith C. Florence Nightingale. New York: McGraw-Hill, 1951

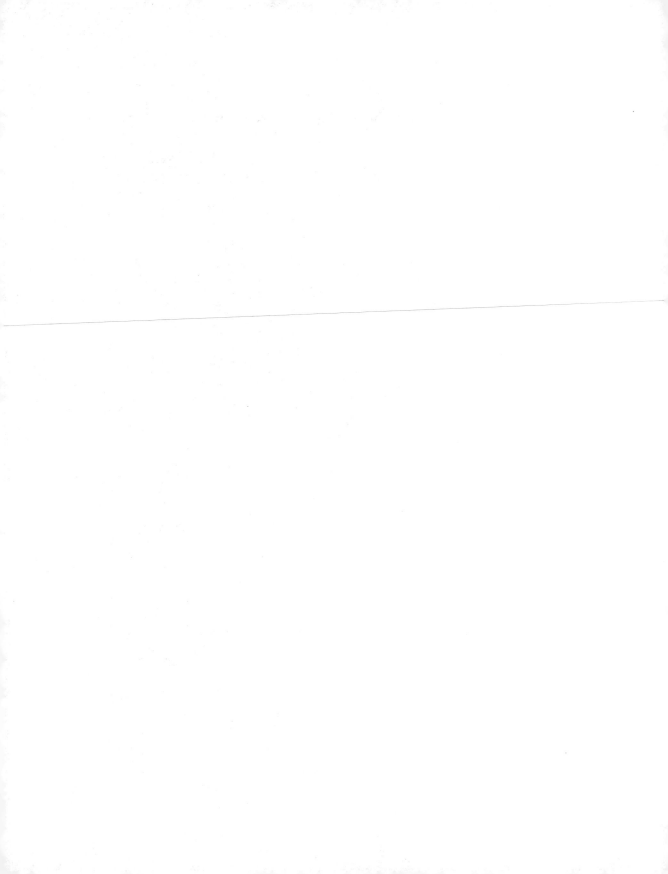

Nursing as a Developing Profession

Only when we grant love, passion, feeling, and imagination the same legitimacy that we grant reason, logic, and techniques; only when we restore our sense of community and reclaim our place as active participants in our world; only then will we be healthy as individuals, a profession, and a world community. (Moccia, 1988)

Objectives

After completing this chapter, you should be able to:

1. Analyze the reasons the profession has had difficulty defining nursing.
2. Describe how nursing differs from medicine.
3. Formulate a personal definition of nursing and identify a theorist who defines nursing similarly.
4. Identify the seven characteristics which social scientists use to evaluate professions.
5. Discuss the application of these seven characteristics to nursing as a profession.
6. Compare and contrast the terms profession and professional.
7. Explain how the image others hold of nursing affects the profession and the role of the nurse.
8. Analyze areas of nursing about which studies have been conducted and discuss why each is important.
9. Describe some of the traditions in nursing and consider why they became traditions.

KEY TERMS

Body of specialized knowledge
Code of ethics
Formal characteristics
Image
Institutions of higher education
Lifetime commitment
Medicine
Nursing

Occupation
Profession
Professional
Professional policy
Professional activity
Service to the public
Studies about nursing
Traditions

What is nursing? Is nursing an art or a science? If it is both, which category should receive the primary emphasis? How can "hunches," "gut feelings," and "intuition" be useful in a world surrounded by scientific rationale, steeped in protocol, and immersed in critical thinking and clinical pathways? Should nursing be considered a profession or an occupation? What factors are affecting the emergence of nursing as a profession? Does nursing possess a unique body of knowledge? Is the nurse a professional? If so, what educational background qualifies the nurse for professional standing? Should the educational preparation for nursing occur in a variety of settings that award different degrees? How will the skills of graduates from various programs be differentiated in practice? Do different levels of competence exist in the practice of clinical nursing? What is the position of the nurse in relation to other members of the health care team? What is the role of the nurse in preventive care? What is the exclusive role of the nurse? What forces have had a hand in the development of that role? What is the future of that role? What should we remember from our past that will assist in the development of nursing in the future?

These are only a few of the questions being asked by nurses today. Not all the questions have clear answers. Some of the answers result in debate and dialogue among nurses, health care providers, and health care consumers. As a novice, joining the ranks of those who have preceded you, you will want a grasp of the issues that have challenged, and in some instances plagued, nurses over the years. You will want to develop pride in nursing's heritage that can be gleaned only by gaining an understanding of the nurses who helped to shape the profession. As a nurse in the 21st century, you may have many opportunities to directly influence some of the answers to these questions.

NURSING DEFINED

When you entered the nursing program in which you are now enrolled, what was your perception of nursing as a profession? During the time that you have been studying nursing, has that perception of nursing changed? Defining nursing can be difficult. Nurses themselves cannot agree on a single definition, partly because of nursing's background. Little is known about the work of the nurse in prehistory, yet, Donahue (1996, p. 2) writes, "From the dawn of civilization, evidence prevails to support the premise that *nurturing* has been essential to the preservation of life. Survival of the human race, therefore, is inextricably intertwined with the development of nursing."

Distinguishing Nursing From Medicine

The formulation of clear and concise definitions of nursing have also been hampered by the lack of an obvious distinction between nursing and medicine. For example, it is not unusual to hear a prospective nursing student say, "I've always been interested in the medical field, so I decided to go into nursing." Something of an interdependence exists between medicine and nursing, and they have somewhat paralleled one another in historical development. However, anyone who has been involved in the profession of nursing for any period of time will be quick to assure you that distinct differences exist. The primary differences are the purpose and goal of each profession, and the education needed to fulfill each role. We must also acknowledge that historically medicine has been perceived as a profession for men, and nursing a profession for women. Though we can dismiss these stereotypes today, they had an influence on the development of both professions.

In general, medicine is concerned with the diagnosis and treatment (and cure, when possible) of disease. Nursing is concerned with caring for the person in a variety of health-related situations. The caring aspects of nursing are well documented in nursing literature (Benner & Wrubel, 1989; Bevis & Watson, 1989; Carper, 1979; Watson, 1979). We think of medicine as being involved with the cure of a patient, and nursing with the care of that patient. The role of the nurse in patient care (today we often refer to this as client care) also involves teaching about health and the prevention of illness as well as the care of the ill individual. Nursing takes place in the community and in the home, in hospice centers, ambulatory care environments, schools, day care centers and rehabilitation facilities; in all environments, nurses play a key role in promoting higher standards of health.

With advancing technology in the health care fields, the diverse areas of specialization, the different routes to educational preparation, and the distinct practice settings and roles occupied by the nurse, it is critical that nurses provide clear information for themselves as well as for the public. To state that you are a registered nurse says little about what you do. It conveys nothing about where you are employed or your educational background. For example, as a registered nurse, you might be employed in a community hospital or in a long-term care facility, you might have a significant role in a critical care unit, you might have earned additional credentials and be working in advanced practice, or you might be a nurse educator.

Thus, you can see that the words ''nurse'' and ''nursing'' have been applied to a wide variety of health care activities, in many different settings, performed by people with a variety of different educational backgrounds. The old adage ''A nurse, is a nurse, is a nurse'' is out of place in a highly technical health care delivery system that struggles to keep ''high touch'' and ''high tech'' compatible.

The Effect of Technology on the Definition of Nursing

Technological advances have significantly affected the definition of nursing and the role of the nurse. They have also significantly reshaped the methods by which care is delivered. The acute care hospital cares for sicker patients who are diagnosed with conditions they could not have survived twenty-five years ago. Today, recovery is anticipated after careful evaluation and treatment that may require diagnostic procedures (eg, angiography, sonography, or tomography), delicate medical procedures, and specialized critical care nursing that requires a host of variously prepared health care providers. Critical thinking skills are needed to perform the diverse tasks expected of a nurse. Nurses in many positions have been required to assume ever greater levels of responsibility. Only recently have they been given the official authority, autonomy, and recognition that should accompany those responsibilities.

Early Definitions of Nursing

A nurse is a person who nourishes, fosters, and protects—a person who is prepared to care for the sick, injured, and aged. In this sense "nurse" is used as a noun and is derived from the Latin *nutrix*, which means "nursing mother." The word "nurse" has also referred to a woman who suckled a child (usually not her own)—a wet nurse. Dictionary definitions of nurse include such descriptions as "suckles or nourishes," "to take care of a child or children," "to bring up; rear." In this way "nurse" is used as a verb, deriving from the Latin *nutrire*, which means "to suckle and nourish." With such an origin it is understandable that people generally have associated nursing with women.

References to "the nurse" can be found in the Talmud and in the Old Testament, although the role of the nurse in these references is not clearly defined. The nurse in these texts was probably more similar to the wet nurse than to someone who cared for the sick.

And Jacob came to Luz, that is Beth-el, which is in the land of Canaan, he and all the people who were with him. And he built there an altar, and called the place El-beth-el; because there God had revealed himself to him when he when he fled from his brother.
And Deborah, Rebekah's nurse died, and she was buried under an oak below Beth-el: so the name of it was called Allon-bacuth. (Genesis 35:6-8, Revised Standard Version of the Holy Bible)

Slowly, over the centuries, the word "nurse" has evolved to refer to a person who tends to the needs of the sick. Florence Nightingale, in her *Notes on Nursing: What It Is and What It Is Not*, described the nurse's role as one that would "put the patient in the best condition for nature to act upon him" (Nightingale, 1860, p. 133).

It is more than just a coincidence that the development of nursing as a profession has been inextricably tied to the role that women have played in society at various times in history, and to the forces that have had an impact on that society. In the past, nurses were undoubtedly more concerned about carrying out their responsibilities than about defining the role of the nurse. Throughout the years, we have seen the concept of the nurse grow and evolve from one of the nurse as mother, nourishing and nurturing children, to one of the nurse, without specific reference to gender, with responsibilities encompassing ever-expanding and challenging services to people needing health care.

Definitions of Nursing Theorists

As nursing has grown into a profession, many nursing theorists have developed definitions of nursing consistent with their conceptual frameworks. Table 5-1 presents the definitions of some of the theorists.

In 1958, Virginia Henderson was asked by the nursing service committee of the International Council of Nurses to describe her concept of basic nursing. Hers is one of the most widely accepted definitions of nursing:

The unique function of the nurse is to assist the individual, sick or well, in the performance of those activities contributing to health or its recovery (or to peaceful death) that he would perform unaided if he had the necessary strength, will or knowledge. And to do this in such a way as to help him gain independence as rapidly as possible (Henderson, 1966, p. 15).

TABLE 5-1. Definitions of Nursing by Major Theorists		
Theorist	**Major Theme**	**Definition**
Florence Nightingale (1859)	Environment/Sanitation	The goal of nursing is to put the patient in the best condition for nature to act upon him, primarily by altering the environment.
Hildegard Peplau (1952)	Interpersonal Process	Nursing is viewed as an interpersonal process involving interaction between two or more individuals that has as its common goal assisting the individual who is sick or in need of health care.
Virginia Henderson (1966)	Development/Needs	Nursing's role is to assist the individual (sick or well) to carry out those activities . . . he would perform unaided if he had the necessary strength, will, or knowledge.
Faye Abdellah (1960)	Nursing Problems	Nursing is a service to individuals, families, and society based on an art and science that molds the attitudes, intellectual competencies, and technical skills of the individual nurse into the desire and ability to help people cope with their health care needs, and is focused around twenty-one nursing problems.
Ernestine Wiedenbach (1964)	Nursing Problems Model	Nursing is a helping, nurturing, and caring service rendered with compassion, skill, and understanding, in which sensitivity is key to assisting the nurse in identifying problems.
Myra Levine (1969)	Conservation and Adaptation	Nursing means the nurse interposes her skill and knowledge into the course of events that affect the patient. When influencing adaptation favorably, the nurse is acting in a therapeutic sense. When the nursing intervention cannot alter the course of adaptation, the nurse is acting in a supportive sense.
Ida Jean Orlando (1972)	Interpersonal Process	Nursing's unique and independent role concerns itself with an individual's need for help in an immediate situation for the purpose of avoiding, relieving, diminishing, or curing that individual's sense of helplessness.
Dorothea Orem (1980)	Self-Care	Nursing is concerned with the individual's need for self-care action, which is the practice of activities that individuals initiate and perform on their own behalf in maintaining life, health, and well-being.
Dorothy E. Johnson (1980)	Systems Approach	Nursing is an external regulatory force that acts to preserve the organization and integration of the patient's behavior at an optimal level under those conditions in which the behavior constitutes a threat to physical or social health, or in which illness is found.
Imogene M. King (1981)	Open Systems Approach	The focus of nursing is the care of human beings resulting in the health of individuals and health care for groups who are viewed as open systems in constant interaction with their environment.
Betty Neuman (1982)	Systems Approach	Nursing responds to individuals, groups, and communities who are in constant interaction with environmental stressors that create disequilibrium. A critical element is the client's ability to react to stress and factors that assist with reconstitution or adaptation.

(continued)

TABLE 5-1. Definitions of Nursing by Major Theorists *(continued)*		
Theorist	**Major Theme**	**Definition**
Sister Callista Roy (1984)	Adaptation	The goal of nursing is the promotion of adaptive responses (those things that positively influence health) that are affected by the person's ability to respond to stimuli. Nursing involves manipulating stimuli to promote adaptive responses.
Martha E. Rogers (1984)	Science of Unitary Man	Nursing is an art and science that is humanistic and humanitarian directed toward the unitary human, and concerned with the nature and direction of human development.

Nursing as Defined by Organizations

In 1965, the American Nurses Association (ANA) published the "First Paper on Education for Nursing," which identified significant aspects of nursing. It stated that "essential components of professional nursing practice include care, cure, and coordination" (American Nurses Association, 1965, p 107).

Many would stress that any definition of nursing must indicate that it is both an art and a science. It is an art in the sense that it is composed of skills that require expertness and proficiency for their execution. It is a science in the sense that it requires systematized knowledge derived from observation, study, and research.

In 1980, the ANA, through its Social Policy Statement, provided yet another definition of nursing: "Nursing is the diagnosis and treatment of human responses to actual or potential health problems" (American Nurses Association, 1980, p 9). That definition had a widespread effect, and we see its application in the language used in nursing diagnoses today.

In 1994, the National Council of State Boards of Nursing (NCSBN) again revised a Model Nurse Practice act that was first developed in 1982 and revised in 1988. The single most important part of any nurse practice act is the legal definition of nursing practice (see Chapter 7). This legal definition is critical because it provides the foundation and guidelines for education, licensure, scope of practice, and, when necessary, the basis for corrective actions against people who violate the practice act. Although early publications of the Model Nurse Practice Act reflected the difficulty the committee experienced in arriving at a precise and succinct definition, the 1994 revision was clear. It stated, "The 'Practice of Nursing' means assisting individuals or groups to maintain or attain optimal health, implementing a strategy of care to accomplish defined goals, and evaluating responses to care and treatment" (Model Practice Act, National Council of State Boards of Nursing, 1994).

Another factor that has made it difficult to define nursing is that it is taught as encompassing both theoretical and practical aspects, but it is pursued (and continues to be defined) primarily through practice, an area little studied. Benner (1984) states, "Nurses have not been careful record keepers of their own clinical learning . . . . This failure to chart our practices and clinical observations has deprived nursing theory of the uniqueness and richness of the knowledge embedded in expert clinical practice." She further discusses the differences between "knowing that" and "knowing how." When attempting to define nursing we often stumble over these two concepts and how to combine the distinct and unique aspects of both.

As the profession grows and responsibilities change, undoubtedly we will continue to redefine and refine our definition of nursing. By being responsive to changes, nursing has become more closely aligned with professions such as law, theology, and education, in which changing practices have required greater precision and refinement of definitions of the profession. Recent challenges facing the Task Force on Workforce Regulation of the Pew Health Professions Commission regarding the scope of nursing practice as defined in state practice acts, will also encourage examination and clarification of nursing's definition.

CHARACTERISTICS OF A PROFESSION

The meaning of professionalism has been a subject of debate for many years. The *Flexner Report*, issued in 1910, was one of a series of papers issued by the Carnegie Foundation about professional schools. The Flexner Report, which focused on medicine, provided the incentive for many future efforts to define and discuss the characteristics of a profession (Table 5-2).

TABLE 5-2. Criteria for a Profession

Flexner (1915)	Bixler & Bixler (1959)	Pavalko (1971)
• Activities must be intellectual (as opposed to physical)	• Utilizes a specialized body of knowledge	• Work is based on a systematic body of theory and abstract knowledge
• Activities, because they are based on knowledge, can be learned	• Enlarges the body of knowledge it uses and improves its techniques of education and service by the use of the scientific method	• Work has recognized social value
• Activities must be practical rather than academic		• Requires a special amount of education to attain specialization
• Profession must have teachable techniques	• Entrusts the education of its practitioners to institutions of higher education	• Provides service to the public
• Must have a strong internal organization of members	• Applies its body of knowledge in practical services which are vital to human and social welfare	• Group has freedom to regulate and control its own work behavior (autonomy)
• Practitioners must be motivated by altruism (a desire to help others)	• Functions autonomously in the formulation of professional policy and in the control of professional activity	• Members are committed toward work as a life-time or long-term pursuit rather than a stepping stone to another profession
	• Attracts individuals of intellectual and personal qualities who exalt service above personal gain and who recognize their chosen occupation as a lifework	• Members share a common identity and possess a distinctive subculture
	• Strives to compensate its practitioners by providing freedom of action, opportunity for continuous professional growth, and economic security	• There exists a code of ethics

When nursing and nursing education were evolving in the United States, no one questioned whether nursing qualified as a profession or whether it was more occupational in nature. As a matter of fact, evidence suggests that from an early date the word "profession" was associated with nursing. Strauss (1966) gives as an example a magazine article entitled "A New Profession for Women" that appeared in 1882. The article described nursing reform, and carried with it a picture of Isabel Hampton. Strauss (1966) also refers to the writings of Lizabeth Price, published in 1892, in which nursing was discussed as a profession.

From approximately the 1950s through the 1970s or mid-1980s, nursing periodically was reviewed against the characteristics of a profession that had been established in the sociological literature. The activities for which nurses were responsible, the legal ramifications of practice, and particularly the education of future nurses, were subjected to the scrutiny of sociologists and nursing leaders who found it challenging to examine nursing against established standards.

Some critics challenge that nursing falls short of meeting these criteria. Some of nursing's leaders would also claim that nursing falls short of fulfilling a professional role (Schlotfeldt, 1987; Newman, 1990). Amid these challenges, other nurses are working to advance the standing of nursing through the development of a code of ethics, standards of practice, and peer review. In light of the challenges, it might be helpful to explore how major criteria could be applied to nursing (Fig. 5-1).

A Body of Specialized Knowledge

A primary criticism leveled at nursing is that nursing has no "body of specialized knowledge" that belongs uniquely to nursing. Critics state that nursing borrows from biologic sciences, social sciences, and medical science, and then combines the various skills and concepts to call it "nursing." Nursing leaders and theorists disagree as to whether nursing is a unique profession or one borrowed from other disciplines. In fact, this amalgamation and synthesis of some areas with application to another may be one of the unique qualities of nursing. Nursing researchers are also working to develop an organized body of knowledge that is unique to nursing. Nursing theorists are challenging one another to identify and describe the general principles that govern nursing practice. (See Chapter 6 for more information on nursing theories.) As a result of these efforts, nursing should emerge as a profession with an established body of knowledge.

Use of the Scientific Method to Enlarge the Body of Knowledge

Critical to any profession is its ability to grow and change as the world changes. Equally important is the method by which those changes occur. They cannot take place in a haphazard, random, or hit-or-miss fashion. In other words, they must be well thought out. Data must be systematically gathered and carefully analyzed, the problem(s) must be correctly identified, alternative solutions must be sought, the best approach selected and implemented, and the results thoroughly evaluated. As a student of nursing you already recognize that

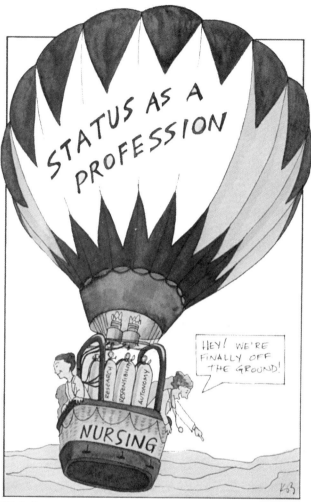

FIGURE 5-1
Some continue to question whether nursing truly can support the title of "profession."

this has been applied to nursing practice through the nursing process and through critical thinking. Tangible proof of this growth is the quick turnover in nursing textbooks. One seldom finds a clinical text in use in a quality program that has not been published within the last 4 years. Accreditation criteria set down for nursing programs by the national accrediting agencies require that libraries be stocked with up-to-date texts and periodicals. Nursing knowledge also increases because of nursing research and nursing practice. The number of nurses involved in nursing research continues to grow. Similarly, the number of nursing journals devoted to reporting nursing research results is increasing in number. All of this reflects the continued growth of the body of knowledge in nursing through the use of the scientific method.

Education Within Institutions of Higher Education

Perhaps no issue in nursing has been more controversial than the education of its practitioners. Nursing's heritage, like that of medicine, was founded in apprenticeship. Students were assigned to experienced practitioners who taught the skills with which they were familiar. Once those skills were acquired, the student moved into the world of employment. Our earliest programs of education were located in hospitals rather than colleges or universities. (See Chapter 4 for more information on the history of nursing education.)

Over time, the settings in which nurses are educated have changed. Today, the majority of nursing programs preparing registered nurses are located in collegiate settings (at either a community college or senior college or university). However, not all nurses today are educated in institutions of higher learning. Hospital-based programs still provide an avenue to nursing education. Controversy over the length of nursing education programs (2-year versus 4-year) and the "technical" aspects of patient care continues.

Control of Professional Policy and Professional Activity

Most critics reviewing professions against professional standards place an emphasis on the ability of any group to develop its own policy and to function autonomously. Some would suggest that this is an area in which nursing has always been weak, although current health care reform may assist the profession in achieving the full autonomy it has been seeking. Traditionally the nurse worked under the direction of the patient's physician, often in a hospital setting. The physician wrote the orders for medical care to be implemented by the nurse, and the agency or hospital set the policies under which that care was delivered. Only in the last 50 years has nursing made significant inroads in defining the unique role of the nurse in "care" as opposed to "cure" of the patient. Today nurses are responsible for planning and implementing the nursing care patients receive, and nurses are also accountable for the care provided. Nursing committees establish policies and protocols. Nursing diagnosis, once challenged as an inappropriate responsibility for nurses, has become a standard of good nursing care. In some practice settings, nurses are eligible for third-party payment; that is, they can be reimbursed by insurance companies for the care they have provided, a situation that will continue to improve with health care reform. Although nurses continue to carry out the medical regimen outlined by physicians, a more collaborative relationship is beginning to occur, and the contribution of the nurse is receiving more recognition. The practice acts of an increasing number of states provide prescriptive authority to nurses who have completed the necessary educational preparation.

All health care professions are changing in response to public demand. Consumers are represented on licensing and accreditation boards, protocols exist for managing conditions and situations, and fees may be established by outside groups. Society is no longer willing to give any profession total autonomy.

A Code of Ethics

The general standard for the professional behavior of nurses in the United States is the ANA Code for Nurses. This document was developed by the ANA and is periodically revised to address current issues in practice. The International Council of Nurses, housed in Geneva,

Switzerland, has also developed a code for nurses that reiterates many of the behaviors outlined in the ANA code. The international code sets the standards for ethical practice by nurses throughout the world. Copies of both of these codes and more discussion regarding the ethical conduct of nurses are found in Chapter 9.

Nursing as a Lifetime Commitment

Bixler and Bixler (1945) emphasized in their list of criteria for professions that a profession should attract people of certain intellectual and personal qualities, who exalt service above personal gain and who consider their chosen occupation to be their life work. Pavalko (1971) also identified as a significant criterion the commitment members have toward work as a lifetime or at least a long-term pursuit rather than a stepping stone to another profession. Studies indicate that most people who prepare for a career in nursing remain within the profession, but the "burnout" that occurs from stress (see Chapter 11) has become a concern. Most individuals who have been nurses continue to identify themselves as nurses long after they have retired. Today there is a greater likelihood that individuals who enter the profession of nursing at one educational level will continue to advance in practice and education by pursuing additional degrees (and experience). The concept of "articulation" between variously positioned degree-granting institutions is in the forefront of nursing today. More discussion of articulation in nursing education is found in Chapter 6.

Service to the Public

Some theorists list altruism, service to the public, and dedication among criteria for professions. Some suggest that altruism, or the desire to provide for the good of society, must be the worker's motivating force. Nurses have long struggled with the ambiguity that can result from this concept. Possessing a history with a strong religious heritage, the giving of oneself at all costs helped frame the image of nursing and nurses. As nursing has come of age as a profession, we have recognized that "giving away" one's services should not be considered professional. Because nurses expect appropriate remuneration for services rendered does not suggest that they are less than dedicated to the patients for whom they are caring. Providing service to the public should not mean sacrificing one's financial security. Medicine, law, dentistry, and engineering are some examples of professions in which practitioners are amply rewarded financially for the services they provide. Collective bargaining, once viewed as the antithesis of professionalism, is becoming an acceptable method of negotiating work-related issues for many professions. Greater discussion of nurses and collective bargaining is included in Chapter 12.

DIFFERENTIATING BETWEEN THE TERMS *PROFESSION* AND *PROFESSIONAL*

Nursing involves activities that may be performed by many different caregivers. These people include nurse aides or assistants, orderlies, practical nurses, and registered nurses prepared for entry into nursing through any of several educational avenues (see Chapter 6).

Each of these caregivers is contributing to nursing as a profession. To meet the nursing needs of the public, it is essential that caregivers function at various levels of practice. This has led to confusion about the use of the terms *profession* and *professional*. Is there a difference between looking at the practice of nursing in its totality and at the practice of "professional" nursing?

A popular view of a profession involves the approach a person has to the role that is required. Most professionals are serious about their activities, strive for excellence in performance, and demonstrate a sense of ethics and responsibility in relationship to their careers. Such people consider their work a lifelong endeavor rather than a stepping stone to another field of employment. They place a positive value on being termed professional, and perceive being termed nonprofessional or technical as an adverse reflection on their status, position, and motivation.

Some people think that professionalism has a great deal to do with attitude, dress, conduct, and deportment. The attributes that are considered professional vary according to the personal values and stereotypes of the person doing the evaluating. For example, an early concept of the "truly professional" nurse was that of a person dressed in a starched white uniform and cap, whose hair was off her collar, and whose shoes were freshly polished. Some individuals would continue to support this concept of the "professional nurse." Others might perceive the "professional nurse" as one who is open and kind in interpersonal relationships, who focuses on the needs of others, and who is tactful and skillful in interview techniques.

In at least one instance, federal legislation has helped to establish a list of the characteristics of a professional. Public Law 93-360 (Labor Management Relations Act, 1947 [amended, 1959, 1974]), which governs collective bargaining activities, defines the professional employee as follows:

(a) any employee engaged in work (i) predominantly intellectual and varied in character as opposed to routine mental, manual, mechanical, or physical work; (ii) involving the consistent exercise of discretion and judgment in its performance; (iii) of such a character that the output produced or the result accomplished cannot be standardized in relation to a given period of time; (iv) requiring knowledge of an advanced type in a field of science or learning customarily acquired by a prolonged course of specialized intellectual instruction and study in an institution of higher learning or a hospital, as distinguished from a general academic education or from an apprenticeship or from training in the performance of routine mental, manual, or physical processes; or

(b) any employee, who (I) has completed the courses of specialized intellectual instruction and study described in clause (iv) of paragraph (a), and (ii) is performing related work under the supervision of a professional person to qualify himself to become a professional employee as defined in paragraph (a).

The sociological and legal definitions are much more restrictive than the popular definition of the term *professional*. A communication block can result from people using the term in different ways. When one person is using a restrictive, sociological definition and the other person responds from a standpoint of personal belief and feeling, agreement is almost impossible. Styles offers a refreshing approach. She has used the word *professionhood* rather than professionalism and suggests that nurses would be better served by a set of internal beliefs about nursing (that force us to pay attention to our own image as the dominant figure) than by a set of external criteria about professions (Styles, 1982).

THE IMAGE OF NURSING TODAY

During the late 1970s and early 1980s, a great deal of time and energy was invested in studying the image of nursing. Much of this work was done by Beatrice and Phillip Kalisch, who have written prolifically about the topic. Much of their writing deals with segments of an overall study of the image of the nurse in various forms of mass media, including radio, movies, television, newspapers, magazines, and novels. They believe that popular attitudes and assumptions about nurses and what nurses contribute to a patient's welfare can greatly influence the future of nursing. It is their contention that since the 1970s, the popular image of the nurse has not only failed to reflect changing professional conditions but has been based on derogatory stereotypes that have undermined public confidence in and respect for the professional nurse. Nurses should be concerned about negative or incorrect images because such images can influence the attitudes of patients, policy-makers, and politicians. Negative attitudes about nursing may also discourage many capable prospective nurses, who will choose another career that offers greater appeal in stature, status, and salary.

Television and Motion Pictures

From studying nurses on television (one of the most important source of information in the country), Kalisch and Kalisch found that nurses often had no substantive role in the television stories. Often the nurse was part of the hospital background in programs that focused on physician characters, whose careers were viewed as more important and who scored high on such attributes as ambition, intelligence, rationality, aggression, self-confidence, and altruism. When a nurse was the focus of a program, the story line involved the nurse's personal problems, rather than her role as a nurse. The nurse frequently was portrayed as the ''handmaiden'' to the physician, and scored high on such attributes as obedience, permissiveness, conformity, flexibility, and serenity. It is interesting to note that nurses ranked lower than physicians on such items as humanism, self-sacrifice, duty, and family concern, all of which are values traditionally ascribed to nurses (Kalisch & Kalisch, 1982a).

Kalisch and Kalisch found a rise and fall in the image of nurses in motion pictures, with the high point occurring during the war years of the 1940s and the low point occurring in the 1970s, when the nursing profession was denigrated and satirized in many films (Fig. 5-2). This latter fact will have an impact on the attitudes of prospective nurses because the largest proportion of moviegoers each year are adolescents. The earlier, positive images of nurses usually came from films that were biographies of outstanding nurses such as Sister Kenny, who worked with polio patients, or Edith Cavell, a World War I heroine who was shot by the Germans for helping Allied soldiers escape from occupied Belgium. For a time the nurse–detective was a popular theme in films; such nurses were portrayed as intelligent, perceptive, confident, sophisticated, composed, tough, and assertive. During the 1970s, however, nurses in films often were portrayed as malevolent and sadistic (eg, the roles of Nurse Ratched in *One Flew Over the Cuckoo's Nest* and Nurse Diesel in *High Anxiety*). This was the lowest point for the image of nurses in the history of film; nurses in film were lacking in such values as duty, self-sacrifice, achievement, integrity, virtue, intelligence, rationality, and kindness. Few films centered on the individual achievement or personal autonomy of the nurse. When compared with the physician's role, the nurse's role was seen as less

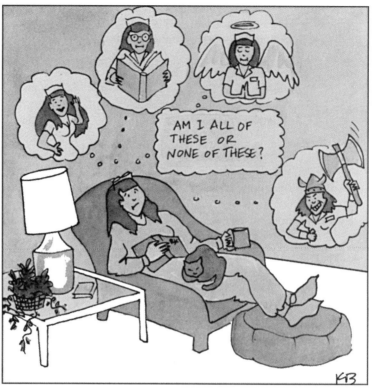

FIGURE 5-2
Nurses should be concerned about negative or incorrect images because these are sure to influence the attitudes of patients, policymakers, and politicians.

important (Kalisch & Kalisch, 1982b). There may be hope that this trend is reversing, however; a recent film, "The English Patient," which received the Oscar as Best Picture of the Year in 1997, added credibility to the role of the nurse by portraying the nurse character as caring, thinking, and involved.

The Image of the Nurse in Print

To study the image of nursing in novels, Kalisch and Kalisch analyzed 207 books. As with film and television, they found that the nurse in the novel was almost always female, single, childless, white, and younger than the age of 35.

Because nurses almost always have been depicted in novels as women, emphasis has also been on traditional female roles (ie, wife, mistress, mother). Three nurse stereotypes have resulted:

1. The nurse as man's companion
2. The nurse as man's destroyer
3. The nurse as man's mother or the mother of his children

The man in the novel is often a physician. Novelists of the 1970s and 1980s have often maligned their nurse characters, ignoring the nurses' professional motivations and health care perspectives (Kalisch & Kalisch, 1982c).

Muff (1988) has analyzed feminine myths and stereotypes and has elaborated on nursing stereotypes. After reading books about nurses written for school-aged children (eg, Cherry Ames, Sue Barton, Kathy Martin, and Penny Scott), she has made the following conclusions:

- Nursing is described as glamorous.
- Medicine and nursing are imbued with a sense of mystery and elitism.
- Nursing is simplistic.
- Nurses move from job to job.
- Nurses are subservient and deferential, following orders, running errands, and idolizing the physicians for whom they work.

All of the nurses in these books were educated in hospital-based diploma programs, earning the ''R.N.'' only after hours of hospital service, even though the Martin and Scott series were both written in the 1960s.

Muff (1988) has also examined the role of the nurse as it is captured in the romance novel. In many instances appearances (eg, the color and condition of the nurse's hair) were most important, and the nurse was portrayed as a ''pure'' girl, dressed in white, whose main aim was to get a man, usually a doctor. Women who were not looking for husbands were in nursing for altruistic reasons, and duty and self-sacrifice were glamorized. Muff also found that the image of the nurse in the novel usually could be placed into one of the following categories: ministering angels, handmaidens, battle-axes, fools, and whores. She stated that the stereotypes of nursing presented in television and film also usually fit one of these categories. When reviewing the nurse image on get-well cards, she had to add a new category, that of ''token torturer.''

Only newspapers and news magazines have tended toward realism rather than fantasy. News articles have examined the shortage of nurses, discussing reasons for it (such as working conditions, salaries, benefits, and hardships). Special feature articles have also provided information about new or unique nursing roles, such as those of nurses in Vietnam (Muff, 1982). With the outbreak of war in the Middle East in 1991, nurses received positive recognition by the media. Nurses serving in reserve status with branches of the military were among the first called up when the conflict began. As our society recognizes the need to honor women as well as men for their contributions, nurses are often singled out for special recognition—especially during wartime. For example, Clara Maass was commemorated on a U.S. postage stamp, the first of many nurses to be honored in this way. This 25 year-old Spanish American War nurse was so moved by the suffering of her patients with yellow fever that she volunteered to be bitten several times by the disease-carrying mosquito in an effort to determine how the disease was transmitted. Although she survived the first bite, she died of yellow fever from a subsequent exposure.

The nurses who served during the Vietnam war have received recognition for their contributions in the form of a monument in Washington D.C. The monument, located near the well-known memorial honoring Vietnam veterans, is the first national memorial honoring nurses. Although some might argue that nurses have better things to do than to worry about how the nurse is portrayed in the media, a consistently misrepresented image can negatively affect the way the public thinks about nurses. Therefore, nurses have responded to television advertisements or programs that portray nurses and nursing in a negative light with letters and telephone calls. Boycotts on the purchase of products that appear in negative advertisements has proved to be a fairly effective way to bring about change. Actions such as these were responsible for the cancellation of a television show that cast nursing in an inaccurate and demeaning light.

During the 1980s, various nursing organizations waged campaigns to enhance the image of nursing. In 1981, the National League for Nursing (NLN) took an active role in developing media that portrayed nursing in a positive light. The National Commission on Nursing Implementation Project was responsible for initiating an advertising campaign on television and radio that emphasized nursing as a prestigious, desirable, and respected career. Some hospital associations, such as the Texas Hospital Association, also launched recruiting operations that focused on the desirability of nursing as a career.

STUDIES FOR AND ABOUT NURSING

Early in this century, the quality of many nursing schools and their graduates was poor, and many of Florence Nightingale's admonitions regarding nursing education were forgotten. Nurses, doctors, friends, and critics of nursing became concerned about the inadequate preparation being offered. Before the problem could be corrected, it was necessary to learn more about the programs and how nurses were being used in the employment market. To accomplish this, studies about nursing and nurses were initiated.

We recognize that many students in nursing are not excited by studies, especially not by those conducted years ago. However, the development of nursing as a profession has been affected by them, and it seems important to discuss significant studies. We think you will recognize some recurring themes that remain relevant today.

Although the first nursing studies were not begun until the early 1900s, the number of studies since the 1950s has been voluminous. It is impossible to pick up any professional nursing publication and not find mention of some new study in progress. In an effort to classify and catalog references to these studies, Virginia Henderson prepared *A Nursing Studies Index*. In 1952, a group of nurses, under the sponsorship of the Association of Collegiate Schools of Nursing, launched a new journal called *Nursing Research*, which was designed to disseminate information about nursing research.

Many of the early studies were conducted by a single individual with a particular purpose in mind. Over the years, studies have often taken the form of a "report" by a special group of individuals, often appointed by a governmental or professional agency. Although by no means inclusive of all studies and reports, Table 5-3 highlights some of the major significant studies of nursing that have provided benchmarks to the profession. Following is a discussion of some of the major studies and their impact on nursing.

Early Studies

One of the earliest nursing studies was carried out under the guidance of M. Adelaide Nutting in 1912. Published by the U.S. Bureau of Education, it was entitled "The Educational Status of Nursing." The study investigated what and how nursing students were being taught, and under what conditions students were living. Although it did not receive

TABLE 5-3. Major Studies About Nursing

Date	Name of Study	Primary Investigator/Sponsor	Focus and Recommendation
1912	*The Educational Status of Nursing*	M. Adelaide Nutting/U.S. Bureau of Education	What and how students were being taught and conditions under which they were living. Began to establish nursing as a profession.
1923	*Winslow-Goldmark Report on Nursing and Nursing Education in the United States*	Josephine Goldmark/Rockefeller Foundation	The educational preparation of students including public health nurses, teachers, and supervisors. It pointed out fundamental faults in hospital training schools and resulted in the establishment of the Yale University School of Nursing.
	Committee on the Grading of Nursing Schools—a three-part study	Francis Payne Bolton and contributions of thousands of nurses	
1928	*1) Nurses, Patients, and Pocket Books*	May Ayres Burgess/statistician	An inquiry into the supply and demand for nurses. Demonstrated that there was an over-supply of nurses.
1934	*2) An Activity Analysis of Nursing*	Ethel Johns and Blance Pfefferkorn	Looked at the activities that constitute nursing as a basis for improving curricula.
1934	*3) Nursing Schools Today & Tomorrow*	Ethel Johns	Described the nursing schools of the period and made recommendations about professional schools.
1937	*A Curriculum Guide for Schools of Nursing—* Not truly a study of nursing, but often referred to as one because of its far reaching effects.	National League for Nursing Education	A revision of a 1917 publication, it outlined the curricula for a 3-year course, emphasizing sound educational teaching procedures. Followed by many schools of the time.
1948	*Nursing for the Future*	Esther Lucille Brown/Carnegie Foundation, the Russell Sage Foundation, and the National Nursing Council	Done to determine society's need for nursing. Described inadequacies in nursing schools. Resulted in recommendations that nursing education be placed in universities and colleges and encouraged recruitment of large numbers of men and members of minority groups into nursing schools.
1948	The Ginzberg Report or *A Program for the Nursing Profession—*a report of the discussions of the Committee on the Functions of Nursing	Eli Ginzberg/Columbia University	Reviewed problems centering around the shortage of nurses. Recommended that nursing teams consisting of variously educated nurses be developed.
1950	*Nursing Schools at the Mid-Century*	Margaret Bridgman/National Committee for the Improvement of Nursing Services—Russell Sage Foundation	Studied the practices of over 1000 nursing schools (including organization, costs, curriculum, clinical resources, and student health) and stimulated improvement in baccalaureate schools.

(continued)

TABLE 5-3. Major Studies About Nursing *(continued)*

Date	Name of Study	Primary Investigator/Sponsor	Focus and Recommendation
1955	*Patterns of Patient Care*	Francis George and Ruth Perkins Kuehn/University of Pittsburg	Assessed the amount of nursing service needed by a group of medical/surgical patients and determined how much of that care could be delegated to nursing aides and other nonprofessional people.
1958	*Twenty Thousand Nurses Tell Their Story*	Everett C. Hughes/ANA and American Nurses Foundation	Looked at nurses, what they were doing, their attitudes toward their jobs and job satisfaction. Formed basis for development of nursing functions, standards, and qualifications.
1959	*Community College Education for Nursing*	Mildred Montag/Institute of Research and Service in Nursing Education— Teachers College, Columbia University	Reported the findings of a 5-year study of 8 2-year nursing programs. Led to the establishment of more Associate Degree Programs.
1963	*Toward Quality in Nursing: Needs and Goals*	W. Allen Wallis—Consultant Group on Nursing—a panel of nurses in the health field/U.S. Public Health Service	A report requested by the U.S. Surgeon General to determine funding priorities. Advised on the need for nurses, recruitment concerns, need for nursing research, and improvement of nursing education.
1970	*An Abstract for Action* (a report of the National Commission on Nursing and Nursing Education)	Jerome Lysaught/ANA, ANF, NLN, Mellon and Kellogg Foundations	Looked at current practices and patterns of nursing. Suggested joint practice committees, master planning for nursing education, funding for nursing education and research.
1979	*The Study of Credentialing in Nursing*	Inez Hinsvark/ANA	A review of credentialing—especially of nursing. Resulted in the appointment of a Task Force. Supported a free-standing credentialing center for nursing.
1983	*National Institute of Medicine Study*	Katherine Bauer/DHHS	Required by the Nursing Training Act of 1979, determined the need for continued outlay of federal money for nursing education. Resulted in 21 specific recommendations. Found that the shortage of nurses of the 1960s and 1970s no longer existed, that federal support of nursing education should focus on graduate study, and that the federal government should discontinue efforts to increase "generalist nurses."
1988	*Secretary's Commission on Nursing*	Lillian Gibbons/DHHS	Responded to serious nursing shortage. Validated the shortage. Recommended increased financial support of education and improved status and working conditions for nurses.

(continued)

TABLE 5-3. *(continued)*

Date	Name of Study	Primary Investigator/Sponsor	Focus and Recommendation
1990	*Secretary's Commission on the National Nursing Shortage*	Caroline Burnett/DHHS	Appointed for 1 year to advise on implementation of 1988 report. Had three main foci: recruitment and retention, restructuring of nursing service, and use of nursing personnel and information systems.
1991	*Report of the National Commission of Nursing Implementation Project (NCNIP)*	Vivian De Back/ANA, NLN, AACN, AONE, Kellogg Foundation	Looked at nursing education, practice, management and research and developed recommendations for the future of nursing.
1993	*Health Professions Education for the Future*	E.H. O'Neill/Pew Health Professions Commission— Pew Charitable Trusts	Reinforced the belief that the education of health professions was not adequate to meet the health needs of America. Identified competencies for 2005 and emphasized the need for nurse-midwives, nurse practitioners, and the role of nurses in health promotion.
1995	*Reforming Health Care Workforce Regulation*	Pew Health Professions Commission	Had as its mission assisting schools preparing health professionals to understand the changing nature of health care, the needs for the future, and how to design and implement the programs preparing these workers. Recommended reform of the licensing process, specifically elimination of exclusive scopes of practice.

the attention it probably deserved, it began to establish nursing as a profession, suggesting that schools of nursing be independent from hospitals and leading the way to more studies.

The Winslow-Goldmark Report, sometimes called the Goldmark Report, followed in 1923. This was also referred to as ''The Study of Nursing and Nursing Education in the United States'' (Winslow-Goldmark Report, 1923) and was the work of a committee composed of physicians, nurses, and lay people. The report focused on the preparation of public health nurses, teachers, administrators, the clinical learning experiences of students, and on the financing of schools. Subsequently, the Yale University School of Nursing and the Vanderbilt University School of Nursing were established, funded by an endowment from the Rockefeller Foundation.

A three-part study, sponsored by the Committee on the Grading of Nursing Schools (a 21 member group of representatives from a variety of nursing and medical professional organizations), was conducted between 1928 and 1934. The first part, which was socioeconomic in nature and entitled ''Nurses, Patients, and Pocketbooks,'' attempted to determine if there was a shortage of nurses in the United States; the second part, an ''Activity Analysis of Nursing,'' examined those nursing activities that could be used as a basis for improving the curricula in nursing schools; part three, "Nursing Schools Today and Tomorrow," described the schools of the period and made recommendations for professional schools.

In 1932, the National League for Nursing Education (later to become the National League for Nursing) conducted its first study, a comparative study of the bedside activities of graduate and student nurses. Conducted by Blanche Pfefferkorn, the Director of the NLNE Department of Studies, the study indicated that nursing care should be given by graduate nurses rather than students, and provided information about the number of tasks assigned to nursing students that had nothing to do with acquiring a nursing education.

The last of the early nursing studies that we mention was not really a study, but often is referred to as one because of its far-reaching impact. *A Curriculum Guide for Schools of Nursing*, published in 1937, was a revised version of a document published in 1917. It outlined the curricula for a 3-year course, emphasizing sound educational teaching procedures. It was read and followed by many schools that were operating programs at that time.

Midcentury Studies

By the 1950s studies about nurses and nursing were numerous and dealt with many aspects of the profession. Only a few of those studies are mentioned here.

Of particular significance was a study published in 1948 entitled "Nursing for the Future." Conducted by Esther Lucille Brown, a social anthropologist, the study is also known as the Brown report. Funded by the Carnegie Foundation, the study was done to determine society's need for nursing, and recommendations were made for higher education for nurses. It prompted serious examination of professional education and pointed out weaknesses in the existing educational programs. The investigators recommended that basic schools of nursing be placed in universities and colleges, and encouraged the recruitment of large numbers of men and minorities into nursing schools. This report set the stage for studies of nursing education that followed in the 1950s and 1960s, and for recommendations that were to continue into the 1990s.

The Ginzberg report was published the same year. A report rather than a study, it reviewed problems centering around the current and prospective shortage of nurses. The conclusions and recommendations were published in the book entitled *A Program for the Nursing Profession*. The report recommended that nursing teams consisting of 4-year professional nurses, 2-year registered nurses, and 1-year practical nurses be developed. This would ease the nursing shortage by enabling each member of the team to function in the role for which he or she was educationally prepared.

In 1958, a study entitled "Twenty Thousand Nurses Tell Their Story" was published. It was part of a 5-year research project that was conceived by the ANA and financially supported by nurses throughout the country. The report was prepared by Everett C. Hughes, a professor of sociology at the University of Chicago. The study looked at nurses, what they were doing, their attitudes toward their jobs, and their job satisfaction. As a result, nurses learned a great deal about themselves.

Another significant study was initiated by Mildred Montag and was published in 1959. This study on "Community College Education for Nursing" resulted in the creation of associate degree nursing education (see Chapter 6).

Significant Studies of the 1960s and 1970s

In 1961, the Surgeon General of the U.S. Public Health Service appointed a 25-member panel called the Consultant Group of Nursing. This group was to advise him on nursing needs and identify the role of the federal government in assessing nursing services to the nation. In 1963, this group presented a report entitled "Toward Quality in Nursing," which recommended a national investigation of nursing education that would place emphasis on the criteria for high-quality patient care.

After publication of "Toward Quality in Nursing," the ANA and the NLN appropriated funds and established a joint committee to study ways to conduct and finance a national inquiry of nursing education. It was decided that the study would expand to consider probable requirements in professional nursing to occur over several decades to come, as well as to examine changing practices and educational patterns of the present time. W. Allen Wallis, president of the University of Rochester, headed the study. Financing was obtained from the American Nurses Foundation, the Kellogg Foundation, the Avalon Foundation, and an anonymous benefactor. To conduct the study, the National Commission for the Study of Nursing and Nursing Education was set up as an independent agency and functioned as a self-directing group. The 12 commissioners were chosen for their broad knowledge of nursing, for their skills in related disciplines, or for their competencies in relevant fields, with no commissioner representing a particular interest group or position. In August 1967, at the first meeting of the commission, Jerome P. Lysaught was appointed director of the planning and operation of the inquiry.

The study focused on the supply and demand for nurses, nursing roles and functions, nursing education, and nursing as a career. The commission found it necessary not only to examine these key concerns but also to relate these issues to the social system that provides care to the public.

The final report of the commission, "An Abstract for Action," was published in 1970. It included 58 specific recommendations and concluded with four central recommendations. It also listed three basic priorities:

1. Increased research on both the practice and education of nurses
2. Enhanced educational systems and curricula based on research
3. Increased financial support for nurses and for nursing

In 1973, a progress report from the National Commission for the Study of Nursing and Nursing Education concerning the implementation of the recommendations of the original report was published under the title "From Abstract into Action." The commission believed that it was imperative that nursing achieve the goals established in the recommendations so that nursing could emerge as a full profession and assist in providing optimal health care for this country.

Studies of the 1980s

One of the major studies of nursing conducted in the 1980s was that of the National Commission on Nursing. This group was composed of a forum of 30 commissioners from disciplines such as nursing, hospital management, business, government, education, and medicine—all of whom were concerned about the current nursing-related problems in the health care system, especially the apparent shortage of nurses. The commission was sponsored by the American Hospital Association, Hospital Research and Educational Trust, and the American Hospital Supply Corporation. Its chairman was H. Robert Cathcart. The group began its work in September 1980 and focused on areas that dealt primarily with the environments in which nurses worked, the relationship between nursing education and nursing practice, nursing issues, and the status of nursing as a profession (National Commission on Nursing, 1981).

The commission began systematically to examine and evaluate data sources, including journal articles, state studies, and policy documents. A series of public hearings held in six major cities across the nation and two open forums provided the opportunity for input about nursing issues from each region of the country. The highlights of the findings, along with the commission's recommendations and future action plans, were published in the initial report of the group in September 1981. The final recommendations were published in 1983. Although the findings and recommendations are too lengthy to be included in this chapter in their entirety, it is important to mention the five major categories of issues identified by the study (National Commission on Nursing, 1981, p 5):

1. The status and image of nursing, which includes changes in the nursing role
2. The interface of nursing education and practice, including models of education for preparing to practice
3. The effective management of the nursing resource, including such factors as job satisfaction, recruitment, and retention
4. The relationship among nursing, medical staff, and hospital administration, including nursing's participation in decision-making
5. The maturing of nursing as a self-determining profession, including defining and determining the nature and scope of practice, the role of nursing leadership, increasing decision-making in nursing practice, and the need for unity in the nursing profession

Many of the commission's findings were not surprising to people who were involved with nursing. Included were findings indicating that physicians and health care administrators often did not understand the role of nurses in patient care, and that traditional and outdated images of nurses (including Victorian stereotypes and traditional male–female relationships) impeded acceptance of current roles. Some physicians and administrators thought that nurses were overeducated, and did not support an increase in the nurse's authority to make decisions concerning health care.

The findings that individuals and nursing groups are not unified in defining fundamental, professional goals for nursing, and that nursing, as a profession, lacks cohesiveness and a clear understanding of its role and direction, were not a revelation to many seasoned nurses. These same nurses were also not astonished to learn of the numerous and diverse associations that represent nursing but lack a way to determine common goals for nursing education, practice, and credentialing. The disagreement and confusion about educational preparation for nurses, and the controversy about entry into practice were identified as further obstacles to the advancement of the profession. Clearly there is a need for a system of nursing education that promotes realistic expectations, provides appropriate support for practice and advancement, and includes educational mobility in nursing. As we approach the 21st century, nursing continues to grapple with many of these issues. A number of the issues are ones with which nursing has struggled for years; most of them will not be completely resolved in the next decade. As a new graduate, you will have the opportunity to influence their outcome.

Following in the footsteps of the National Commission of Nursing was the National Commission on Nursing Implementation Project, which began in 1985. Funded by the W. K. Kellogg Foundation for 3 years, the project was cosponsored by the NLN, the ANA, the American Organization of Nurse Executives, and the American Association of Colleges of Nursing. Administered by the American Nurses' Foundation, it had as its purpose to provide leadership in seeking consensus about the appropriate education and credentialing for basic nursing practice, effective models for the delivery of nursing care, and the means for developing and testing nursing knowledge. The aim of this project was to lay the groundwork and take action wherever possible to support effective, high-quality nursing care delivery in the immediate and long-range future.

The results of another nursing study were released in January 1983. This 2-year study, mandated under the 1979 Nurse Training Amendments, was conducted by the Institute of Medicine Committee on Nursing and Nursing Education and was funded by the Department of Health and Human Services at a cost of $1.6 million. The objectives of the study were:

- To provide advice regarding federal support for nursing education
- To gain more information about nurses; to learn, for example, why they do not seek employment in medically underserved areas and why they leave the profession
- To make recommendations regarding measures to improve the supply and use of nursing resources.

The study made 21 specific recommendations to Congress. Because the study found that the shortage of nurses in the 1960s and 1970s had largely disappeared, it was recommended that the federal government discontinue efforts to increase the supply of ''generalist nurses.'' (I.O.M. study sees need for funds . . . , 1983).

The fallacies in these findings soon became apparent. Across the nation, nursing enrollments plummeted in the late 1980s. This drop in enrollment occurred at a time when nurses were assuming expanded roles and more nurses than ever were needed for the delivery of health care throughout the nation. The result was a serious national shortage of nurses, especially in certain settings and in specific areas of care such as long-term care.

Studies of the 1990s

Responding to the need for more nurses, many of the studies of the early 1990s focused on the roles of nurses in the delivery of health care, on educational patterns that would encourage capable individuals to choose nursing as a career, and on programs that would facilitate educational mobility. Issues related to the nurse's image and the nursing shortage merged. A new Commission on the National Nursing Shortage replaced the Federal Commission on Nursing, and $275,000 was budgeted to assist in its function. This commission developed strategies to decrease the nursing shortage, which focused on recruitment, retention, restructuring of nursing services for the most effective utilization of nursing personnel, and gathering data about nursing and the information systems used in nursing.

The Pew Charitable Trust funded the Pew Health Professions Commission originally composed of 21 members. The first report, issued in 1991, declared that the education and training of health professionals was not adequate to meet the needs of the public. The work of the Pew Commission continued with another report in 1993, *Health Professions Education for the Future: Schools in Service to the Nation Study*, that discussed the need for change in the allied health professions, dentistry, medicine, nursing, pharmacy, public health, public health administration, and veterinary medicine. In 1995, the Pew Commission, now comprised of 20 members (four of whom were nurses) issued two more reports. One, entitled *Critical challenges: Revitalizing the Health Professions for the Twenty-first Century*, again emphasized that the education of health professionals was not in step with the health needs of the American people. The report cited the closure of as many as half of the nation's hospitals, massive expansion of primary care in ambulatory and community settings, a surplus of both physicians and nurses, a greater demand for public health professionals, and a fundamental alteration of the health profession schools (de Tornyay, 1996).

The report also made a number of recommendations regarding nursing education, which included the following:

- Recognizing the value of the multiple entry points of professional practice
- Consolidating professional nomenclature so that there is a single title for each level of nursing preparation and service
- Determining the practice responsibilities associated with different levels of nursing education
- Reducing the size and number of nursing education programs (with the suggestion that the reductions occur in associate degree and diploma programs)
- Expanding the number of masters level nurse practitioner programs.

The second report issued by the Pew Commission in 1995 was entitled *Reforming Health Care Workforce Regulation.* The report made several assumptions about what constitutes an appropriate regulatory system; that it be standardized, accountable, flexible, and effective and efficient (see Chapter 7 for more detail on assumptions).

A major recommendation of this study was that scopes of practice be eliminated. Scopes of practice describe the authority each state gives to the health professionals who practice in that state; for example physicians are allowed to perform certain procedures and nurses to perform others. This recommendation would mean that each state licensing authority would identify which specific health care services could be dangerous to the public and therefore could be safely performed only by members of specific professions. If the members of any of the regulated professions could demonstrate that they could safely perform acts not ordinarily listed in their professional practice act, then, (with Board endorsement) those acts could be included in their practice (Curtin, 1995). Essentially the elimination of scopes of practice would mean that each state would base authority to practice on the practitioner's demonstrated ability to perform certain health care services. This meant that differently trained and differently named professions could deliver the same services if they were able to demonstrate competence. Competence would be demonstrated through a combination of training, experience and skills (Finocchio, Dower, McMahon & Gragnolo, p 13, 1995). Additionally, any licensed or unlicensed personnel would be permitted to perform any health care services that were not included in the list of restricted acts if they were deemed competent by the employer. The regulatory responsibility for all health care delivery would essentially be moved from the state to institutional providers of health care services, with the exception of those skills identified legislatively as ''potentially dangerous acts.''

In Ontario, Canada the regulatory system was reworked to make it more flexible and accountable to the public. Through this process, thirteen ''controlled acts'' were identified that are potentially dangerous to the public. Twenty-four companion laws were written that cover the regulated professions. Each law contains individual scopes of practice and identifies the authorized acts that may be performed by individuals licensed under that law. For example, physicians have been granted authority to perform 12 of the 13 controlled acts, midwives may perform seven of the acts, and massage therapists may not perform any of the 13 controlled acts (Pew Health Professions Commission, p. 13–14, 1995).

As this book goes to press, the recommendations to eliminate the scopes of practice are generating considerable discussion among health care professionals. As a new member of one of these groups, you will have an opportunity to speak to the issues being discussed. It is critical that you remain knowledgeable and informed about such matters.

TRADITIONS IN NURSING

Because of its history, nursing has developed a number of traditions. Some of these traditions are being questioned or eliminated, primarily because they are not practical in today's workplace (eg, the wearing of a nursing cap). It is worthwhile, however, to reflect just a little on the development of these traditions and to discuss their relationship to nursing.

The Nursing Pin

The nursing pin may date back to the time of the Crusades when Crusaders marched to Jerusalem to recover the Holy Land. Among the Crusaders were the Knights Hospitallers of St. John of Jerusalem. Their uniform, introduced by a man named Gerard, included a black robe with a white Maltese cross. This Maltese cross became a familiar site on the battlefields of the Holy Land. Following the capture of Jerusalem in 1099, some of the Crusaders noted the excellent nursing care provided by the Hospital of Saint John and decided to join the nursing group. The Maltese cross is an eight-pointed cross formed by four arrowheads joining at their points. The eight points signified the eight beatitudes that knights were expected to exemplify in their works of charity. When the Knights Templars and the Knights of the Teutonic Order were formed in 1118 and 1190, respectively, this symbol was carried forward. The Maltese cross was later to become a symbol of many groups who cared for the sick, including the United States Cadet Nurse Corps.

The actual symbolism of the pin relates to customs established in the 16th century, when the privilege of wearing a coat of arms was limited to noblemen who served their kings with distinction. As centuries passed, the privilege was extended to schools and to craft guilds, and the symbols of wisdom, strength, courage, and faith appeared on buttons, badges, and shields. It was probably this spirit that Florence Nightingale attempted to capture when she chose the Maltese cross as a symbol for the badge worn by the graduates of her first nursing school.

As nursing developed as a profession, each school chose a unique pin, awarded on completion of the program, that was a public symbol of work well done. Many of the early schools, particularly those associated with hospitals supported by religious groups, have incorporated the cross into their pin. The first Nightingale School of Nursing in the United

States was at Bellevue Hospital and is credited with developing the first school badge or pin, which was presented to the class of 1880 (Kalisch & Kalisch, p. 82.) A crane in the center symbolized the nurse's vigilance, an inner circle of blue suggested constancy, and an outer circle of poppy capsules symbolized mercy and the relief of suffering.

The Nursing Cap

The history of the nursing cap is less certain. Several explanations of the origin of the cap have been suggested. It probably evolved during the period of time when nursing was greatly influenced by religion. It may have originated in the habit worn by the Sisters of Charity of St. Vincent de Paul, who established the first modern school of nursing in Paris in 1864. Another opinion suggests that the cap was influenced by the Institute of Protestant Deaconesses, founded by Pastor Theodore Fleidner at Kaiserwerth in Germany, where Florence Nightingale studied. The white cap of the deaconesses of the early Christian era and the nun's veil of the Middle Ages have been said to be the forerunners of the nursing cap as we know it today (Mangum, 1994). The veil was modified to become a cap and was associated with service to others. We need to remember, also, that in Florence Nightingale's day every lady wore a cap indoors. If you look at pictures of Queen Victoria you will notice the cap of plain white stiffened muslin framing her face. It was considered proper for women to keep their heads covered, thus, the cap would be viewed as the proper dress for a young woman of the day. The cap worn by students at Kaiserwerth when Florence Nightingale was a student was hood shaped, had a ruffle around the face, and tied under the chin. A final conjecture is that the cap was originally designed to cover the long hair that was fashionable in the late 19th century, when short hair cuts were not acceptable for women and the use of a head covering helped to control the hair.

As women's hair styles changed and hair was worn shorter, the head covering became smaller and lost its scarf or veil in the United States and Canada. (The hair covering aspect remained a part of the cap in many areas of England and Europe.) As hospitals developed nursing education programs, they each created their own cap and nursing pin as a symbol of that particular hospital and nursing school. Some of these were rather "frilly" and were fashioned after the ether cone through which ether was dropped. As hair styles changed, the size of the cap also changed, until it became one of individual taste or preference. A "capping" ceremony was part of the ritual of the nursing student and will be discussed later.

As the role of nurses changed and as high technology became a significant part of the hospital work environment, nurses found that caps were bothersome as they tried to carry out their duties. They were knocked askew by curtains, equipment, and tubing. By the 1980s, many hospitals were no longer requiring the cap as a part of the uniform. Nursing programs responded by dropping the cap as a required article of dress. If students wished to have a cap, it was purchased from a local uniform store and had no particular identification with the program (Fig. 5-3).

The Nursing Uniform

Like the nursing cap, which is actually a part of the early nursing uniform, the requirement for special dress came from the religious and military history of nursing and has always

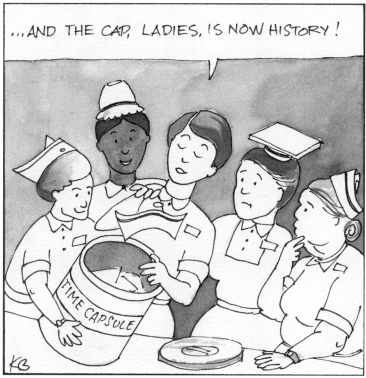

FIGURE 5-3
By the 1980s many nurses were no longer wearing the cap as part of the nursing uniform.

been significant in nursing. This is due in part to the fact that dress provides a strong nonverbal message about one's image. The nurse attired in a white uniform, at least in the 1950s and 1960s, communicated an impression of confidence, competence, professionalism, authority, role identity, and accountability. As nurses have adopted more casual dress, some of this identity has been lost, and hospital committees, nursing programs, and nurses have spent considerable time discussing appropriate attire.

Early uniforms were long, usually stiffly starched, and had detachable collars and cuffs. A full uniform often included a long cape that would cover the uniform. Kalisch and Kalisch (1995, p. 80–81) credit the New York Training School for Nurses at Bellevue Hospital with being the first school to adopt a standard uniform for student nurses in 1876. The uniform consisted of a gingham apron worn in the morning and a white apron worn in the afternoon over a dark woolen dress. A well-bred young woman, Euphemia Van Rensselaer is credited with updating the basic uniform which students were opposed to wearing. Given two days' leave of absence to have a uniform made for herself, she created a tailored uniform consisting of a long gray dress for winter and a calico version for summer, both worn with a white apron and cap. The attractiveness of her appearance resulted in other students accepting the uniform as standard dress. Later, a more easily laundered dress that could be worn throughout the year replaced the grey dress for winter.

A regulation uniform became a distinguishing mark of each nursing school by the end of the 19th century. Typically the uniform consisted of a bodice and skirt of white material, adjustable white cuffs, a stiff white collar, and a white cap. To maintain the feminine hourglass image popular at the time, a tightly laced corset was worn beneath the uniform and ankles were to be hidden from view. Some suggest that the adoption of a distinctive and attractive uniform played a significant role in developing a professional image for nursing, giving it status, respect and authority.

By the 1900s, the uniform became more functional and the hemline was raised. By the mid-1960s, pantsuits became accepted and nurses in certain settings, particularly psychiatric and pediatric units, were challenging the appropriateness of uniforms, especially if they were all white. By 1970, significant changes were occurring in uniforms, with the acceptance of styles that were designed to ''make the nurse more approachable.'' In psychiatric settings, ''no uniform'' became the standard of the day. Today athletic shoes have become acceptable in many institutions, and ''scrubs'' have become so accepted that they are featured in pamphlets advertising uniforms. In 1987, the Springhouse Corporation conducted a survey of nurses throughout the United States and found that most nurses prefer scrubs or lab coats worn over street clothes. The result of this change has been that nurses today are no longer identifiable by uniform. The stethoscope worn around the neck gives the consumer some clue to a person's position (ie, that the person is a health care worker rather than a maintenance person), and hospital identification badges provide further information, but may not include the person's full name.

Today there is controversy over the appropriate attire for nurses. Mangum and Associates (1991) recommend that nurses wear clothing that clearly distinguishes them as professional nurses. Although they do not suggest that nurses wear a cap, they have advocated the use of the more traditional white dress or pantsuit. Others argue that what nurses wear matters less than what they know. Perhaps compromise is necessary.

Ceremonies Associated With Nursing Programs

Long-standing traditions embraced by nursing include the ceremonies that mark various points along the educational paths of nursing students. Primary among these are the ''capping'' and the ''pinning'' ceremonies.

Capping ceremonies are not as common today as pinnings, probably because most nurses and nursing students no longer wear caps. Historically the cap was awarded to students after they completed a certain part of the program. In some instances it was awarded on completion of the probationary period, but more often is was given after the completion of the first year. Often held in a nearby church, a special ceremony was planned, to which students invited family and others who were interested in their progress. The director of the school, assisted by other school dignitaries and faculty, solemnly placed the cap on the head of each student. Students proudly wore the cap throughout the remainder of the program. Often a stripe was added to one corner of the cap to signify completion of the second year of study, and a black band was added at the time of graduation.

The second traditional ceremony in nursing, the pinning, was of even greater signifi-

DISPLAY 5-1
The Nightingale Pledge

I solemnly pledge myself before God and in the presence of this assembly:

To pass my life in purity and to practice my profession faithfully;

I will abstain from whatever is deleterious and mischievous and will not take or knowingly administer any harmful drug; I will do all in my power to maintain and elevate the standard of the profession, and will hold in confidence all personal matters committed to my keeping and all family affairs coming to my knowledge in the practice of my calling;

With loyalty will I endeavor to aid the physician in his work, and devote myself to the welfare of those committed to my care.

Gretter, 1893

cance, and is continued by many schools today. The pinning heralded the completion of the program. Amid much pomp and circumstance, family and friends gathered to watch as the nursing director ceremoniously "pinned" each new graduate. Graduates often recited, in unison, the Nightingale Pledge (Display 5-1), written in 1893 by Lystra E. Gretter, superintendent of Harper Hospital school in Detroit (Calhoun, 1993). This tradition is often repeated in nursing schools today, although the original pledge is in some cases modified.

As nursing education has moved into institutions of higher education, some of the traditional ceremonies have been discontinued. Some argue that the ceremony recognizing program completion in the collegiate environment is the college commencement, and that "special" celebrations for students of particular areas of study are not appropriate. However, in many of the large universities, the various disciplines now have separate ceremonies or an additional ceremony for their members. In other cases, the tradition is continued although there is some tendency for graduates not to purchase a pin.

KEY CONCEPTS

- In its development as a profession, nursing has struggled with its definition, its image, and its role in the health care delivery system. The role in the health care delivery system has probably never been more critical than it is today.
- The position nursing occupies as a profession is often judged against sociologically developed characteristics of a profession. Not everyone agrees that nursing meets those standards.
- The standards of a profession typically include seven requirements: that it possess a well-defined and well-organized body of knowledge; enlarge a systematic body of knowledge and improve education; educate its practitioners in institutions of higher learning; function autonomously in the formulation of policy; develop a code of ethics; attract professionals who will be committed to the profession for a lifetime; and compensate practitioners by providing autonomy, continuous professional development, and economic security.

- Nursing has also struggled with the terms profession and professional. At times the characteristics of the ''professional'' become confused with the formal concept of a profession.
- Nursing has struggled with its image. Various groups have waged campaigns to improve the image of nursing and thus make it a more attractive profession.
- Since the beginning of the 20th Century, nursing has been a much studied profession. Early studies dealt with nursing education; later studies dealt with the image of nursing, nurses themselves and with nursing's role in health care delivery.
- Nursing as a profession has many traditions, some of which are being challenged today. Among the traditions are the pin, the cap, the uniform, and nursing ceremonies.

Critical Thinking Activities

1. Analyze the definitions of the major nursing theorists. Develop your own definitions of nursing and compare it to those of the theorists.
2. Select one of the characteristics of a profession that you believe nursing does not completely meet. Describe the actions that you believe should occur in the profession to fully meet that criterion.
3. Interview five of your friends who are not nurses. What is their image of nursing? What do they understand of the role of the nurse? Do they view nursing positively?
4. Identify at least three areas in nursing that you believe need further study and describe how you would begin to conduct those studies. Who would you involve?

REFERENCES

Abdellah FG. Patient-Centered Approaches to Nursing. New York: Macmillan, 1960

American Nurses Association. Nursing: A Social Policy Statement. Kansas City, MO: American Journal of Nursing Co, 1980

American Nurses Association. First Position on Education for Nursing. Am J Nurs 65(12):106–111, 1965

Benner P, Wrubel J. The Primacy of Caring. Menlo Park, CA: Addison-Wesley, 1989

Bevis EO, Watson J. Toward a Caring Curriculum; a New Pedagogy for Nursing. New York: National League for Nursing, 1989

Bixler GK, Bixler RW. The professional status of nursing. Am J Nurs 45(9):730, 1945

Calhoun J. The Nightingale Pledge: A commitment that survives the passage of time. Nurs Health Care 14(3):130–136, 1993

Carper BA. The Ethics of Caring. ANS3:11–19, March, 1979

Curtin LL. Your license and mine. Journal of Nursing Education 26(12):7–8, 1995

de Tornyay, R. Critical challenges for nurse educators. J Nurs Educ, 35(4) 146–147, 1996

Donahue MP. Nursing: The Finest Art, 2nd ed. St Louis: CV Mosby, 1996

Flexner A. In Bernard LA, Walsh M: Leadership: The Key to the Professionalization of Nursing. New York: John Wiley & Sons, 1981

Finocchio LJ, Dower CM, McMahon T, Gragnolo CM, and the Taskforce on Health Care Workforce Regulation. Reforming Health Care Workforce Regulation: Policy Considerations for the 21st Century. San Francisco, CA: Pew Health Professions Commission, December 1995

Henderson V. The Nature of a Science of Nursing. New York: Macmillan, 1966

I.O.M. study sees need for funds in graduate, specialty areas. Am J Nurs 83(3):343, 344, 454, 1983

Johnson D. The behavioral system model for nursing. *In* Riehl JP, Roy C: Conceptual Models for Nursing Practice, 2nd ed. East Norwalk, CT: Appleton-Century-Crofts, 1980:207—216

Kalisch PA, Kalisch BJ. Nurses on prime-time television. Am J Nurs 82(2):264, 1982a

Kalisch PA, Kalisch BJ. The image of the nurse in motion pictures. Am J Nurs 82(4):605, 1982b

Kalisch PA, Kalisch BJ. The image of nurses in novels. Am J Nurs 82(8):1220, 1982c

King IM. A Theory for Nursing: Systems, Concepts, Process. New York: John Wiley & Sons, 1981

Labor Management Relations Act (1947) as amended by Public Laws 86–257 (1959) and 93–360 (1974), Section 2

Levine ME. Introduction to Clinical Nursing. Philadelphia: FA Davis, 1969

Mangum, S. Uniforms and caps: Do we need them? *In* Strickland OL, Fishman DJ: Nursing Issues in the 1990s. Albany, NY: Delmar Publishers, 1994:46–66

Mangum S, Garrison C, Lind C, Thackeray R, Wyatt M. Perception of nurses' uniforms. Image: The Journal of Nursing Scholarship 23:127–130, 1991

Moccia P. Curriculum Revolution: Agenda for Change. New York: National League for Nursing, Inc. 1988

Muff J. Handmaiden, battle ax, whore. *In* Muff J: Socialization, Sexism and Stereotyping. Prospect Heights, IL: Waveland Press, Inc. 1988:113–156

National Commission for the Study of Nursing and Nursing Education: Summary, Report and Recommendations. Am J Nurs 70(2):279, 1970

National Commission on Nursing. Initial Report and Preliminary Recommendations. Chicago: Hospital Research and Educational Trust, 1981

National Council of State Boards of Nursing, Inc. Model Practice Act. Chicago, Il: The Council, 1994

Neuman B. The Neuman System Model: Application to Nursing Education and Practice. East Norwalk, CT: Appleton-Century-Crofts, 1982

Newman MA. Professionalism: Myth or reality. *In* Chaska NL: The Nursing Profession: Turning Points. St Louis: CV Mosby, 1990:49–52

Nightingale F. Notes on Nursing: What It Is, and What It Is Not. (An unabridged republication of the first American edition, as published by D. Appleton and Company in 1860.) New York: Dover Publications, 1954

Orem D. Nursing: Concepts of Practice, 2nd ed. New York: McGraw-Hill, 1980

Orlando IJ. The Discipline and Teaching of Nursing Process. New York: GP Putnam's Sons, 1972

Pavalko RM. Sociology of Occupations and Professions. Itasca, IL: Peacock Publishers, 1971

Peplau HE. Interpersonal Relations in Nursing. New York: GP Putnam's Sons, 1952

Revised Standard Version of the Holy Bible, 35 Genesis 6–8

Rogers ME. Science of Unitary Human Beings: A Paradigm for Nursing. Paper presented before the International Nurse Theorist Conference, Edmonton, Alberta, May 1984

Roy C. Introduction to Nursing: An Adaptation Model, 2nd ed. Englewood Cliffs, NJ: Prentice-Hall, 1984

Schlotfeldt RM. Resolution of issues: An imperative for creating nursing's future. J Prof Nurs 3:136–142, 1987

Strauss A. The structure and ideology of American nursing: An interpretation. *In* Davis J: The Nursing Profession. New York: John Wiley & Sons, 1966:60–108

Styles M. On Nursing: Toward a new endowment. St. Louis: CV Mosby, 1982

Watson J. Nursing the Philosophy and Science of Caring. Boston: Little Brown, 1979

Wiedenbach E. Clinical Nursing, A Helping Art. New York: Springer Publishing Co., 1964

Winslow-Goldmark Report. The Study of Nursing and Nursing Education in the United States. New York: Macmillan, 1923

FURTHER READING

Aaronson LS. A challenge for nursing: Reviewing a historic competition. Nurs Outlook 37(6):274–279, 1989

Backer BA. Lillian Wald: Connecting caring with activism. Nurs Health Care 14(3):122–129, 1993

Bunting S, Campbell JC. Feminism and nursing. Adv Nurs Sci 12(4): ll–24, 1990

Bullough VL, et al. The Emergence of Modern Nursing. New York: Macmillan, 1969

Christy T. Equal rights for women: Voices from the past. Am J Nurs 2(2):288–293, 1971

Christy T. First fifty years. Am J Nurs 9(9):1778–1784, 1971

Christy T. Portrait of a leader: Lavinia Lloyd Dock. Nurs Outlook 17(6):72–75, 1969

Christy T. Portrait of a leader: M. Adelaide Nutting. Nurs Outlook 17(1):20–24, 1969

Christy T. Portrait of a leader: Isabel Hampton Robb. Nurs Outlook 17(3):26–29, 1969

Christy T. Portrait of a leader: Isabel Maitland Stewart. Nurs Outlook 17(10):44–48, 1969

Dolan JA. Nursing in Society: A Historical Perspective, 14th ed. Philadelphia: WB Saunders, 1978

Gamer M. The ideology of professionalism. Nurs Outlook 27(2):108–111, 1979

Griffin GJ, Griffin JK. Jensen's History and Trends of Professional Nursing, 7th ed. St Louis: CV Mosby, 1973

Hanson KS. The emergence of liberal education in nursing education, 1893–1923. J Prof Nurs 5(2): 83–91, 1989

Kalisch PA, Kalisch BJ. The Advance of American Nursing, 3rd ed. Philadelphia: J.B. Lippincott Co., 1995

Kalisch BJ, Kalisch PA. Heroine out of focus: Media images of Florence Nightingale: I. Popular biographies and stage productions. Nurs Health Care 4(4):181–187, 1983

Kalisch BJ, Kalisch PA. The nurse–detective in American movies. Nurs Health Care 3(3):146–153, 1982

Kalisch BJ, Kalisch PA, Scobey M. Reflections on a television image. Nurs Health Care 5(5):248–255, 1981

Larisey MM. Attic treasures: A look at nursing history. Nurs Forum 25(1):20–24, 1990

Melosh B. Not merely a profession: Nurses and resistance to professionalization. Am Behav Scientist 32(6):668–679, 1989

Parsons M. The profession in a class by itself. Nurs Outlook 34(6):270–275, 1985

Roberts MM. American Nursing: History and Interpretation. New York: Macmillan, 1954

Sleeper R, et al. Issues in Health Care: The Edna A. Fagan Health Care Lecture Series. Publication No. 14-1599. New York: National League for Nursing, 1976

Woodham-Smith C. Florence Nightingale. New York: McGraw-Hill, 1951

6 Educational Preparation for Nursing

Strong educational preparation in the biological and psychosocial sciences, and in nursing arts and science, is the necessary base for advanced skill acquisition, because this knowledge provides the basis for safe care and gives the most advantageous position for gaining a sense of salience. (Benner, 1984)

Objectives

After completing this chapter, you should be able to:

1. Compare and contrast the educational preparation of the nursing assistant, the licensed practical (vocational) nurse, the graduate of a hospital-based program, the associate degree graduate and the baccalaureate degree graduate.

2. Identify the purposes of other forms of nursing education: external degree programs, registered nurse baccalaureate programs, master's preparation, doctoral studies, and nondegree programs.

3. Discuss the concept of articulated programs.

4. Identify factors that have prompted change in nursing education, including studies and sociopolitical events.

5. Discuss the development and effect of the ANA position paper on nursing education, and the arguments for and against it.

6. Explain what is meant by a "grandfather" clause, and the effect of such a clause on proposed changes in licensure.

7. Discuss the concept of differentiated practice and provide a rationale for its development.

8. Identify factors that have influenced changes in nursing education and explain the effect of each.

9. Analyze the ways in which nursing theories serve to advance the profession.

10. Define the continuing education unit, discuss its purpose, and identify the major points supporting mandatory continuing education and the major points supporting voluntary continuing education.

KEY TERMS

Accreditation

Advanced placement

Advanced practice

Articulation

Associate degree

Baccalaureate degree

Career ladder

Community-based

Competencies

Differentiated practice

Diploma

Doctorate

Educational mobility

Entry into practice

External degree

Grandfather clause

Home health aide

Hospital-based program

Internship

Interstate endorsement

Mandatory continuing education

Nursing assistant

Position paper

Postsecondary education

Practical (vocational) nurse

Registered nurse

Scope of practice

Theorist/theory

Titling

Voluntary continuing education

Unlike many other professions that provide a single route of educational preparation, the development of nursing as a profession has resulted in three major educational routes that prepare graduates to write the National Council Licensure Examination (NCLEX) for registered nursing. These circumstances have resulted in various alternatives and opportunities for prospective students. In 1995, the Pew Commission recommendations for nursing included recognizing the value of the multiple-entry points to professional practice (Pew Commission, 1995).

Multiple-entry points, however, have resulted in confusion. Health care consumers often find it difficult to understand the various types of nursing credentials—and probably have little interest in credentials as long as the care they receive is satisfactory. Employers have difficulty differentiating among the three major types of registered nurse graduates who, at least initially, enter the work environment performing similar behaviors. This confusion has led to another recommendation from the Pew Commission: that nursing distinguish between the practice responsibilities of each of these different levels of nursing (Pew Commission, 1995).

An educator is charged with the responsibility of graduating a "safe" practitioner, but may lack clear direction as to how the professional preparation provided by the various educational routes should differ in purpose, structure, and outcome. You will find that nursing leaders often vigorously debate aspects of nursing educational preparation such as where it should take place, which tests should measure the various competencies, and which credentials should be awarded.

The three educational avenues that prepare men and women for registered nursing are hospital-based diploma programs, 2-year associate degree programs (primarily found at junior and community colleges), and baccalaureate programs (offered at 4-year colleges and universities). It is also possible for students to begin their nursing education in programs that culminate in a master's degree, and several programs now exist in which a student can earn a doctorate before being eligible to write the state licensing examination for registered nursing. In the following section we will discuss the various educational routes to nursing.

At least two other groups of caregivers are identified with nursing: the nursing assistant, who is certified, and the practical (vocational) nurse, who is licensed through a separate examination that is different than that taken by the registered nurse. We will briefly discuss the education of each of these groups of caregivers.

THE NURSING ASSISTANT

For years care has been provided to patients in hospitals and long-term care facilities by individuals we have called nursing aides or assistants. In the past, these caregivers were hired without formal preparation for their responsibilities, and were provided ''on-the-job training.'' The use of the nursing aide likely started during World War I, and was certainly reinforced during World War II when approximately 150,000 trained volunteer nursing aides served in wartime hospitals.

In 1987, Congress passed the Omnibus Budget Reconciliation Act (OBRA), which regulates agencies receiving federal funds, and includes the regulation of education and certification of nursing assistants who work in nursing homes. This act stipulated that by October 1, 1990, all people working as nursing assistants in nursing homes (hospitals and assisted living units were not included) would be required to complete a competency evaluation program or approved course of study (Hegner & Caldwell, 1995; Sorrentino, 1994). Certification falls under state jurisdiction, but is guided by federal regulations. These regulations require that an individual complete a minimum of 75 hours of theory and practice, and pass both a theory and practice examination in order to be certified. In many states, the hours of preparation required exceed the 75 hours established by law. Following the federal legislation, the National Council of State Boards of Nursing Inc. developed the Nurse Aide Competency Evaluation Program (NACEP), which identifies the minimum skills a nursing assistant must attain and can be used to guide programs registering or certifying nursing assistants. The state agency responsible for certifying and maintaining the list of nursing assistants varies from state to state; most commonly it is the Board of Nursing or the State Department of Health Services.

The certified nursing assistant (CNA) functions under the direction of the registered nurse or the licensed practical (vocational) nurse. Each state determines the skills that may be performed by the nursing assistant. Typically, these include basic nursing skills, especially in the areas of communication, residents' rights, personal hygiene and grooming, assisting patients with nutritional and elimination needs, and mobility. The preparation of the certified nursing assistant emphasizes the importance of a safe environment and includes instruction in the use of side rails and restraints. Some states also require a designated number of hours per year of continuing education. The training occurs in a variety of settings, including high schools, long-term care facilities, hospitals, community colleges, regional occupational programs (ROPs), and privately operated programs. Some consider this preparation the first rung on the ladder of nursing education, and, in some states, the nursing assistant may be exempt from certain classes required in licensed practical (vocational) nursing programs.

PRACTICAL NURSE EDUCATION

The practical nurse is no newcomer to the health care delivery system. In the past, the practical nurse was the family friend or community citizen who was called to the home in emergencies. This person, usually self-taught, learned by experience which procedures were effective and which were not. She would perform basic care procedures such as bathing, and also would cook and perform light housekeeping duties for the family, much as the home health aide does today. Although controls on the licensing of practical nurses and the accreditation of their curricula have been slower to evolve than those regulating professional nursing, states gradually began enacting licensure laws governing practical nursing. By 1945, 19 states and one territory had licensure laws, but licensure of the practical nurse was mandatory in only one state (Kalisch & Kalisch, 1995). When more states began adopting mandatory licensure laws for practical nurses, a large number of individuals who had been functioning in this capacity were granted a license by waiver, and were excused from any formal training (see Chapter 7 on credentialing). Most, if not all, of these people have now retired from nursing practice.

It is not clear when formal preparation for practical nursing began. Some suggest training programs were started in 1897 (Kalisch and Kalisch, 1995). A more popular belief is that the first programs were initiated through the YWCA in Brooklyn, New York, around 1892. The school established through the YWCA was known as the Ballard School, after Lucinda Ballard, who provided the funding to operate the school. The course of study lasted approximately 3 months, and the students, called ''attendants,'' were trained to care for invalids, the elderly, and children in a home setting.

A YWCA may seem to many of us to be a strange place for a practical nursing program. In fact, however, YWCAs were an important source of inexpensive housing for many young women who, in the late 1890s and early 1900s, traveled from their homes to large cities in search of new careers and better lives. Because most of these women were untrained and had no marketable skills, the YWCA was a natural site for a school.

Other early practical nursing programs were offered by the Thompson School, founded in Brattleboro, Vermont, in 1907; the American Red Cross, beginning in 1908; and the Household Nursing Association School of Attendant Nursing, begun in Boston in 1918.

Although only 11 schools were in existence by 1930, the number of programs expanded rapidly during the 1940s. During World War I, and especially during World War II, the need became crucial for people who had some basic nursing skills—and, more importantly, who could be prepared quickly. As this need intensified, the practical nurse, who until this time had practiced primarily in the home, moved out into the world.

In 1941, the Association of Practical Nurse Schools was founded; in 1942 membership was opened to practical nurses and the name was changed to the National Association of Practical Nurse Education and Service (NAPNES). The first planned curriculum for practical nursing was developed in 1942, and in 1945, NAPNES established an accrediting service for schools of practical nursing. The National Federation of Licensed Practical Nurses (NFLPN) was organized in 1949. In 1957, this group, working with the American Nurses Association (ANA), attempted to clarify the role and function of the practical nurse, just as various groups throughout the nation have worked at delineating the roles of other nursing program graduates. The Council on Practical Nursing was established by the National

League for Nursing (NLN) in 1957. In 1966, the Chicago Public School Program became the first practical nurse program to be accredited by the NLN.

The general curriculum for practical nurses, which takes between 9 months and one year to complete, varies considerably from state to state and even from school to school. In many instances the education is measured in clock hours instead of credit hours, as in the professional registered nursing programs. Most of today's practical nursing educational programs stress clinical experience, primarily in structured care settings such as hospitals and nursing homes. Basic therapeutic knowledge and introductory content from biologic and behavioral sciences correlate with clinical practice; usually one third of the time is spent in the classroom and two thirds in clinical practice.

The educational preparation of the practical nurse takes place in a great variety of settings. Programs may be offered by high schools, trade or technical schools, hospitals, junior or community colleges, universities, or independent agencies. There has been a movement to incorporate practical nursing and associate nursing degree programs in the community college, as part of a *career ladder* approach to nursing education. All nursing students in these colleges are grouped together for *core* courses during the first academic year. At the end of this time, a student has the option of stopping the educational program to seek licensure as a practical nurse, or continuing for an additional year to become a registered nurse. Many students opt to do both. Graduates of these core programs in practical nursing usually have a broader and more in-depth understanding of the biologic sciences, and sometimes the social sciences (often also a part of the core curriculum), especially if these are taught in college-level courses that are transferable to a 4-year institution. Because issues related to *educational mobility* and *articulation* between programs have been receiving much attention (to be discussed later in this chapter), these combined programs have become popular.

Graduates of practical nursing programs take the NCLEX-PN; if they pass the exam, they use the title of licensed practical nurse (LPN) or, in California and Texas, the title of licensed vocational nurse (LVN). The scope of their practice focuses on meeting the health care needs of clients in hospitals, long-term care facilities, clinics, and the home. LPNs or LVNs work with clients whose conditions are considered stable. Their work is supervised by a registered nurse or a licensed physician.

As with the associate degree and hospital-based diploma programs for registered nurses, the educational preparation for practical nurses—and the future of practical nursing—have been topics of much discussion. There are those who advocate two levels of nurses: the practical nurse prepared with an associate degree, and the registered nurse prepared with a baccalaureate degree. Others would eliminate practical nursing altogether. In 1987, North Dakota became the first state (and to date the only state) to require all candidates taking the licensure examination for practical nursing to have completed an associate degree in practical nursing (see discussion later in this chapter). With the ''graying'' of America, and the growing need for nurses in home health care and in long-term care facilities, practical nurses will continue to play a significant role in health care delivery.

DIPLOMA EDUCATION

The earliest type of nursing education in the United States took place in diploma programs administered by hospitals. The first hospital with a nurse training school was the New England Hospital for Women, which accepted five probationers on September 1, 1872 (Kalisch and Kalisch, 1995). The history of these hospital-based programs is discussed in detail in Chapter 4.

By the late 1940s and early 1950s, many hospital-based nursing schools had affiliated with nearby colleges and universities; these schools adopted general education requirements such as anatomy, physiology, sociology, and psychology as part of the curriculum. During this time the National League of Nursing Education (later to become the NLN) was assuming an active role in curriculum guidance and accreditation. Nursing programs gained a stronger educational foundation because they were required to align themselves more closely with other types of *postsecondary education.*

Thus, diploma schools in operation today have sound educational programs that meet the criteria necessary for accreditation. They employ qualified faculty who have developed clinical learning experiences that meet the student's learning needs rather than the hospital's service needs (which so often took priority in the past). The length of these programs varies from twenty-seven to thirty-six months. Many diploma schools are affiliated with a college or university so that postsecondary credit can be formally awarded. Graduates have been provided with a foundation in the biologic and social sciences, and may have taken some courses in the humanities. There is a strong emphasis in diploma programs on client experiences. The course of study also includes experience in nursing management (for example, being in charge of a nursing unit). Graduates work in acute, long-term, and ambulatory health care facilities.

During the mid-1960s, there was a significant decline in enrollment in diploma schools. As more nursing education programs were moved to institutions of higher education, many hospital-based schools elected to discontinue their programs. Some merged with a local community college or university that assumed administrative responsibility for managing the nursing program, and awarded an associate or baccalaureate degree when graduation requirements were satisfied. The elimination of hospital-based programs has occurred most extensively in the western part of the United States, where only one such program remains in existence.

Finances have also played a role in this change. With increasing constraints on funding, many hospitals have found that the costs associated with supporting a nursing program are too great. Many diploma programs that exist today have strong endowments and private funding support.

ASSOCIATE DEGREE EDUCATION

The movement toward associate degree education began in 1952. Associate degree nursing (ADN) programs have the distinction of being the first (and, to date, the only) type of nursing education established on the basis of planned research and experimentation. Three events undoubtedly influenced their beginning. First, these programs followed in the wake of the proliferation of community colleges in the United States—particularly the organization and growth of 2-year community colleges that not only offered the first 2 years of a traditional 4-year college program, but also brought to the community many vocational and adult education programs. The goal of the community college was to make some form of college education available to everyone. Second, the cadet nurse program, which was created during World War II, demonstrated that qualified students could be adequately educated in less than the traditional 3 years. Finally, the development of associate degree education was influenced by the studies conducted on nursing education in the United States, as discussed in Chapter 5.

Associate degree programs helped to solve the nursing shortage of the 1960s and the 1980s. These programs, which focused on preparing graduates skilled in bedside nursing, rapidly increased in number. Associate degree programs particularly appealed to men, minorities, and older students, who had not traditionally pursued educational preparation in nursing. Because most programs were located in community colleges, they tended to be more geographically accessible than the baccalaureate programs located in 4-year colleges and universities.

Characteristics of Associate Degree Education

Associate degree education began with the Cooperative Research Project in Junior and Community College Education for Nursing at Teachers College, Columbia University. The original project, which was directed by Mildred Montag, included seven junior and community colleges and one hospital school, located in six regions of the United States. This type of nursing education has expanded from only three schools in 1952 to almost 850 in 1997.

The four basic characteristics of associate degree education include (NLN, 1973):

1. Encompassing the nursing program as an integral part of the college that controls and finances the program
2. Ensuring the members of the nursing faculty the same privileges and responsibilities granted to other faculty
3. Organizing a curriculum with a clearly stated philosophy, rationale, and conceptual framework, designed to be completed in 2 years
4. Ensuring that nursing students are treated the same as other community college students with regard to admission, progression, and graduation requirements

The programs are designed to award an associate degree on completion, and graduates are eligible to write the state licensing examination for registered nursing.

Approximately half of the credits needed for the associate degree must be fulfilled by general education courses such as English, anatomy, physiology, speech, psychology, and sociology; the other half must be fulfilled by nursing courses. Clinical learning experiences are carefully selected to correspond with the content delivered in classroom lectures; the pre- and postconferences help to reinforce the relationship between the two.

Competencies of the Associate Degree Graduate

In 1990, the Council of Associate Degree Programs of the NLN revised and retitled a document published in 1978 that described the abilities of the associate degree graduate. Retitled "Educational Outcomes of Associate Degree Nursing Programs: Roles and Competencies," this document condensed what was previously five roles into three. These are: Role as Provider of Care, Role as Manager of Care, and Role as Member Within the Discipline of Nursing. The competencies, which focus on these three roles, describe the behaviors the associate degree graduate demonstrates on graduation, and the competencies the graduate is expected to demonstrate 6 months following graduation. These last competencies are identified as "anticipated competencies" (NLN, 1990).

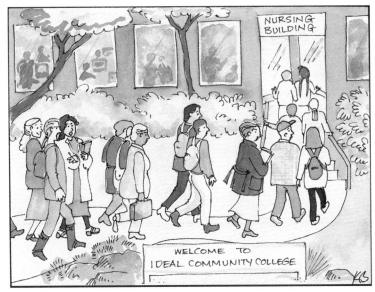

FIGURE 6-1
Associate degree programs attract older people, married women, minorities, men, and students with a wider range of educational experiences and intellectual capabilities.

The advent of associate degree education in nursing has brought with it greater diversity in the students who enroll in nursing programs (Fig. 6-1). Nursing students were traditionally a homogeneous group— typically consisting of single white women, ranging in age from 18 to 35, who graduated in the upper third of their high school classes. Associate degree programs (although they sometimes impose selective admission policies on the "open door" philosophy of the community colleges) attract older people, married women, minorities, men, and students with a wider range of educational experiences and intellectual abilities. People who already possess baccalaureate or higher degrees in other fields sometimes seek admission to an associate degree program, often because it can be completed in a shorter period of time than would be needed to earn another baccalaureate degree.

Concerns Facing Associate Degree Education

Associate degree education, like other educational programs, has experienced change. With these changes have come some concerns.

THE ISSUE OF CREDIT-CREEP

As programs have developed, there has been a growing tendency to place more emphasis and time on nursing courses than on general education courses. Faculty, prepared with master's degrees in nursing, have difficulty defining *essential content.* They often try to comply with requests from advisory committees for graduates who will need shorter orientation programs, and who will possess greater knowledge in certain specialty areas (eg, coronary care). The 1990 changes in the role of the graduate have necessitated the inclusion of management principles and skills in the curriculum. Changes that some colleges have made in the basic requirements for the associate degree have increased the number of credits nursing students must complete; the concept of "core courses" that are taken by all students who graduate from a college has become popular. More content and a greater number of credit hours, coupled with selective admission criteria (that give preference to students who have completed general education course work), have resulted in programs that can take as many as 3 to 5 years to complete.

The recent shift to community-based practice also offers a challenge to associate degree educators. What part of the current curriculum should be cut to provide community experiences? How are those experiences to be supervised? What should be the balance between acute care and community experiences?

According to the criteria for accreditation of these programs, established by the accredited schools that are members of the Council of Associate Degree Programs of the NLN, 108 quarter hours or 72 semester credits is the maximum number of credits for any program (NLN, 1991). Many schools have difficulty meeting this criterion.

THE SELECTIVE ADMISSION PROCESS

Another concern facing educators is the growing number of students seeking admission to associate degree programs. When enrollments in nursing programs dropped throughout the nation in 1986, associate degree programs were the least affected. Today, although another drop in applicants to nursing programs is predicted, most associate degree programs continue to have many more applicants than openings in beginning nursing classes. In response to this problem, faculty have developed selective admission processes. Some schools use a "waiting list," which honors the concept of "first come—first served." Other schools use systems similar to a lottery. Also popular are "factoring" or "point" systems that award points for courses completed, past work experience, cumulative grade point average, or a combination of all of these. These factoring systems often require that a student spend at least a year in college before starting nursing courses to secure a position in the beginning nursing class.

MISUNDERSTANDINGS ABOUT ASSOCIATE DEGREE EDUCATION

For many years, associate degree education was poorly understood by employers, the public, and to some extent, nursing educators in general. Although this route to nursing education is now firmly established as credible preparation for a nursing career, it has continued to receive some unfavorable publicity—with rumors surfacing periodically that the programs will be discontinued. Although it has lost much of its original passion and dissension because of the nurse shortage of the later 1980s and early 1990s, the controversy regarding "entry into practice" and the preparation needed for "professional" nursing, (which will be discussed later in this chapter) is renewed intermittently. Thus, advocates for associate degree education continue to find themselves clarifying facts and emphasizing the contributions made by graduates of the programs.

BACCALAUREATE EDUCATION

The first school of nursing to be established in a university setting was started at the University of Minnesota in 1909. The program existed as a quasi-autonomous branch of the university's school of medicine. The program was not very different from the 3-year hospital-based program; nothing was required in the way of higher general education, and graduates were prepared for the registered nurse certificate only. Education took place predominantly through apprenticeship, and students provided service to hospitals in exchange for education. However, nursing education did become a part of an academic organization, and by 1916 nursing programs had been developed at 16 colleges and universities.

Most of the early programs offering a baccalaureate degree in nursing extended over a 5-year period. This allowed for the 3 years of nursing school curriculum similar to that of the hospital-based programs, and for an additional 2 years of liberal arts. In 1924, the Yale School of Nursing became the first to be established as a separate department within a university; Annie W. Goodrich was its dean. However, the proliferation of these schools was not rapid.

Although the development of baccalaureate education for nurses may not seem like a major step to young people today, you need to remember that it was not until 1920 that the 19th Amendment to the Constitution of the United States granted women the right to vote. Many people considered nursing to be a less than desirable occupation: vocational in its orientation; overshadowed by militaristic, religious, and technical characteristics; and confined to women. Liberal education, scholarship, and knowledge were thought to be incompatible with the female personality, and capable of interfering with marriage. The nursing curriculum, with its emphasis on the performance of skills rather than on the philosophical and theoretical approaches used in the humanities, was not well accepted by universities. Opposition to collegiate education for nurses also came from physicians, who argued that nurses would be "overtrained." Physicians were not certain that a sound knowledge base was as important as the acquisition of technical skills and manual dexterity that could be acquired with brief training at the bedside. Physicians also argued that a baccalaureate education would make nursing services too expensive.

Many nursing leaders have advocated for baccalaureate education as the minimum educational preparation for supervisory and administrative nursing roles. Baccalaureate education also provides the background needed for public health positions, including school nursing, and the educational base for entry into graduate education in nursing. In 1965, the ANA recommended baccalaureate preparation in nursing as the minimum educational preparation for entry into professional nursing practice, an issue that will be discussed later in this chapter. The American Nurses' Credentialing Center, which offers certification in 24 specialty areas, now requires a baccalaureate degree for initial basic certification in a nursing specialty, and requires a master's degree for initial certification as a clinical specialist or nurse practitioner. Those certified before these new requirements took effect are permitted to maintain their certification. Some of the other nursing specialty organizations that provide certification do not require a baccalaureate degree for certification.

Characteristics of Baccalaureate Education

Baccalaureate nursing programs are located in 4-year colleges and universities. When the program of studies includes an upper division (junior and senior years) baccalaureate nursing major that is built onto 2 years of liberal arts and science courses taken during the freshman and sophomore years, it is known as a *basic* or *generic* baccalaureate program.

Applicants to such programs must meet the entrance and graduation requirements established by the university, and those of the nursing school. The admission requirements usually specify academic preparation at the high school (or preadmission) level, including courses in foreign language and higher-level mathematics and science, and a high cumulative grade point average. Relatively high scores on college admission tests may also be required.

During the freshman and sophomore years of study, students who pursue a nursing education take liberal arts, biology, and physical science courses with college students who are preparing for other majors. In some schools, these courses may be completed on a part-time basis; however, this extends the overall course of study beyond 4 years. The number of required liberal arts and science courses may vary from program to program, but usually constitutes about one half the total number of credits specified for graduation—typically 120 semester credits or 180 quarter credits. Students usually begin their study of nursing content in their junior year, thus the term ''upper-division major'' in nursing. Nursing theory can be taught so that it builds on an understanding of the physical and biologic sciences and liberal arts studied the previous 2 years.

Recently, some schools offering baccalaureate nursing education have begun to introduce nursing content at some point in the sophomore year of study. Nursing courses offered at this point often include an overview of the nursing profession and some of the fundamental nursing skills.

Students in baccalaureate nursing programs learn basic nursing skills. They also learn concepts of health maintenance and promotion, and disease prevention; supervisory and leadership techniques and practices are also taught, along with an introduction to research. Clinical course work includes experience in public health nursing, community health settings, and as nursing team leaders within the acute care hospital. Emphasis is placed on developing skills in critical decision-making, on exercising independent nursing judgments that call for broad background knowledge, and on working in complex nursing situations in which the outcomes are often not predictable. Acting as a client advocate, the graduate of a baccalaureate nursing program collaborates with other members of the health care team in structured and unstructured settings, and supervises those with lesser preparation. Baccalaureate graduates often work with groups as well as with individuals.

Changes in Baccalaureate Education

In recent years, the nature of baccalaureate education has changed. Some schools, seeking to add an advanced component, have included courses that permit a degree of specialization at the baccalaureate level (eg, supplemental courses in coronary or critical care nursing).

Other schools are providing more grounding in research, either as preparation for graduate school or for a more varied role in nursing. There is another interesting variation in baccalaureate education in California. In that state, the rules and regulations for schools of nursing stipulate that all courses required by the Board of Nursing for licensure as a registered nurse be offered within the first 36 months of full-time training, the first six academic semesters, or the first nine academic quarters, whichever is shortest (California Board of Registered Nursing, 1994). This means that all educational preparation required for application for licensure in California must be completed by the end of the junior year. This leaves the senior year open for specialty experience, preceptorships, or whatever a school might deem appropriate education. This variation in the licensure law has caused problems. Some students complete their junior year and successfully pass the licensing examination; these students may elect to drop out of school and work as registered nurses. Although they are licensed in the state of California in a category of nongraduates, these students have no educational credentials. This creates problems if they seek licensure in another state, because all other states (at the present time) require a degree or diploma for licensure. Table 6-1 provides a comparison of the major avenues to registered nurse licensure.

MASTER'S AND DOCTORAL PROGRAMS THAT PREPARE FOR LICENSURE

Our discussion of the various educational programs for registered nursing would be incomplete without mention of the generic master's program. The concept of the master's degree in nursing developed at Yale and several other schools of nursing, where students admitted with a baccalaureate degree in another area were granted a master's degree in nursing after completing an established 2-year program of study that prepared them for registered nurse licensure. Case Western Reserve University initiated the first program in which the student earns a doctorate in nursing (ND) before being eligible to write the licensing examination. Most of the graduates of these programs are engaged in teaching and research.

These types of programs reflect the thinking of some nursing leaders that the minimum preparation for professional nursing should be the master's degree. These programs also provide a higher degree to those people who possess basic baccalaureate preparation in another area of study and are making a career change. With increasing emphasis being placed on the need for a baccalaureate degree for professional practice, this type of program is certainly a credible option . When programs of this type are not available, many students with degrees in other disciplines choose to pursue a 2-year associate degree in nursing. Even when other options are available, some people with degrees in other disciplines opt for the 2-year degree because it requires less time and expense.

SIMILARITIES AMONG ENTRY-LEVEL PROGRAMS

Currently there are as many similarities in the various avenues to nursing education as there are differences. These similarities may be grouped into several broad classifications that include academic standards, administrative concerns, and areas relating to students.

Academic Similarities

In the academic realm, several similarities stand out:

1. All graduates write the NCLEX for registered nursing in their state. All writers must meet the same minimum cutoff score to pass the test and become licensed.
2. All schools preparing graduates for licensure must meet the criteria established for state board approval and (in many instances on a voluntary basis) the criteria developed for national accreditation.
3. All faculty are pushed to develop curricula responsive to the needs of today's health care delivery system, which demands greater efficiency, an ability to work in a highly technical environment, knowledge of new protocols, community experiences, and greater responsibility and accountability.
4. The recruitment of faculty possessing master's and doctoral degrees is an ongoing effort. Salaries in education have lagged behind those in practice. The graduate with a master's degree can find many challenging positions in hospitals, clinics, and even in private practice that pay more than teaching positions.
5. Members of the faculty are pushed to meet the increasing demands of education, clinical excellence, tenure, and possibly vocational certification or research. The workload and the time invested in performance of professional responsibilities often are greater than for instructors in other disciplines, even though they are considered colleagues in the educational setting.

Administrative Similarities

From an administrative perspective, two similarities are noted among entry-level programs:

1. Adequate financial support is a major concern. All nursing programs are relatively expensive to operate in comparison with other forms of education provided in colleges and universities. Federal and state agencies, as well as colleges and universities, are limiting funding and are demanding greater accountability. In tough economic times, the nursing program—like the one at the University of California, Los Angeles (UCLA)—may be the one chosen to be phased out. Less financial assistance is available to students in the form of scholarships and loans than in the past. Tuition costs are rising.
2. Finding appropriate learning experiences is a challenge. Most programs find themselves searching and competing with other schools for learning experiences in clinical agencies. To some extent, this competition is caused by changes in societal values and in the health care delivery system. Families are electing to have fewer children and, more recently in some areas, to deliver these children at home. The result has been fewer clients in the obstetric units of hospitals. Pediatric clients are managed on an outpatient basis as much as possible, and hospitalization, when required, is kept to a minimum. The management of the client with psychiatric disturbances is moving from institutions to community mental health centers whenever feasible. The increase in the number and size of schools in urban areas creates a high demand for clinical facilities in those areas. Finally, there have been changes in the attitudes of the consumer and the agency toward having students

provide care. The concept of the "teaching" hospital is not as viable as it once was. Consumers paying for the high cost of care want that care provided by qualified nurses rather than by students who are still learning.

Similarities Relating to Students

Three similarities relating to students are noted:

1. Selection of students is a major task. All schools must develop sound educational programs while balancing student enrollments against faculty recruitment and retention factors. In many instances, the number of applications exceed the positions available in beginning classes. At the same time, schools must be responsive to a culturally diverse population. This has resulted in the development of selective admission policies that must be carefully scrutinized by school officials, and then reviewed by the school's attorney for correct legal form and legal ramifications, before being accepted by the school's policy-making group.

2. Legal concerns are demanding more time and attention. Programs are caught up in more legal concerns than in the past, because applicants and students are seeking their "rights as individuals" and challenging admission and dismissal policies. The National Student Nursing Association Student Bill of Rights and Responsibilities is widely accepted by schools of nursing throughout the country. This bill sets forth the students' basic rights and establishes grievance procedures if a student believes that these rights have been violated (see Chapter 3, Fig. 3-6). Another legal concern relates to malpractice coverage for students. Some collegiate programs, now removed from the umbrella coverage of the hospital, ask that students purchase malpractice insurance as protection against any lawsuits that might arise as the result of errors committed in the learning process.

3. There is greater diversity in the student body. All programs are finding more diversity in the characteristics of applicants seeking admission. Programs are receiving more applications from men, minorities, older adults, and persons who possess degrees in other fields of study. Students with English as a second language are presenting new challenges to nursing faculty in all types of programs.

One usually finds nursing educators united in their efforts to create quality programs that will graduate students who can function satisfactorily in a changing and challenging health care delivery system (see Table 6-1).

OTHER FORMS OF NURSING EDUCATION

Educational offerings in nursing have expanded tremendously since the 1960s. This is partly a result of the changing role of the nurse in health care delivery, and the need for more adequate education to meet the preparation requirements of that role. Another contributing factor is the continuing push to make nursing truly professional. The result is the need for practitioners with master's and doctoral degrees who are interested and competent in research techniques and skills. A third significant reason for advancing nursing education relates to the need for leadership in nursing administration and education. Nurse educators,

TABLE 6–1. Educational Opportunities for Registered Nursing: A Comparison

	Diploma	Associate Degree	Baccalaureate
Location	Is usually conducted by and based in a hospital	Most often conducted in junior or community colleges, occasionally in senior colleges and universities	Located in senior colleges and universities
Length of Study	Requires generally 24–30 months but may require 3 academic years	Requires usually 2 academic or sometimes 2 calendar years	Requires 4 academic years
Requirements for Admission	Requires graduation from high school or its equivalent, satisfactory general academic achievement, and successful completion of certain prerequisite courses.	Requires that applicants meet entrance requirements of college as well as of program	Requires that applicants meet entrance requirements of the college or university as well as those of program
Program of Learning	Includes courses in theory and practice of nursing and in biologic, physical, and behavioral sciences	Combines a balance of nursing courses and college courses in the basic natural and social sciences with courses in general education and the humanities	Frequently concentrates on courses in the theory and practice of nursing in the junior and senior years
	May require that certain courses in the physical and social sciences be taken at a local college or university		Provides education in the theory and practice of nursing and courses in the liberal arts as well as the behavioral and physical sciences
Clinical Component	Provides early and substantial clinical learning experiences in the hospital and a variety of community agencies; these focus on an understanding of the hospital environment and the interrelationship of other health disciplines	Requires as a significant part of the program supervised clinical instruction in hospitals and other community health agencies	Provides clinical laboratory courses in a variety of settings where health and nursing care are given
Opportunity for Educational Advancement	Little or no transferability of courses unless affiliated with a community college or university	Is structured so that some credits may be applied to baccalaureate degree	Provides the basic academic preparation for advancement to higher positions in nursing and to master's degree

(continued)

	Diploma	Associate Degree	Baccalaureate
Competency on Graduation	Graduate is prepared to plan for the care of patients with other members of the health care team, to develop and carry out plans for the care of individuals or groups of patients, and to direct selected members of the nursing team. Has an understanding of the hospital climate and the community health resources necessary for the extended care of patients	Graduate is prepared to plan and give direct patient care in hospitals, nursing homes, or similar health care agencies and to participate with other members of the health care team, such as licensed practical nurses, nurses aides, physicians, and other registered nurses in rendering care to patients	Graduate is prepared to plan and give direct care to individuals and families, whether sick or well, to assume responsibility for directing other members of the health care team, and to take on beginning leadership positions. Practices in a variety of settings and emphasizes comprehensive health care, including preventive and rehabilitative services, health counseling and education, and care in acute and long-term illnesses
			Has necessary education for graduate study toward a master's degree and may move rapidly to specialized leadership positions in nursing as teacher, administrator, clinical specialist, nurse practitioner, and nurse researcher
Licensure	Must successfully complete state licensing examination	Must successfully complete state licensing examination	Must successfully complete state licensing examination

TABLE 6-1. Educational Opportunities for Registered Nursing: A Comparison (continued)

joining the ranks of other professionals in the academic environment, are required to possess equivalent educational backgrounds. Nurses who assume roles in nursing administration have found the need for a solid understanding of management and finance, which are acquired through study at the master's and doctoral levels.

Registered Nurse Baccalaureate Programs

Recently there has been an increase in the number of registered nurse baccalaureate (RNB) programs. These programs are designed for the registered nurse, with either a diploma or an associate degree, who wishes to return to school to complete a baccalaureate degree in nursing. There are also master's degree programs that admit registered nurses with associate degrees who will graduate in 3 years with a master's degree in nursing, receiving a baccalaureate degree part way through the program. Some schools have also added programs designed to admit the licensed practical (vocational) nurse, who will emerge with a baccalaureate degree in nursing. These programs carry different names in different parts of the country, including baccalaureate registered nurse (BRN) programs, two-on-two programs, and, in the Midwest, capstone programs.

There are many reasons for the increase in this form of nursing education, several of which were discussed above. In addition, many highly qualified young men and women are entering associate degree programs because of cost and time factors, and are then planning more education several years after completing the original program. The nursing profession is aiming to increase the number of nurses prepared with baccalaureate and higher degrees.

The RNB programs vary greatly throughout the United States. In some instances they exist in universities that already offer the generic baccalaureate program. The students may be completely integrated with generic baccalaureate students, partially separated from them, or in a totally separate program. Another form of RNB preparation is the two-on-two approach, in which registered nurse students transfer into the college or university with junior standing and complete an additional 2 years of upper-division nursing classes. In some instances, this is the only nursing program offered by a college or university; that is, the college may not offer a basic program that prepares a graduate for licensure. Some schools offer nurse practitioner preparation in conjunction with the baccalaureate degree, although the current trend is to place this at the master's level.

Another general trend is to allow the transfer of credits in the natural and biologic sciences, and in basic courses such as psychology and sociology earned at junior and community colleges. Often some transfer of credit is allowed for nursing courses (eg, 45 quarter credits or 30 semester credits), but the courses may be challenged by examination. Distribution requirements of the particular college or university must be satisfied, and upper-division nursing courses must be completed in such areas as physiologic nursing, community health, and supervision. A minimum of 2 years usually is required for completion of the program, although the time may be shorter or longer, depending on the number of requirements satisfied at the time of entry.

When the programs offering baccalaureate education to registered nurses were first launched, they were criticized by some nurse educators. The criticism seemed to have three central themes. First, the ladder concept in nursing education was slow to develop. Many nurse educators perceived associate degree education as terminal (ending at the associate degree level), and did not accept it as a stepping stone to baccalaureate education.

The second concern related to the problems associated with evaluating and granting credit for previous education. How should one compare nursing process taught at the freshman level in a community college with nursing process taught at the junior level in a 4-year college or university?

A third problem was determining whether additional courses specifically for the registered nurse should be offered. Educators seriously questioned whether the standards, program objectives, and educational structures that had been developed for the generic student were appropriate for the registered nurse. What learning experiences could be included that would help to "socialize" the student for the role of a baccalaureate graduate? What additional nursing courses were needed to form the upper-division major in nursing that would provide a foundation for graduate education?

Because the skills of the various graduates were not clearly delineated, it was difficult to develop a curriculum that would enable the RNB graduate to demonstrate specific terminal behaviors. When attempts were made to develop such programs, baccalaureate educators found themselves confronted with another concern: they were working with adult students. This required them to rethink teaching and learning principles to provide effective education. Students were seeking a learning program that allowed for part-time study, provided more evening and weekend classes, and permitted part- or full-time employment—in other words, a program tailored to their life circumstances.

Recently, RNB education and two-on-two educational programs have gained more acceptance. Schools operating both basic and RNB programs may report graduating more RNB students than basic graduates. At least three factors are responsible for the change in attitude toward RNB education. First, the ANA Commission on Nursing Education has provided a push to increase the availability of baccalaureate programs for registered nurses. Nursing educators are challenged to create and accept more innovative educational strategies.

The second factor comes from pressure within each state itself. A number of states have enacted legislation, sometimes in response to the nursing shortage, that requires the development of a statewide plan for articulation between various types of nursing education programs. In most instances the legislation establishes a date by which the plan will be implemented.

The third factor influencing the development of RNB programs has been a call for increased educational mobility from organizations in the health care arena. The American Medical Association (AMA) House of Delegates has suggested career mobility as one way to alleviate the nurse shortage. Recently the Pew Commission recommended strengthening existing career ladder programs in order to make movement through these levels of nursing as easy as possible (de Tornyay, 1996). Some of the RNB programs currently in operation provide for part-time study or for studies completed through evening courses. The desirability of such an approach for nurses who must work to support their education is obvious. Other innovative RNB programs provide baccalaureate education to people living in areas geographically remote from colleges or universities. These programs have used new technologies for distance learning, including the electronic transmission of information.

The External Degree

The concept of an external degree is not new. Universities in Australia, the Soviet Union, and England have long recognized independent study validated by examination. The University of London has awarded college degrees earned in this fashion since 1836. The major difference between the external degree and the traditional educational experience is that students awarded an external degree are not required to attend classes or follow any prescribed methods of learning (however, they may choose to take some classes). Learning is assessed through highly standardized and validated examinations. This approach to education was not developed in the United States until about the mid-1950s, and then only in selected areas. New York's Empire State College and the University Without Walls consortium were the first schools in the United States to recognize the value of self-directed learning.

The New York Regents External Degree (REX) Program of the University of the State of New York has become part of this movement. The New York Board of Regents established the College Proficiency Examination Program in 1961. Similar to the College-Level Examination Program tests developed by the Educational Testing Service, the examinations allow students to gain credit and meet the regents' external degree requirements without attending classes.

In 1971, the New York Board of Regents authorized an external associate degree program in nursing; the external baccalaureate degree in nursing was to follow in April 1976, with the first baccalaureate degrees awarded in 1979. The W. K. Kellogg Foundation provided funds to support the initiation of the program. The programs have grown in popularity, and both the associate degree program and the baccalaureate program are accredited by the NLN.

The nursing program, like other external degree programs in arts, science, and business, uses an assessment approach and is primarily—although not exclusively—designed for those with some experience in nursing. It is philosophically based on principles of adult learning, which advocate flexible and learner-oriented education. Specifically, the responsibility for demonstrating that learning has occurred is placed on the student, and the responsibility for identifying the content to be learned, and objectively assessing that this has occurred rests with the faculty. The nursing major is divided into cognitive and performance components. The cognitive learning is documented through nationally standardized and psychometrically valid written examinations. Clinical skills are evaluated through four criteria-referenced performance examinations at regional performance assessment centers throughout the country.

Despite objections, alternative and nontraditional avenues to nursing education appeal to the learner, and these programs continue to evolve. Nursing education, like nursing care, should be tailored to fit the consumer's needs.

NURSING EDUCATION AT THE GRADUATE LEVEL

The critical need for nurses with additional preparation to work in educational settings, in supervisory roles, and as clinical specialists, and to fulfill the expanded role of the nurse, has resulted in more programs at the graduate level.

Master's Preparation

There are a variety of models of master's preparation in nursing. Some less traditional approaches include outreach programs; summers-only programs; RN-to-MSN tracks (that provide a direct route to the master's degree for registered nurses who have graduated from diploma or associate degree programs); programs for students with special needs (such as registered nurses with non-nursing baccalaureate degrees, or those seeking preparation as technical nurse educators); and programs that admit non-nurses and foreign graduates. Some schools offer off-campus classes, sometimes rotating sites, and some use telecommunication systems to deliver core content by way of television. In at least one school, all classes are on Fridays. Several unique programs (eg, those at Yale University, Pace University, and the University of Tennessee at Knoxville) offer a master's degree in nursing after completion of a baccalaureate degree in another field. Such programs, called generic master's degree programs, were discussed earlier in the chapter.

Most programs require at least a full year for completion; many have been expanded to 2 years. Master's programs in nursing are typically found in senior colleges and universities that have baccalaureate programs in nursing. They have the option of seeking voluntary accreditation from the NLN.

Doctoral Studies

The number of requests for admission to doctoral study in nursing has greatly increased since the early 1980s. The impetus for this movement stems from the need for advanced study for academic advancement or tenure in the educational setting, and reflects the need in nursing research for the advancement of the profession as a whole.

Before doctorates in nursing were offered, doctoral study in other fields allowed nurses to benefit from post-master's preparation. A doctorate outside the area of nursing was often the only doctorate available to the person seeking further education; doctorates in nursing are relatively new to the educational milieu, as opposed to such degrees in psychology, sociology, anthropology, or physiology. Certainly nursing can and has benefited from other disciplines.

Doctoral programs in nursing offer various degrees such as the doctor of nursing science (DNSc), the doctor of science in nursing (DSN), the doctor of nursing education (DNEd), and the doctor of philosophy (PhD) in nursing. Other types of doctorates are also available to nurses, such as the doctor of education (EdD) and the doctor of public health (DPH).

The difference in the preparation and function of graduates possessing these various degrees is confusing; typically, the nurse with a doctorate assumes a leadership role in education, often serving as a faculty member or the dean or director of a nursing program. These nurses may also choose to be involved in the research and development of a body of nursing knowledge.

Although it plays no role in the accreditation of doctoral programs, the NLN has published a pamphlet entitled "Doctoral Programs in Nursing" that provides information about various programs of doctoral study in nursing.

ARTICULATED PROGRAMS

Today an increasing number of graduates are seeking additional education beyond the associate degree or diploma, and the "ladder" concept in nursing education is growing in popularity. There are more registered nurse baccalaureate and "two-on-two" programs as these graduates demand easier matriculation into 4-year institutions of learning. Programs have been developed that provide direct articulation between lower-level and higher-level programs. In some states legislation has been passed strongly encouraging, and in some instances mandating, articulation plans.

The purpose of an articulated program is to facilitate opportunities for students to start nursing education, stop when some goal is achieved, or keep moving up the educational ladder. A number of states (California, Colorado, Florida, Maryland, Minnesota, Missouri, New Mexico, North Dakota, Texas, Utah, and others) have established state-wide articulation plans that provide the opportunity for registered nurses to transfer to BSN programs. Many allow the majority of work completed at the lower level to meet the requirements of the baccalaureate degree. The University of Washington, and some other schools, have formalized R.N. to master's pathways.

Similar plans exist for articulation between practical (vocational) nurse programs and associate degree programs. Again, the articulated program allows students to move up the career ladder from practical nurse to associate degree nurse, to the nurse with a baccalaureate degree. Students in an articulated licensed practical nurse/associate degree program spend a year preparing to be an LP(V)N, and another year completing the associate degree. If they want to continue after this 2-year period, they can earn a baccalaureate degree at another institution after 2 more years of study. From that point, a student may continue to work toward a master's degree (Fig. 6-2).

Such programs usually involve planning between two or more institutions, but, depending on start and stop points, they may exist within a single institution. Of concern to nurse educators today is whether nursing assistants should be included in this ladder approach and, if so, how they can be accommodated. Some state boards of nursing have already stipulated that a mechanism be established to recognize the previous knowledge acquired by the nursing assistant.

These multiple-entry, multiple-exit programs are not without problems. Initially they

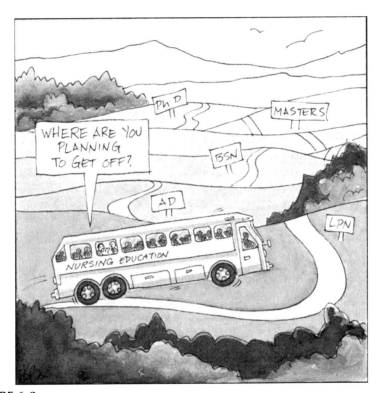

FIGURE 6-2
Among innovations occurring in nursing education over the past decade are programs that provide direct articulation between lower-level and higher-level programs.

are difficult to develop because of the tremendous amount of joint planning they require. Leveling of content in nursing as well as in the supporting areas of the natural and behavioral sciences is critical. Understanding what has been taught and determining how to evaluate current knowledge is also important. This is particularly relevant to articulation between practical nurse programs and registered nurse programs, where graduates of the practical program may know how to perform many of the nursing skills but may lack the theory base of registered nurses. Educators need to speak the same language and develop mutual respect.

NONDEGREE PROGRAMS

Specialized programs have been developed to help to prepare individuals for roles of increased breadth and scope. Some of these programs are incorporated into the preparation leading to a particular degree; others exist as part of a school's continuing education program.

The registered nurse anesthesia and midwifery programs both award a certificate after completion of a standardized and rigorous course of study lasting from 18 months to 2 years. At one time, admission requirements stipulated licensure only; however, the trend is toward making a baccalaureate degree in nursing an admission requirement, and toward awarding a masters degree on completion of the program.

More recent programs offer nurse practitioner and nursing specialist preparation in areas of nursing practice such as pediatrics, gerontology, family health, genetics, and women's health care. Recent health care reform has resulted in an increased emphasis on the role of advanced nursing practice in health care delivery, and more demand for educational programs to prepare these practitioners. The Pew Commission has encouraged the growing number of master's level nurse practitioner training programs (de Tornyay, 1996). Lipman and Deatrick (1994) stipulate that advanced skills in clinical decision making, and coordinating care from the hospital to the community and home, are essential parts of this preparation. Programs that prepare nurse practitioners concentrate study in specific areas over a period of time lasting from several months to a year or more. Requirements for admission vary tremendously. Some programs require licensure for admission, others stipulate the baccalaureate degree, and still others require that the education occur at the post-master's degree level. The American Nurses' Credentialing Center requires the master's degree for all those seeking initial nurse practitioner certification, and some states now require the master's degree for those seeking initial licensure as a nurse practitioner.

The proliferation of such programs has been so great that a complete listing is impossible. A student interested in pursuing such preparation is encouraged to write to the college or university of choice for information about available programs.

INTERNSHIPS AND RESIDENCIES FOR THE NEW GRADUATE

When nursing education moved from hospital-based diploma programs into higher education, a new problem was created. Employers of the new graduates, who expected these graduates to function as experienced and qualified professionals on the day after graduation, complained that the graduates were not prepared to assume staff nurse positions within their institutions.

The changes in nursing education, including changes in diploma education, had resulted in shortened clinical experience. Many graduates of diploma schools in the 1950s would have had as much as 4000 clock hours of clinical experience, albeit more through apprenticeship and service to the hospital than as a learning experience. Graduates of associate and baccalaureate degree programs, with integrated curricula and objective-based learning experiences, joined the work world with clinical learning time of 800 or fewer clock hours. Hospital-based programs also decreased their clinical hours as curricula were reorganized.

Critics employed in nursing service were distressed by a new type of graduate who could think, analyze, and synthesize, but who was inexperienced in "doing." Most graduates needed orientation to the work facility and to their new role, and time to become efficient in the administration of their newly learned skills. Although few would question the need for internships and residencies for new physicians, the need for similar experiences for new nursing graduates was disputed. The new graduates, unable to live up to expectations placed on them, often became frustrated and discouraged; some opted for less stressful situations, sometimes even outside nursing. Nursing educators, in defending the education provided, cited other professions, such as law and engineering, in which graduates needed a period of time to adapt to the world of work.

By the 1970s, it was apparent that something must be done. Although cost was a problem, orientation programs, internships, and residencies for new graduates were instituted by hospitals. The programs were intended to ease the transition from the role of student to that of staff by providing the opportunity to increase clinical skills and knowledge, as well as self-confidence. These programs can last from several weeks to a year, and are designed for graduates of all nursing programs—associate degree, diploma, and baccalaureate. They often include rotations to various units within the hospital, including specialty areas, and they accommodate different shifts. Usually some formal classwork is associated with the experience, but the majority of the time is spent in direct patient care, often under the supervision of a preceptor.

Some direct benefits to institutions, other than a better prepared new employee who remains in employment, have resulted from such programs. Inadequacies in policy and procedure books have been uncovered and, as a result, these books have been rewritten. Performance evaluation tools that are more objective in format have emerged. Nursing practice throughout some agencies has become more standardized. Job satisfaction has increased. It is no longer unusual for hospitals to advertise planned orientation and internships as benefits offered to the new graduate seeking employment.

The major disadvantage voiced by hospitals is the cost of operating such programs. At a time when cost containment is crucial, hospitals are not anxious to deal with the additional costs of such programs. Another problem is the fact that employees who benefit from such programs often resign from their positions soon after completing an internship. This has resulted in hospitals stipulating a period of required employment following the internship.

FACTORS INFLUENCING NURSING EDUCATION

During the 20th century, society has experienced tremendous change. Nursing, as a part of that society, has also experienced enormous change. A number of factors influenced nursing education.

The Brown Report

One of the important early studies of nursing was conducted in 1948 by Esther Lucile Brown, who was not a nurse (see Chapter 5). She was concerned that young women were not choosing nursing as a profession, and believed, as a result of her study, that the majority of nursing schools were not providing a professional education. In "Nursing for the Future," Brown (1948) recommended that nursing education move away from the system of apprenticeship that predominated at the time, and move toward a planned program of education similar to that offered by other professions. She recommended that the schools be operated by universities or colleges, hospitals affiliated with institutions of higher learning, medical colleges, or independently. She also recommended that programs be periodically examined or reviewed, and that a list of accredited schools be published and distributed.

The Brown report attracted the attention of many nursing leaders who shared her concerns about recruiting qualified women into nursing. The study also took place shortly after World War II, and nurses who had been involved in the military were gaining a new sense of autonomy and independence that they were not willing to leave behind. Committees formed to respond to the suggestions put forth in the Brown study, particularly those related to the accreditation of programs. At the same time, the National League for Nursing Education (NLNE), later to become the National League for Nursing (NLN), was recommending that hospital schools of nursing consider transferring control and administration of their programs to educational institutions. The NLNE also urged that federal grants be provided to nursing schools to allow for their improvement.

Development of the State Board Test Pool Examination

Along with the push for the improvement of nursing education, licensing authorities were pressured to establish a uniform licensing examination. The NLNE offered to assist states in developing and adopting machine-scored examination questions that would ensure greater uniformity in testing. Originally only six states participated in the testing developed by the NLNE, but by 1949, 41 states were using this "State Board Test Pool Examination." In 1951, all licensing jurisdictions adopted the test and established a standard passing score. In 1994, the test was first administered via computer. The development of the State Board Test Pool Examination helped all schools to focus on common goals, and laid the foundation for interstate endorsement of licenses. (See Chapter 7 for more information on the development of the licensing examination.)

National Accreditation of Nursing Programs

By 1952, the NLN had a temporary accreditation program in place, and was helping schools to find ways to improve their programs of instruction. The accreditation of programs had a noticeable effect on standards of nursing education. As a result of accreditation activities, schools were forced to look at the educational preparation of faculty, the workload of faculty and students, the structure of clinical teaching, withdrawal rates, and the state board examination scores. The quality of education was enhanced, and graduating from a nationally accredited school meant added opportunities for advanced education or certain types of employment.

Changes in Nursing Service

While changes were occurring in the education of nurses, nurses in the workplace were also experiencing significant changes. With the advent of antibiotics and other major advances in medical protocols, the public was receiving care in hospitals rather than treatment in the home. Infants previously born at home were now being born in hospitals. Federal funds were allocated for the construction of hospitals. Increased hospitalization drove the need for qualified nurses to a new high. Hospitals were desperate to find nurses to fill needed positions, and nurses represented half of all hospital personnel.

The role of the nurse changed in response to changes in the workplace. Nursing staff began assuming responsibilities formerly associated with physicians. Unfortunately, they were also assuming responsibilities that could have been assumed by housekeeping, dietary, laboratory, and pharmacy departments. Nurses began spending more time managing personnel, delegating responsibilities, and carrying out other administrative duties. These changes in practice demanded nurses prepared with higher levels of education (ie, baccalaureate and master's degrees).

The Report of the Surgeon General's Consultant Group

In 1961, the surgeon general of the United States Public Health Service appointed a group to advise him of the federal government's role in providing adequate nursing services to the country. This group was known as the Surgeon General's Consultant Group on Nursing, and they published their report in 1963.

The report emphasized the need for more nurses, and identified the lack of adequate financial resources for nursing education as a major problem. Several other major concerns were also reported, among them the fact that too few schools were providing adequate nursing education, that too few college-bound young people were being recruited into the profession, and that more nursing schools were needed in colleges and universities, were among the other major problems that were reported. Educational preparation at the baccalaureate degree level was recommended as the minimum preparation for nurses assuming leadership roles (U.S. Public Health Service, 1963).

The Surgeon General's Consultant Group on Nursing also made recommendations that federally funded low-cost loans and scholarships be made available to students in both professional and practical nursing programs. It advocated the use of federal funds to construct additional nursing school facilities and to expand educational programs. The Nurse Training Act of 1964 was an outgrowth of these recommendations.

The ANA Position Paper

In the early 1960s, the educational preparation of nurses became a major concern of the American Nurses Association (ANA). The ANA believed that the improvement of nursing practice depended on the advancement of nursing education. In 1962, a committee was appointed to study the issue, and in 1965, this activity culminated in the development and publication of ''A Position Paper on Educational Preparation for Nurse Practitioners and Assistants to Nurses.''

The paper took four major positions:

1. The education of all those who are licensed to practice nursing should take place in institutions of higher education.
2. Minimum preparation for beginning professional nursing practice at the present time should be baccalaureate degree education in nursing.
3. Minimum preparation for beginning technical nursing practice at the present time should be associate degree education in nursing.
4. Education for assistants in the health service occupations should be short, intensive preservice programs in vocational education institutions, rather than on-the-job training programs (American Nurses Association, 1965, p 107).

RESPONSES TO THE ANA POSITION PAPER

No other single action or position affected nursing as much as this position paper. For almost 40 years the profession has been divided over the issues it brought forth. A basic concern related to the fact that roles, functions, and responsibilities (competencies) were not clearly established for graduates of programs offering three different routes to preparation for registered nursing. All graduates performed similar activities when hired as new graduates in acute care facilities. Little has changed since the publication of the position paper.

Associate degree nursing programs in community colleges and hospital-based diploma programs took serious exception to the paper. Both groups saw their graduates as "professionals" and were unwilling to compromise title or licensure. As a result, many individuals associated with these two groups dropped their membership in ANA because they could not support this position.

Because of the dissension the position paper created among nursing groups, little immediate action followed. In 1974, New York became the first state to support the ANA position. By 1986, 48 state nurses' associations had taken positions supporting the change. In January, 1986, North Dakota published and put into effect administrative rules that required nursing programs to develop specific curricula leading to the associate degree for practical nurse programs and to the baccalaureate degree for registered nurse programs. The requirement became effective January 1, 1987. Thus North Dakota became the first, and to date the only, state to require a baccalaureate degree for registered nurse licensure and an associate degree for practical nurse licensure (North Dakota Rule, 1986).

Other nursing organizations also reviewed the tenets of the position paper and endorsed it. The first was the National Student Nurses' Association, which voted in favor of the paper at its 1976 convention. Other groups to support the baccalaureate degree as the minimum educational level for future entry into professional practice included the Association of Operating Room Nurses, the Emergency Department Nurses' Association, The Association of Rehabilitation Nurses, the American Association of Occupational Health Nurses, and the Executive Board of the Nurses' Association of the American College of Obstetricians and Gynecologists (now called the Association of Women's Health, Obstetric, and Neonatal Nursing). All of these groups took this action in 1979.

Several other groups have had more difficulty establishing a position regarding this paper. Because members of the NLN include educational councils representing practical, diploma, associate degree, baccalaureate, and higher degree programs, the organization has voiced support for all types of programs. At the 1987 biennial convention, the membership ''postponed indefinitely'' resolutions addressing this issue, and in 1989 instructed the NLN to put its energies into activities that would promote upward mobility in nursing.

The National Council of State Boards of Nursing and the National Federation of Licensed Practical Nurses (NFLPN) also made decisions about the education required for entry into practice. At an August 1986 meeting, representatives of the state boards voted without debate or opposition to take a ''formal position of neutrality on changes in nursing education requirement for entry'' (Hartung, 1986, p 124). In August 1984, the membership of the NFLPN voted to support increasing the period of study in the practical nurse program to 18 months, and to support awarding an associate degree at the completion of the program of study. To date only North Dakota has begun to implement these NFLPN recommendations.

Problems Associated with Changing Educational Requirements for Licensure

A number of problems are associated with making any changes in educational requirements for licensure. Four major problems are related to titling, scope of practice, grandfathering, and interstate endorsement.

TITLING

One of the most controversial problems associated with changing requirements for licensure involves the use of *titles*. Although the position statement calls for two levels of nursing practice, the titles to be used by persons working at each level have not been specified by most states. Some advocate using ''RN'' for the baccalaureate graduate and ''LPN'' for the 2-year associate degree graduate. Needless to say, this is unacceptable to associate degree graduates and students, who currently may use the RN title if successful on state licensing examinations. It is also upsetting to graduates of current diploma schools, from which no degree is granted. Others have suggested that the 2-year graduates be titled ''associate nurse'' or ''registered associate nurse.'' When a tertiary care hospital in South Dakota implemented differentiated nursing practice, the terms ''associate nurse'' for the associate degree graduate and ''primary nurse'' for the baccalaureate graduate were used. This approach again overlooks the diploma graduate. It is not likely that this issue will be easily resolved.

SCOPE OF PRACTICE

Of equal concern is the description and delineation of the *scope of practice* for the two levels of caregivers. The scope of practice, as will be discussed in Chapter 7, is that section of the Nurse Practice Act that outlines the activities a person with a particular license may legally perform. This would mean the separate testing of each level as currently exists between the R.N. and L.P.N. licensure examination. This problem might be of less concern if the nursing profession could come to agreement on an approach to differentiated practice (which will be discussed later in this chapter). As some states have moved toward plans for two levels of practice, the process of making nursing diagnoses and developing nursing care plans has been included in the scope of practice of the baccalaureate-prepared nurse only, a position totally unacceptable to associate degree advocates. Again the diploma graduate is left out of the discussion.

THE GRANDFATHER CLAUSE

The application of the *grandfather clause* presents another challenge to nurses. Historically, when a state licensure law is enacted, or if a current law is repealed and a new law enacted, the grandfather clause has been a standard feature that allows persons to continue to practice their profession or occupation after new qualifications have been enacted into law. The legal basis for the process is found in the 14th Amendment to the U.S. Constitution, which says that no state may deprive any person of life, liberty, or property without due process of law. The Supreme Court has ruled that the license to practice is a property right. The grandfather clause has been used in nursing at various times in the past. For example, when psychiatric nursing became a requirement of all programs, nurses who graduated and were licensed without psychiatric nursing experiences were "grandfathered" into the new role. In other words, they continued to practice as registered nurses without taking a formal course in psychiatric nursing, and without being required to write a psychiatric examination to maintain their licenses. If nursing began to require a baccalaureate degree for individuals using the registered nurse title, under the provisions of the grandfather clause, all associate graduates licensed prior to the implementation date for the change would continue to use the title "registered nurse." Those licensed after the change would use whatever new title was established. Although this serves to "protect" the title of currently licensed nurses, it does not assure that employers will not write job descriptions stipulating a baccalaureate degree as the minimum educational preparation acceptable for an advertised position. Complicating this matter is the fact that some nurses believe the grandfather clause should be conditional. If it were conditional, nurses licensed before the changes in the licensure law would continue to use their current title for a stipulated period of time—for example, 10 years. At the end of that period, if they had not completed the education mandated in the changes, (or any other conditions that might have been added), they would have to use the title stipulated in the new law for nurses with their educational preparation. Because of the complexity, and the difficulties associated with implementation, it is unlikely that conditional "grandfathering" will ever become a reality.

INTERSTATE ENDORSEMENT

A fourth concern is that of *interstate endorsement.* Nursing is one of the few professions to have developed a process whereby national examinations with standardized scores are administered in each state or jurisdiction. This allows a nurse who has passed the licensing examination in one state to move to another state and seek licensure, without the need to retake and pass another examination. Because nurses have been highly mobile, this has been a great advantage. Changes in one state without similar changes in other states will affect nursing mobility. For example, if a graduate of an associate degree program in New Jersey, who has passed the National Council Licensing Examination (NCLEX) for registered nursing, seeks licensure in North Dakota, additional education is required. North Dakota would issue the graduate a temporary permit to work as a registered nurse in North Dakota under the condition that the graduate enroll in a baccalaureate program. The temporary permit is renewable as long as progress is made toward the degree. A permanent license is issued when the baccalaureate degree is awarded.

When changes do occur in certain states, it is hoped that similar changes will be considered across the nation so that interstate endorsement can be maintained.

DIFFERENTIATED PRACTICE

In the beginning of the 1990s, some nursing leaders began to reassess the entry-into-practice issue. Although its reevaluation may have been encouraged by the nursing shortage of the late 1980s and the push toward cost cutting typical of the 1990s, the reevaluation may also reflect a new thinking regarding the role of nurses and nursing. Many nursing leaders encouraged recognition of the need for different types of practitioners prepared with different types of education—or, differentiated practice. *Differentiated nursing practice* can be defined as "the practice of structuring nursing roles on the basis of education, experience, and competence" (Boston, 1990, p. 2). It has also be defined as "practice expectations that are consistent with expected competencies of graduates from different kinds of education programs" (Harkness, Miller and Hill, 1992, p. 26). Today many groups support the concept of differentiated practice. The report of the Pew Commission (1995) advised that nursing distinguish between the different levels of nursing, recommending associate preparation for the entry level hospital setting and nursing home practice, baccalaureate preparation for hospital-based care management and community-based practice, and master's degree preparation for specialty practice in the hospital and independent practice as a primary provider. The National Commission Nursing Implementation Project (NCNIP) also strongly supported differentiated practice.

The American Association of Colleges of Nursing and the American Organization of Nurse Executives established a Task Force on Differentiated Competencies for Nursing Practice funded by the Robert Wood Johnson Foundation. This group was later expanded to include representatives from The National Organization for Associate Degree Nursing. Their goals are to institute five to ten differentiated education–practice demonstration projects across the country, to develop a core of leaders for the projects, to develop a value-neutral language to describe differentiated nursing practice and education, and to disseminate the work completed in the project (American Association of Colleges of Nursing, 1995).

Competency Expectations and Differentiated Practice

The task of describing and differentiating the competencies and the scope of practice of nurses graduating from various types of programs is one of the major challenges facing nursing today. As stated earlier, graduates of baccalaureate nursing programs, associate degree programs, and hospital-based programs all write the same licensing examination, designed to assure minimum safe practice. This approach fails to recognize the broad range of functions in nursing, and the potential for improving the quality of care given, if different roles and responsibilities were identified. In the work environment of acute and long-term care facilities, little differentiation exists in beginning staff nurse positions.

Realistic statements regarding competencies of each level or category of nursing education are necessary so that each category of graduate can be used effectively and efficiently within the health care delivery system. Validated competencies will also provide a basis for the development of curriculum patterns that will ensure adequate preparation of each category of caregiver, without running the risk of overeducation or undereducation at any one level. The competencies can also serve as a foundation for educational mobility patterns within the profession, job descriptions within the health care system, and responsive reimbursement packages.

The Work of Organizations in Defining Competencies

Some work has been done toward describing the competencies of graduates of different programs in nursing. In 1990, the Council of Associate Degree Programs of the NLN published "Educational Outcomes of Associate Degree Nursing Programs: Roles and Competencies," a revision of an earlier competency statement. The "Characteristics of Baccalaureate Education in Nursing," revised by the Council of Baccalaureate and Higher Degrees of NLN in 1994, accomplishes a similar purpose for baccalaureate education. Similarly, the Council of Diploma Programs of NLN has developed competencies for graduates of hospital-based programs.

Since 1986, the National Council of State Boards of Nursing has conducted several studies aimed at role delineation and job analysis of entry-level registered nurses. The purpose of these studies was to validate the NCLEX-RN. During 1997, the National Council will develop the protocol for conducting a study to identify similarities and differences in the practice of all levels of licensed nurses within and across employment settings, and will conduct the study in 1998 (Issues, 1996).

Special Projects to Differentiate Practice

Several projects have been conducted throughout the United States in an effort to achieve a regional consensus among nursing service persons and educators on differentiated statements of scope of practice for each level of graduate.

THE MIDWEST ALLIANCE IN NURSING PROJECTS

Two projects sponsored by the Midwest Alliance in Nursing (MAIN) have focused on defining competencies. One, entitled "Defining and Differentiating ADN and BSN Competencies and Facilitating ADN Competency Development" was funded by the W.K. Kellogg Foundation. The second, entitled "Continuing Education for Consensus on Entry Skills," was funded by a grant from the Division of Nursing of the Department of Health and Human Services. These studies resulted in the development of general statements on roles and the delineation of specific competencies in the area of direct care, communication, and management (Primm, 1987).

THE HEALING WEB PROJECT

Following in the steps of the MAIN work on competencies, the Healing Web Group was comprised of representatives of nursing education and practice from six midwestern and western states. These individuals had as their goal the design, implementation and evaluation of a variety of educational and practice differentiation activities. The projects were to serve as models for differentiation in both practice and education, as well as to provide the model for collaboration between nursing education and practice. One project site has been in operation for over 6 years.

THE SIOUX FALLS EXPERIENCE

One of the sites for the Healing Web Group was Sioux Falls, South Dakota. Here a detailed project was implemented to differentiate educational design. For one year nursing students in associate and baccalaureate degree programs are provided nursing education simultaneously in concurrent clinical laboratory experiences in which they work as a team with differentiated roles. A differentiated curriculum provides learning experiences specifically targeted to the competencies of the two levels of students. Team learning is directed at establishing the unique goals for the differentiated roles. This is reinforced in joint seminars that involve hospital staff, faculty and students. The success of this project is encouraged by the small number of nursing programs in South Dakota and the fact that the ADN program is located at the University of South Dakota.

Sioux Valley Hospital has reported a significant cost savings through the use of this differentiated practice model, including decreased length of stay, decreased intensive care days, and decreased number of readmissions. The hospital has been identified by *Modern Hospital* as among the ''100 Top U.S. Hospitals—Benchmarks for Success'' (Modern Hospitals, 1994).

THE COLORADO EXPERIMENT

In 1988, the State of Colorado developed two sets of recommendations. First, they asked for a statewide plan to facilitate articulation of nursing education programs, to allow nurses to move from one educational credential to another without unnecessary replication of learning or curricular experience. The second recommendation called for a differentiated model for nursing practice that would facilitate appropriate utilization of nurses with varying educational credentials and degrees of experience. This would be accompanied by a differentiated pay scale to allow appropriate compensation of nursing personnel as career advancement or growth occurred. Movement from one role to another required completion of the appropriate additional degrees, although growth within each role was possible without acquiring formal education.

A complex and detailed set of competency statements, job descriptions, and evaluative tools was developed as a part of this project. The project also facilitated movement from one role to another. Wide-scale implementation of this model has not yet occurred.

FORCES FOR CHANGE IN NURSING EDUCATION

As the nursing profession advances, and as education remains responsive to the changes that are occurring, it is imperative that nursing education undergo modifications. A discussion of some of the most significant challenges follows.

Establishing Programs That Provide for Educational Mobility

One of the challenges to nursing educators has been the growing emphasis on educational mobility in nursing. Students begin their education at one level and wish to continue into a program that prepares them for a higher level of client care and responsibility. Students want to advance from one level to another with minimal repetition of course work. Educational mobility has received impetus in some states from legislative mandates that stipulate that plans for articulation from one type of nursing program to another must be developed and implemented within a given period of time. More recently, one of the recommendations of the Pew Commission (1995) included strengthening the existing career ladder programs in order to make movement through these levels of nursing as easy as possible. Thus we see associate degree programs articulated with practical (vocational) nursing programs, increased efforts to facilitate transfer of associate degree graduates into baccalaureate programs, and the emergence of LPN to BSN and ADN to Master's pathways.

Increasing Community-Based Practice Experiences

Another significant change in nursing practice is the trend toward community-based practice. Most nursing programs, especially hospital-based and associate degree programs, have a history of being strongly oriented toward the hospital as the primary clinical teaching environment. "Community," as it was used in nursing education, was associated with public health nursing and was to be found in baccalaureate education only.

Earlier hospital discharge to the home and an increasing emphasis on prevention has created new demands on nursing. Nurses are expected to provide care in clients' homes, the workplace, schools, nursing homes, community health agencies, clinics, shelters, and community gathering places. As the arena in which nursing is practiced begins to shift, nursing educators are being challenged to define what part of the nursing curriculum should be taught in a community setting. Often this requires different clinical teaching strategies and approaches. Faculty, who received most if not all of their education in acute care hospitals, believe that students do not spend enough time on hospital clinical units and are therefore unwilling to further shorten the amount of time. Most are uncertain as to how a community experience should be provided and how it can be evaluated. Others worry about the legal ramifications associated with having students in many different environments and in less controlled situations. Tremendous strides have been taken in developing innovative approaches to community-based nursing; more will follow.

Increasing Emphasis on the Use of the Computer

Today's health care settings could not operate without computers and computerized equipment. Computers are used for business operations, for medical records, for collection of clinical data such as vital signs and hemodynamic values, for voice activated charting at the bedside, for nursing care plans, for communication from the physicians' office to nursing stations, and for many other facets of operation. Most of the equipment used in today's modern hospital is also computerized. New graduates move into a highly technical world when they seek their first nursing positions (Fig. 6-3).

The computer plays a major role in nursing education. It is as essential to the operation

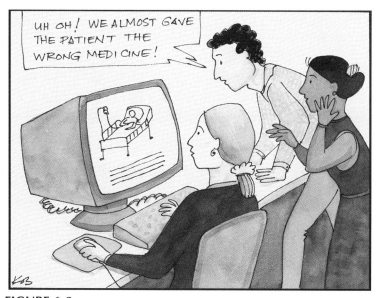

FIGURE 6-3
CAI can include interactive and linear programs, patient simulations, drill and practice routines, problem solving programs, and tutorials.

of colleges and universities as it is to the operation of hospitals. Additionally, it serves as a major instructional tool. The computer offers a variety of approaches to instruction that are appealing and helpful to a diverse student population. Classroom lectures and presentations are augmented by computer assisted instruction (CAI) that takes the form of interactive and linear video programs, patient simulations, drill and practice routines, problem-solving programs, and tutorials, to name a few examples. Faculty use computers for word processing, literature review, and the development and scoring of tests. Some faculty use computers in the classroom to augment their lectures and discussions. E-mail and the Internet are also a part of most teaching environments. Some instructional programs are delivered to sites distant from the main campus through distance learning modalities incorporating computerized technology. At the end of their program of study, all students demonstrate their ability to practice safely on computerized licensing examinations in the form of computerized adaptive testing (CAT). Although only cognitive abilities are tested currently, it is conceivable that early in the 21st century, a candidate taking the National Council Licensing Examination (NCLEX) for registered nursing might receive a two-part examination that would include clinical simulations measuring clinical decision making skills.

Computer literacy among students and faculty is no longer an issue—it is the current state of the art. Of concern to nursing educators, however, is the cost of the equipment and programs needed for this instruction, and the increasing cost of keeping both equipment and programs current. At a time when the budgets of educational institutions are experiencing severe cuts, people responsible for the purchase of supplies and equipment increasingly must find creative ways to acquire needed items. Another challenge to faculty is finding time to evaluate the existing software and integrate it into the approved curriculum.

Increasing Emphasis on Nursing Theories and Research

As the nursing profession continues to grow, one of the areas receiving more emphasis is nursing theory and research. This emphasis will undoubtedly continue. As nursing education keeps pace with the advancement of nursing knowledge, there is a push to develop curricular patterns that respond to the work of nursing theorists. Most approval bodies, state and national, now stipulate that a nursing program must have a coherent organizational framework or conceptual framework around which the program of learning is developed. Many programs have chosen to select the approach of a particular nursing theorist, and have structured the program of learning around that theorist's work. The program in which you are enrolled may reflect this trend. Perhaps one of the hospitals to which you are assigned for clinical experience also uses the principles of a nursing theory to structure the delivery of care, although this is less common than the use of a theory in curriculum development.

A theory is a "scientifically acceptable general principle which governs practice or is proposed to explain observed facts" (Riehl and Roy, 1974, p 3). Because nursing as a developing profession is seriously involved in research, to build a sound body of nursing knowledge, theories are valuable to us. They provide the bases for hypotheses about nursing practice. They make it possible for us to derive a sound rationale for the actions we take. If the theories are testable, they will then allow us to build our knowledge base and to guide and improve nursing practice (Fig. 6-4).

Today there are many published nursing theories. In an attempt to structure and organize those theories, various authors have categorized or classified them. Not all are classified similarly. Included are general classifications such as the art and science of humanistic nursing, interpersonal relationships, systems, and energy fields. Other categories include growth and development theories, systems theories, stress adaptation theories, and rhythm theories.

Examples of growth and development theories with which you are probably familiar are those of Maslow, Erikson, Kohlberg, Piaget, and Freud. Most basic nursing texts incorporate a discussion of the concepts developed by these theorists. The theories are so named because they focus on the developing person. They have the common characteristic of arranging this development in terms of stages through which a person must pass to reach a particular level of development. They allow nurses to monitor progress through the various stages and evaluate the appropriateness of that progress. You will recognize Maslow for his approach to self-actualization, Erikson for his psychosocial development, Kohlberg for his theories of moral reasoning, Piaget for his approach to cognitive development, and Freud for psychosexual theories on which medicine later based the school of psychoanalysis. These theories are not truly theories of nursing, however, because they were not developed for the purpose of explaining, testing, and changing the practice of nursing. They represent some of the "borrowed" knowledge around which we build our profession.

Most nursing theories are developed around a combination of concepts. Among these concepts, four approaches usually are included:

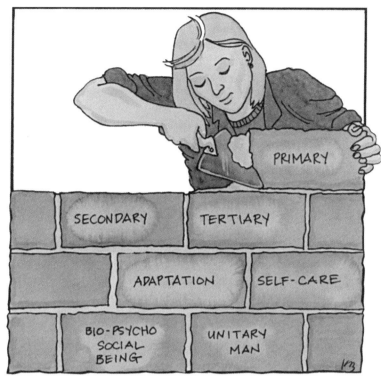

FIGURE 6-4
Nursing is in the process of building a body of scientific knowledge.

1. An approach to the human person
2. An approach to health/illness
3. An approach to the environment (or society)
4. An approach to nursing

Nursing theories are usually classified with regard to the structure or approach around which they are developed.

Theories that speak to the art and science of humanistic nursing were among the earliest pure nursing theories developed. Some authors have looked back at the contributions of Florence Nightingale and have included her work in that grouping. Among others are Virginia Henderson and her *Definition of Nursing*; Faye Abdellah and the *Twenty-one Nursing Problems*; Lydia Hall and her *Core, Care, and Cure* Model; and Madeleine Leininger's *Transcultural Care Theory*.

Interpersonal process theories deal with interactions between and among people. Many of these theories were developed during the 1960s. Included in this grouping could be Hildegard Peplau's *Psychodynamic Nursing,* Joyce Travelbee's *Human to Human Relation-*

ship, Ernestine Wiedenbach's *The Helping Art of Clinical Nursing,* and Imogene King's *Dynamic Interacting Systems* model, although the last could also be classified as a systems theory.

Systems theories are so named because they are concerned with the interactions between and among all the factors in a situation. A system is usually viewed as complex and in a state of constant change. It is defined as a whole with interrelated parts and may be a subsystem of a larger system as well as a suprasystem. For example, a person may be viewed as a system composed of cells, tissue, organs, and the like. The person is a subsystem of a family, which in turn is a subsystem of a community. In a systems approach, the person is usually considered as a ''total'' being, or from a ''whole'' being viewpoint. Systems theories also provide for ''input'' into the system and ''feedback'' within the system. The systems approach became popular during the 1970s. Included in this group of theorists would be Dorothy Johnson, Sister Calista Roy, and Betty Neuman.

Stress adaptation models are based on concepts that view the person as adjusting or changing (adapting) to avoid situations (stressors) that would result in the disturbance of balance or equilibrium. The adaptation theory helps to explain how balance is maintained and therefore directs nursing actions. Included in this group one often finds Sister Calista Roy's adaptation model and Betty Neuman's work, but both may also be considered systems models, as mentioned above.

One of the most recent classifications of theories is by energy fields. These theories, although developed earlier, received growing recognition during the 1980s. Included in this group are the works of such persons as Myra Levine, Joyce Fitzpatrick, Margaret Newman, and Martha Rogers.

It is not our purpose to discuss and critique all the many approaches to nursing theory. The student who wants to pursue nursing theorists further is encouraged to consult the section on further reading at the end of the chapter. Table 6-2 outlines the approaches of a number of the current nursing theorists.

CONTINUING EDUCATION

Continuing education programs are widely publicized in today's nursing literature. They are frequently presented just prior to and during major nursing conventions. Some professional meetings carry continuing education credit. Other continuing education programs exist as extensions of nursing programs at colleges and universities.

Continuing education in nursing is defined as ''planned learning experiences beyond a basic nursing educational program. The learning experiences are designed to promote the development of knowledge, skills, and attitudes for the enhancement of nursing practice, thus improving health care to the public'' (American Nurses Association, 1974).

Like so many other areas of nursing, this is not new. In an article entitled ''Nursing the Sick,'' written around 1882, Florence Nightingale wrote:

Nursing is, above all, a progressive calling. Year by year nurses have to learn new and improved methods, as medicine and surgery and hygiene improve. Year by year nurses are called upon to do more and better than they have done. It is felt to be impossible to have a public register of nurses that is not a delusion (Nightingale, as cited in Seymer, 1954, p 349).

TABLE 6–2. Nursing Theories and Theorists

	Theory or Model
Lydia Hall	Viewed illness and rehabilitation as learning experiences in which the nurse's role was to guide and teach the patient through personal caregiving. Role involves therapeutic use of self (core), the treatment regimen of the health care team (cure), and nurturing and intimate bodily care (care).
Dorothy Johnson	A behavioral systems approach that focuses on health viewed as a state of equilibrium that the nurse assists in maintaining or balancing.
Imogene King	A model in which three open systems interact with the environment: personal, individual, and social. Nurse's role is to assist individual to perform daily activities and includes health promotion and maintenance. Involves goal attainment.
Madeleine Leininger	Focused on a caring model that must be practiced interpersonally. Emphasized a transcultural approach.
Myra Levine	Developed around the four concepts of conservation of energy, structural integrity, personal integrity, and social integrity. Supports a holistic approach to nursing based on recognition of the total response of the person to the interaction between the internal and external environment.
Betty Neuman	A systems model which is influenced by Gestalt theory, stress and level of prevention. Employs lines of resistance and lines of defense in creating a healthy being. Nurses are to identify the stressors and assist the individual to respond. Involves primary, secondary and tertiary prevention.
Dorothea Orem	Recognized as a self-care theory of nursing, supports the concept that each person has a need for the provision and management of self-care actions in order to achieve "constancy." When the individual is unable to provide these, a self-care deficit exists. The role of the nursing system is to help eliminate the self-care deficit through wholly compensatory, partially compensatory, or supportive-educative actions.
Martha Rogers	Includes complicated approaches to health that involve helicy, resonancy, and complementarity. The holistic individual moves through time and space as part of an expanding universe with potential states of maximum well-being. Nurses act to promote symphonic interaction between man and the environment by repatterning the human and environmental fields.
Sister Calista Roy	Identified as an adaptation model which conceives of the individual as being in constant interaction with a changing environment, thus requiring adaptation. Four adaptive modes, or ways in which a person adapts, are identified through: 1) physiological needs, 2) self-concept, 3) role function, and 4) interdependence relations. The nurse's role is to assess a patient's adaptive behaviors and the stimuli that may be affecting the person and to manipulate the stimuli in such a way as to allow the patient to cope or adapt.

The first continuing education courses for nurses probably would be considered post-graduate instruction today. In 1899, Teachers College at Columbia University instituted a course for qualified graduate nurses in hospital economics. Nursing institutes and conferences were first offered to nurses in the 1920s; often these were given to make up for deficiencies in basic nursing curricula. Hospital in-service or staff development programs were also beginning to be discussed in nursing literature around this time. Today most hospitals employ someone who is responsible for the staff education program. By 1959, federal funds became available for short-term courses, giving much thrust to continuing education. In 1967, the ANA published "Avenues for Continued Learning," its first definitive statement on continuing education; and in 1973, the ANA Council on Continuing Education was established. The Council, which is responsible to the ANA Commission on Education, is concerned about standards of continuing education, accreditation of the programs, transferability of credit from state to state, and development of guidelines for recognition systems within states. In 1974, "Standards for Continuing Education in Nursing" was published by the ANA, and the federal government altered the Nurse Traineeship Act of 1972 to include an option that would provide continuing education as an alternative to placing more students into programs receiving federal capitation dollars.

By the 1970s, almost all nursing publications had something to say about continuing education for nurses. Practically all states were organizing or planning to organize some method by which the nurse could receive recognition for continued education. These systems were called continuing education approval and recognition programs, or continuing education recognition programs, and most state systems followed the guidelines and criteria prepared by the ANA.

The continuing education unit (CEU) became a rather uniform system of measuring, recording, reporting, accumulating, transferring, and recognizing participation in nonacademic credit offerings. The definition of a CEU was developed by the National Task Force on the Continuing Education Unit, which represented 34 educational groups. Although nursing was not one of the groups, the definition has been accepted by the profession. Ten hours of participation in an organized continuing education experience under responsible sponsorship, with capable direction and qualified instruction, is equal to one CEU. Many states and organizations however, simply report clock hours of instruction (Fig. 6-5).

Today colleges, universities, hospitals, voluntary agencies, and private proprietary groups are all offering continuing education courses to registered nurses. The cost of this education varies tremendously. Nurses may earn continuing education credits for merely attending meetings and conferences. Little attempt is made to assess whether learning has occurred. Professional journals are including sections of programmed instruction that can be completed in the comfort of one's living room. These have an evaluation mechanism. Telecourses are offered by television. Workshops, institutes, conferences, short courses, and evening courses abound. Yet some nurses do not feel the need to keep up with these current offerings.

A system for accreditation and approval of continuing education in nursing was developed and implemented by the ANA in 1975. Accreditation was awarded for a period of 4 years and assured the public that the continuing education offerings provided consistent quality. A new system, put into operation August 1, 1987, allows organizations that offer continuing education to seek accreditation as either a provider or an approver. A provider is any organization that is responsible for the development, implementation, and evaluation of courses. An approver could be the state nurses' association, a specialty organization, or a federal nursing service that has been designated to approve the continuing education process. Organizations can be both approvers and providers. This program made the system

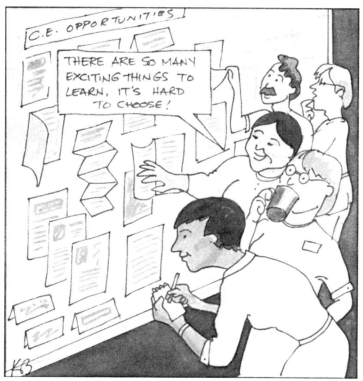

FIGURE 6-5
Today colleges, universities, hospitals, voluntary agencies, and private proprietary groups are all offering continuing education courses to registered nurses.

more accessible to groups seeking approval of courses or classes by bringing the process closer to the membership and to those offering the programs.

An issue today is whether continuing education should be mandatory or voluntary. Mandatory continuing education affects licensure; that means that any nurse renewing a license in a state requiring (mandating) continuing education will have to satisfy that requirement. Voluntary continuing education is not related to relicensure. Government agencies and state legislatures are exerting pressure on nurses, as they have on physicians, attorneys, dietitians, dentists, pharmacists, and other professionals, to provide evidence of updated knowledge before license renewal.

A position supporting mandatory continuing education raises some questions. How should the learning be measured? Who should accredit the programs? How can quality be ensured? By whom and where should records be retained? Who should bear the cost? What should be the time frame for continuing education? How many hours, courses, and credits should be required?

You can write directly to a state board of nursing for information on specific requirements for that state (see Appendix A for addresses).

KEY CONCEPTS

- Three major avenues to preparation for licensure as a registered nurse exist in the United States: the hospital-based diploma, the university-based baccalaureate degree and the associate degree (usually offered in community colleges). Many similarities exist among these programs. In addition, various nontraditional approaches to nursing education have evolved.
- Educational programs prepare nursing assistants and licensed practical (vocational) nurses for roles in the health care delivery system. As these programs have grown, greater oversight of the programs by approval bodies has occurred.
- The nursing shortage that occurred in the 1990s has resulted in decreased dissension regarding educational preparation for nursing, and greater creativity and collaboration in educational approaches.
- Master's and doctoral programs that prepare nurses for leaderships positions within the profession continue to grow. The actual doctoral degree awarded varies.
- One of the most rapidly growing areas is that of advanced practice; this growth was accelerated by health care reform. Recommendations from major commissions have urged continued expansion of advance practice programs.
- Many changes are anticipated in nursing education. These include more emphasis on articulation and career ladder programs, an increase in computer literacy, and a shift in educational settings from acute care facilities to community-based experiences.
- Nursing theories continue to influence nursing and nursing education. Nursing theories assist us in building a body of nursing knowledge and describing and defining nursing practice.
- Nursing education has been influenced by the ANA Position on Nursing Education that advocated the baccalaureate degree as the minimum educational preparation for professional practice. Many nursing educators, particularly those in diploma and associate degree programs, disagreed with this position.
- Models for differentiated practice are being encouraged; these models recognize and utilize graduates according to the competencies inherent in the program from which they graduated.
- Continuing education, whether it is represented by further education that results in a higher degree, or whether it takes the form of classes, seminars, or workshops that update and increase expertise, is being encouraged by more and more organizations. Staying current in practice is critical to safe client care.

Critical Thinking Activities

1. Imagine that you could restructure nursing education for an ideal world. Where would you begin? How many levels of nursing education would you incorporate in your model? Would each level be terminal or articulated with others? Where would general education fit into your model? How would you see the graduate of each program functioning on the health care team? How would you see each level reimbursed for services?

text continued

Critical Thinking Activities   (continued)

2. If nurse practitioners are to work in a collaborative way with physicians, and as primary care providers, what type and level of education do you believe they should complete? How would you go about ensuring that this would occur? What standards regarding continuing education should be mandated?

3. Given the situation we have today, with three routes to preparation for registered nursing, how would you differentiate the skills of the graduate of each program? How should that influence nursing practice? How would you go about implementing differentiated practice on the unit on which you are currently working?

4. Take a stand on the ANA Position on Nursing Education. Provide a rationale for the position you have taken. What do you see as the outcome of the position paper? How would your position be implemented in the future? What implications might it have for nursing practice? Do you believe the salaries of nurses educated at different levels and practicing at differentiated levels should differ? Why or why not? If so, how?

5. Select one nursing theorist. Describe what you find interesting and attractive about her nursing theory. Give a rationale for your decision and describe how using her theory might affect your practice of nursing.

6. Do you believe continuing education should be a mandatory requirement for the renewal of one's license? Why or why not? How would you go about the record-keeping aspect if your answer is yes? Who do you believe should keep the records? How would you go about ensuring competence if your answer is no?

REFERENCES

American Nurses Association's first position on nursing education. Am J Nurs 65(12):106–111, 1965

American Nurses Association. Standards for Continuing Education for Nursing. Kansas City, MO: American Nurses Association, 1974

Benner P. From Novice to Expert. Menlo Park, CA: Addison-Wesley Publishing Co., 1984

Boston C. Differentiated practice: An introduction. In Boston C: Current issues and perspectives on differentiated practice (pp 1–3). Chicago, IL: American Organization of Nurse Executives, 1990

Broad-based research agenda addresses regulatory issues faced by member boards. Issues 17(1):1, 4–6, 1996

Brown EL. Nursing for the Future. New York: Russell Sage Foundation, 1948

California Board of Registered Nursing. Laws Relating to Nursing Education Licensure: Practice with Rules and Regulations. Sacramento: California Board of Registered Nursing, 1994

de Tornyay R. Critical challenges for nurse educators. J Nurs Ed 35(4):146–147, 1996

Hartung D. Organizational positions on titling and entry into practice: A chronology. In: Looking Beyond the Entry Issue: Implications for Education and Service, NLN Publication No. 41-2173, New York: National League for Nursing, 1986

Hegner BR, Caldwell E. Nursing Assistant: A Nursing Process Approach, 6th ed. Albany, NY: Delmar Publishers, 1995

Kalisch PA, Kalisch BJ. The Advance of American Nursing, 3rd ed. Philadelphia: JB Lippincott, 1995

Lipman TH, Deatrick JA. Enhancing specialist preparation for the next century. J Nurs Educ 33(2): 53–58, 1994

National League for Nursing. Criteria and Guidelines for Accreditation of Associate Degree Program, 7th ed. Publication No. 23-2439, Council of Associate Degree Programs. New York: National League for Nursing, 1991

National League for Nursing. Educational Outcomes of Associate Degree Nursing Programs: Roles and Competencies. Publication No. 23-2348, Council of Associate Degree Programs. New York: National League for Nursing, 1990

National League for Nursing. Characteristics of Associate Degree Education in Nursing. Publication No. 23-1500, Council of Associate Degree Programs. New York: National League for Nursing, 1973

Nightingale F. Nursing the sick. *In* Seymer LR: Selected Writings of Florence Nightingale. New York: Macmillan, 1954

Pew Health Professions Commission. Critical challenges: Revitalizing the health professions for the twenty-first century. San Francisco, CA: UCSF Center for the Health Professions, 1995

Primm PL. Differentiated practice for ADN- and BSN-prepared nurses. J Prof Nurs 3(4):218–225, 1987

Riehl JP, Roy SC. Conceptual Models for Nursing Practice. New York: Appleton-Century-Crofts, 1974

Sorrentino, SA. Textbook for Nursing Assistants, 3rd ed. St. Louis: Mosby-Year Book, 1994

100 Top U.S. hospitals-benchmarks for success. Mod Hosp 24(3):8, 14, 1994

U.S. Public Health Service. Toward quality in nursing: Needs and goals. Report of the Surgeon Generals Consultant Group on Nursing. Washington D.C.: U.S. Government Printing Office, 1963

Valuing difference—Creating community: A model for differentiated nursing practice. American Association of Colleges of Nursing: Washington D.C., 1995

FURTHER READING

A call for reform of our nursing education system. The AONE update. Nurs Management 24(1):33, 1993

Allen VO, Sutton C. Associate degree nursing education: Past, present, and future. Nurs Health Care 2(9):496–497, 1981

American Association of Colleges of Nursing. Guidelines for Baccalaureate Education in Nursing for Registered Nurse Students in Colleges and Universities. Publication Series 79, No. 3. Washington, DC: American Association of Colleges of Nursing, 1980

American Nurses Association. A Case for Baccalaureate Preparation in Nursing, ANA publication No. NE-6 15M. Kansas City, MO: American Nurses Association, 1979

Bersky AK, Yocum CJ. Computerized clinical simulation testing: Its use for competence assessment in nursing. Nurs & Health Care 15(3):120–127, 1994

Bersky A, Brady D. A new generation of competence assessment in nursing: Computerized clinical simulation testing (CST). Issues 14(1):1–8, 1993

Bramble K. Nurse practitioner education: Enhancing performance through the use of the objective structured clinical assessment. J Nurs Educ 33(2):59–65, 1994

Brubaker BH. A faculty learns to make self-pacing work. Nurs Health Care 11(2):74–77, 1990

Craver DM, Sullivan PP. Investigation of an internship program. J Contin Educ Nurs 16(4):114–118, 1985

Cross utilization of nursing staff. The AONE update. Nurs Management 24(7):38–39, 1993

Davids SL, Laeger E. Developing a BSN program across two institutions: Arizona State University West Campus/Glendale Community College—the adjuvant model. Nurs Health Care 11(2):84–87, 1990

Fishman DJ. Nursing informatics: The electronic information revolution in education and practice. *In* Strickland OL, Fishman DJ: Nursing Issues in the 1990s. Albany, NY: Delmar Publishers, 1994:471–488

Frik SM, Pollack SE. Preparation for advanced nursing practice. Nurs Health Care 14(4):190–195, 1993

Kasprisin CA, Young WB. Nurse internship program reduces turnover, raises commitment. Nurs Health Care 6(3):137–140, 1985

Koerner J. Differentiated practice: The evolution of professional nursing. J Nurs Ed (8):335–341, 1992

Koerner J, Karpiuk K. Implementing Differentiated Nursing Practice: Transformation by Design. Gaithersburg, MD: Aspen, 1994

Kurzen CR. Contemporary Practical/Vocational Nursing. Philadelphia: JB Lippincott, 1989

Lambert C, Lambert VA. Relationships among faculty practice involvement, perception of role stress, and psychological hardiness of nurse educators. J Nurs Educ 33(4):171–179, 1993

Mead ME, Berger S, Nicksic E. Contracts for continuing education. J Contin Educ Nurs 16(4):121–126, 1985

Montag ML. Community College Education for Nursing. New York: McGraw-Hill, 1959

NLN seeks compromise on entry: ADNs hold out for RN licensure. Am J Nurs 87(1):113, 124–125, 1987

NLN members agree to shelve entry issues and call for steps to spur career mobility. Am J Nurs 89(8):1082–1083, 1989

Parkinson CF, Parkinson SB. A comparative study between interactive television and traditional lecture offerings for nursing students. Nurs Health Care 10(9):498–502, 1989

Primm PL. Entry into practice: Competency statements for BSNs and ADNs. Nurs Outlook 34(3):135–137, 1986

Pruitt RH, Campbell BF. Educating for health care reform and the community. Nurs Health Care 15(6):308–311, 1994

Schwartz MD. An introduction to interactive video systems. Computers Nurs 2(1):8–13, 1984

Seymer LR. The Nightingale training school: One hundred years ago. Am J Nurs 60(5):658–661, 1960

Sharp N. Second license for the advanced practice nurse? Nurs Management 23(9):28–29, 1992

Simpson RL. The new careers in nursing informatics. Nurs Management 23(10):26–27, 1992

State boards declare "neutral stance: in entry-level debate. Am J Nurs 86(10):1180, 1896

Smith PL. Non-nurse college graduates in a specialty master's program: A success story. Nurs Health Care 10(9):494–497, 1989

Tanner CA, Hartshorn J, Rosenfeld P. Critical care nursing in baccalaureate programs. Nurs Health Care 10(9):482–488, 1989

Town J. Changing to computerized documentation—plus! Nurs Management 24(7):44–48, 1993

Trofino J. Voice-activated nursing documentation: On the cutting edge. Nurs Management 24(7):40–42, 1993

Yoder ME. Preferred learning style and educational technology: Linear vs. interactive video. Nurs Health Care 15(3):128–132, 1994

Legal and Ethical Accountability for Practice

As we examine legal, ethical, and bioethical issues in health care, we will first explore the issue of credentials for health care providers. Understanding some of the basic concerns related to credentialing, and the rationale for the existence of credentials, will help to focus your attention on the responsibility of health care providers to the public.

The entire realm of law that guides the practice of any health occupation is a particular concern in a society where individuals often attempt to solve problems in a courtroom. A beginning understanding of rights and responsibilities from the viewpoint of a health care provider is important to you.

Ethical and bioethical issues associated with health care constantly challenge us as professionals and as members of our society. Each new technological advance brings additional concerns to our attention. In this unit we try to provide you with a general background that will help you address legal, ethical, and bioethical concerns. In addition, we present some specific problems with the hope that considering them before you become directly involved will help you to address the issues more comfortably.

Unit III

Credentials for Health Care Providers

As the legal profession becomes increasingly aware of the education and experience of the professional nurse, as well as the unique role a nurse plays in the health care delivery system, it is anticipated that nurses will become more legally accountable for their actions. (Fiesta, 1988)

Objectives

After completing this chapter, you should be able to:

1. Define and discuss the concept of credentialing.
2. Differentiate between a diploma, certification, accreditation, and licensure as credentials.
3. Outline the history of nursing licensure, including the concepts of permissive and mandatory licensure.
4. Identify the major topics found in nursing practice acts.
5. Outline the role of the State Board of Nursing or other state regulatory authority.
6. Differentiate between licensure by examination and licensure by endorsement.
7. Discuss the disciplinary process in regard to a nursing license.
8. Discuss the process of nursing licensure for graduates of foreign nursing schools.
9. Explain the various uses of certification in nursing.
10. Discuss current trends in credentialing within the health care workforce.

KEY TERMS

Accreditation
Advanced practice
Computerized adaptive testing (CAT)
Computerized simulation testing (CST)
Credentialing
Criticality
Disciplinary action
Enacted (statutory) law
Grandfathering
License
Licensure by endorsement

Mandatory licensure
Multistate licensure
NCLEX-PN
NCLEX-RN
Nurse practice act
Permissive licensure
Revocation
Rules and regulations
Sunset laws
Telenursing

redentials are written proof of qualifications. They communicate to others the nature of one's competence and provide evidence of one's preparation to perform in a specific occupation. The basic rationale for credentials in health care occupations is that the safety of the public is protected by providing a standard mechanism for judging competence. Further, those who are engaged in careers in health occupations want to be assured that the standards of practice in their discipline will remain high, and that they will not be replaced by people with less educational preparation who are willing to work for lower wages (Fig. 7-1).

TYPES OF CREDENTIALS IN HEALTH CARE

There are many types of health care credentials; examples include accreditation, diplomas, degrees, licenses, and certificates. Each of these serves a different purpose. Not all are available for each different health occupation.

Accreditation

Accreditation is a process whereby educational institutions or programs are surveyed and evaluated. Some accreditation recognizes the entire educational institution, such as the ac-

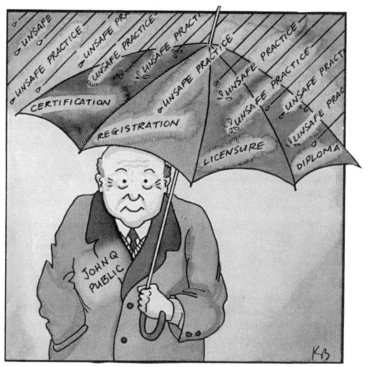

FIGURE 7-1
Various forms of credentiating ensure the public of qualified caregivers.

creditation offered by regional bodies for colleges and universities. If an institution's programs meet published standards, it is awarded accreditation. An associate, baccalaureate, or master's degree awarded by this institution would then reflect a standard of postsecondary education that has been approved by the accrediting organization. Although a non-accredited institution might award a degree, there is no guarantee that the degree meets educational standards; therefore, the degree might not be accepted as adequate evidence of qualifications. Many educational credentials are acknowledged only if offered by an accredited educational institution.

Some accreditation is "specialized," meaning that it only applies to a particular special program within an institution, or to a particular type of technical–professional education. This accreditation requires that the specific program meet professional standards for excellence. An educational institution might have general accreditation for its degrees, but still not have specialized accreditation. Sometimes this is because of the cost of the accreditation process, or because of a philosophical stance that additional accreditation is not needed if the institution has general accreditation. Certain educational organizations are not degree-granting institutions, and therefore are not eligible for general accreditation, but they are still eligible for specialized accreditation. This is true of hospital-based diploma schools of nursing.

The national accreditation of nursing programs is a specialized accreditation provided by the National League for Nursing Accrediting Commission, a subsidiary organization related to the National League for Nursing. This organization provides separate specialized accreditation processes for practical nursing programs, diploma nursing programs, associate degree nursing programs, and baccalaureate and higher degree nursing programs. Nurse practitioner organizations also provide specialized accreditation for institutions offering nurse practitioner programs. The American Association of Colleges of Nursing is developing its own accrediting system for baccalaureate and higher degree nursing programs.

Diplomas and Certificates of Graduation

A school or business offering instruction awards a diploma or certificate to those who complete a designated program of study. An example is the diploma awarded on graduation from high school or college. A business that provides instruction in using computer programs might present certificates to those who complete the course. When only a diploma or educational certificate is available, it is necessary to know about the educational institution and the specific educational program to evaluate the person's abilities.

Licensure

A *license* is a legal credential conferred by an individual state. A wide variety of health professionals are licensed in different states. Most states restrict licensing to those who have more direct contact with clients. Physicians, dentists, pharmacists, and nurses are licensed in all states. The licensing of other health care workers varies.

Mandatory licensure is a requirement that all individuals must obtain a license in a particular jurisdiction in order to practice. There is mandatory licensure for physicians and dentists in all states, and mandatory licensure for nurses in all states but one. Mandatory licensure is instituted when there is a compelling public interest in licensure to protect the public.

Permissive licensure is a system whereby an individual may choose to become licensed to provide evidence of competence, but a license is not required to practice. Permissive and mandatory licensure are discussed in greater detail later in this chapter. Eligibility for licensure and the type of testing required are determined by an individual state or province. Most licensing laws specify completion of a state-approved educational program, and also require the successful completion of a written examination prescribed by the state. Some professions, such as dentistry, require candidates to pass a practical examination as well as a written examination. Nursing is unique in having a standard licensure process in every state and territory in the United States. This was developed through the cooperative action of the state boards of nursing. A national examination may exist for other professions, but its application may vary. For example, there is a national licensing examination for pharmacy, but California prepares and administers its own examination and does not use the national pharmacy examination. There are national medical board examinations, but some states administer independent medical examinations. Even when the same examination is used for licensure, as in pharmacy, some states require that a person new to the state retake the licensing examination when applying for a license in that state.

Some states require completion of continuing education to renew a health care license. Pharmacists were one of the first groups required to pursue continuing education to remain licensed. Continuing education is required for relicensure of nurses and physicians in many states. The cost of monitoring continuing education has been a barrier to its adoption in some states. (see Chapter 6).

Certification

For some groups a standard credential is available in the form of certification provided by a nongovernmental authority, usually a professional organization. Workers with this type of credential are referred to as "certified" or sometimes as "registered." This type of credential should not be confused with a legal license. Certification usually is granted on completion of an educational program and the passing of a standardized examination, both of which are prescribed by a professional organization.

Some organizations provide certification for several related occupational groups. One such organization is the National Accrediting Association for Clinical Laboratory Sciences (NAACLS). Members of the various professional groups involved in laboratory science cooperated in setting up this association. The organization is incorporated as a private, voluntary entity and is not a governmental institution or department. The purpose of this organization is to make the laboratory science credentialing system more independent, and as objective as possible. This organization awards the title medical laboratory technician (MLT) or medical technologist (MT) to those who have met the educational standards and passed the certification examination. These credentials are recognized by all groups in the field of laboratory science as professional credentials. Some states have made certification by this body the required criterion for practice in clinical laboratory sciences.

While some professional organizations conduct their own certification, in most instances they have established an independent national entity with the sole purpose of credentialing. There are several reasons for this. First, the public generally has not trusted the objectivity of professional groups that do not have consumer input; the creation of an independent credentialing body ensures that those currently practicing a profession are not the sole arbiters in determining who enters the field. Secondly, by setting up a separate organization, which must be self-supporting through fees for its services, professional groups are relieved of the financial burden that can result when an accrediting program grows rapidly and costs escalate. The third justification for creating an independent credentialing body is to provide a broader base of support from many related organizations for the credentialing process. A fourth reason relates to the complex federal laws governing nonprofit organizations and their tax-exempt status.

THE HISTORY OF CREDENTIALING IN NURSING

Nursing leaders historically have maintained an ethical position that accountability to the public for quality nursing care is essential. The public, however, often has no method for evaluating the competence of an individual nurse. Therefore, the nursing profession has tried to ensure that nurses have credentials that can be recognized by everyone.

Credentials were not always available for nurses. Before the Nightingale schools became prevalent in England, and nursing schools were established in the United States, little training was available to those who wanted to provide nursing care. Nurses with some training and those without any typically worked side by side. After schools of nursing became common, a rudimentary means of identifying the qualifications of a caregiver was the certificate of completion that was issued by the nursing school. This was the first true nursing credential.

However, because the quality of education offered in the nursing schools varied greatly—programs varied in length from 6 weeks to 3 years—it became apparent that a completion certificate was not an adequate guarantee of competence. Nursing leaders were concerned about this situation; they believed that clients had no way to judge a particular nurse's competence, or whether they might suffer from the care administered by a poorly prepared nurse.

In 1896, the Nurses' Associated Alumnae of the United States and Canada was created. This organization later evolved into the American Nurses Association (ANA). One of the major concerns of the association was the establishment of legal licensure for nurses. The route toward legal licensing for credentialing was long and difficult. Nurses, legislators, and the public had to be educated about the value of licensure for the profession and encouraged to support it. Display 7-1 presents a chronology of nursing licensure.

Permissive Licensure for Nursing

The ANA campaigned vigorously for the adoption of state licensing laws. These early laws provided for permissive licensure. The requirements for permissive licensure included graduating from a school that satisfied certain standards and passing a comprehensive examination. Only those who had met these standards could use the title "registered nurse." An employer or a member of the public could then differentiate between a registered nurse and an individual who used the title "nurse," but had not met the standards required to be registered. Under this system no one was required to have a license to practice nursing.

DISPLAY 7-1
The History of Nursing Licensure

1867	Dr. Henry Wentworth Acland first suggested licensure for nurses in England.
1892	American Society of Superintendents of Training Schools for Nurses organized and supported licensure in the United States.
1901	First nursing licensure in the world: New Zealand.
1903	First nursing licensure in the United States: North Carolina, New Jersey, New York, and Virginia (in that order).
1915	ANA drafted its first model nurse practice act.
1919	First nursing licensure in England.
1923	All 48 states had enacted nursing licensure laws.
1935	First mandatory licensure act in the United States: New York (effective 1947).
1946	Ten states had definitions of nursing in the licensing act.
1950	First year the same examination used in all jurisdictions of the United States and its territories: State Board Test Pool Examination.
1965	Twenty-one states had definitions of nursing in the licensing act.
1971	First state to recognize expanded practice in the nursing practice act: Idaho.
1976	First mandatory continuing education for relicensure: California.
1982	Change to nursing process format examination: National Council Licensure Examination for Registered Nurses (NCLEX-RN).
1986	First state to require baccalaureate degree for initial registered nurse licensure and associate degree for licensed practical nurse licensure: North Dakota (effective 1987).
1994	Computer adapted testing initiated nationwide.

The community benefited from these standards because an established credential attested to a registered nurse's level of competence. The individual who was licensed as a registered nurse profited in regard to job availability and salary when employers differentiated between those who were licensed and those who were not licensed.

The first law providing for permissive licensure was passed in 1903 by North Carolina. By 1923, all the existing 48 states had permissive licensure laws. Alaska and Hawaii passed licensure laws while they were still territories, and continued to recognize these laws when they became states. The set of laws regulating the practice of nursing is termed the *Nurse Practice Act.*

Mandatory Licensure for Nursing

After permissive licensure laws came into being, nurses' activity regarding licensure became less intense because most individuals graduating from nursing schools sought and received licenses to practice. However, there was still concern that some persons were practicing nursing without having demonstrated skill and knowledge. The majority of those functioning without licenses were nursing school graduates who had failed the licensing examinations; they were referred to as graduate nurses, rather than registered nurses. Other nurses who practiced without licenses included individuals who had been educated as nurses in foreign countries.

To end this situation and provide greater protection to the public, many nurses began to call for *mandatory* licensure. Mandatory nursing licensure requires that all persons who wish to practice nursing meet established standards for education, pass standardized examinations, and secure a license to practice in the state, province, or territory in which they wish to work.

The first mandatory licensure law took effect in New York in 1947. Since then, more states have changed their laws relating to the practice of nursing and required licensure. Today, mandatory licensure is the standard in the United States and Canada, and in most other countries. Therefore, if you wish to work as a nurse in any state, territory, province, or other country you must obtain a license there before you begin working. Even though you are licensed to practice in one place, that does not allow you to practice elsewhere without seeking a new license in that jurisdiction (Fig 7-2).

CURRENT NURSING LICENSURE LAWS

The authority for establishing a licensure law lies with the legislature of each jurisdiction. However, new legislation regarding nursing licensure is most often initiated through the

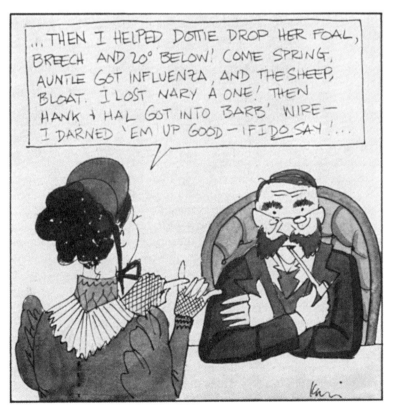

FIGURE 7-2
A standard credential makes hiring easier.

nurses' association or through the State Board of Nursing at the instigation of the nursing community. The group initiating the action may spend months preparing and planning the content of the bill and gaining the support of legislators for its passage.

A proposed change in the law enters the legislative process through an elected member of the legislature who has been persuaded that the change is in the best interest of the public. The proposal must go through the entire legislative committee review, a public hearing, and a legislative voting procedure before it can become a law. When finally passed by the legislature, the legislation becomes part of the licensure law.

During the legislative process, individuals and organizations may affect the content of the proposed legislation by influencing the legislators. In 1974, for example, a bill was introduced in New York that would have changed the educational requirements for entry into nursing practice; the bill indicated that the minimum requirement for practice should be a baccalaureate degree. During the legislative process a great deal of lobbying occurred, and changes were made in the bill. Overall, the support for the bill diminished. The result was the defeat of the bill; the proposed change in educational requirements was not enacted.

Rules and Regulations

Each state has its own set of administrative rules and regulations to carry out the provisions of laws regulating nursing. These rules and regulations are established by an administrative body, usually the *State Board of Nursing*, that is given responsibility for administering the Nurse Practice Act. This responsibility is authorized within the Nurse Practice Act itself. (See the section on the Role of the Board of Nursing.) Most states require that public hearings be held in regard to proposed rules and regulations, but the board has the authority to make the final decision. The rules and regulations must be within the scope outlined by the legislation that was passed. Those that are accepted by the appropriate board have the force of law unless they are challenged in court and are found not to be in accord with the legislature's intent. These rules are termed the administrative law.

In some states, the Nurse Practice Act is detailed and specifies most of the critical provisions regarding licensure and practice. In other states, the practice act is broad, and the administrative body is given a great deal of power to make decisions through rules and regulations.

The difference between what is contained in the enacted law and what is contained in rules and regulations is illustrated by the educational requirements for licensure in each state. In some states the enacted law specifies that a diploma, an associate degree, or a baccalaureate degree is acceptable preparation for registered nursing. In those states, the enacted law would have to change in order for the educational requirements to change. In other states, educational requirements are not in the enacted law—they are established by the Board of Nursing through rules and regulations. In North Dakota, for example, the requirement for the registered nurse license was changed to the baccalaureate degree through state regulations. Thus, both the Nurse Practice Act and state rules and regulations govern nursing in your state.

Nursing Licensure Law Content

In the early 1900s, the ANA, assuming its leadership role in nursing licensure, formulated a model nurse practice act to be used by state associations when planning legislation (Snyder

& LaBar, 1984). The most recent revision of this model was in 1990 by the ANA Congress for Nursing Practice (ANA, 1990). The National Council of State Boards of Nursing (NCSBN) also developed a model nurse practice act (NCSBN, 1982). The NCSBN continues to update its model act as part of its role in supporting the state boards of nursing, with the most recent revision being published by the National Council in 1994 (NCSBN, 1994c). In addition, the NCSBN has written the Model Nursing Administrative Rules, which was also updated in 1994 (NCSBN, 1994d).

Most state nurse practice acts are periodically rewritten to more accurately reflect modern nursing practice. Often the state nurses' association provides legislators with the primary stimulus to reconsider nursing legislation. We recommended that you carefully read the Nurse Practice Act for the state in which you will be practicing. A copy of the act may be obtained from the State Board of Nursing (see Appendix A for addresses).

In some states, one act addresses both practical nursing and registered nursing; other states have two separate, but similar, acts. Historically, the role of the nursing assistant was not outlined in nursing laws. As federal legislation mandating classes and certification for nursing assistants (in long-term care) takes effect, some states are modifying laws, and rules and regulations, to address the role of the nursing assistant. In other states regulations governing nursing assistants rest within a different department of the state government.

The following general topics are usually covered in state licensure laws:

PURPOSE

The purpose of regulating the practice of nursing is twofold: regulations protect the public and make individual practitioners accountable for their actions. Note that the protection of the status of the licensed individual is not the reason for licensure. With this in mind, you can better understand the inclusion of some other topics in the act.

DEFINITIONS

All of the significant terms in the act are defined for the purpose of carrying out the law. This is where the legal definition of nursing and the scope of practice are spelled out.

The NCSBN has given the following definition: ''the 'practice of nursing' means assisting individuals or groups to maintain or attain optimal health, implementing a strategy of care to accomplish defined goals, and evaluating responses to care and treatment. This practice includes, but is not limited to, initiating and maintaining comfort measures, promoting and supporting human functions and responses, establishing an environment conducive to wellbeing, providing health counseling and teaching, and collaborating on certain aspects of the health regimen. This practice is based on understanding the human condition across the lifespan and the relationship of the individual within the environment.'' (NCSBN, 1994, p.3) The National Council document then proceeds to distinguish between registered nurse practice and licensed practical/vocational nurse practice.

No state adopts the exact wording of any recommended definition, but most states include references to performing services for compensation, the necessity for a specialized knowledge base, the use of the nursing process (although steps may be named differently), and components of nursing practice. Several states include some reference to treating human responses to actual or potential health problems; this was first addressed in New York State's license law and was later incorporated in the ANA's "Nursing: A Social Policy Statement" (1980). Most states refer to the execution of the medical regimen, and many include a general statement about additional acts that recognize that nursing practice is evolving and that the nurse's area of responsibility can be expected to broaden.

Definitions of practical (vocational) nursing are more restrictive, and usually state that the individual must function under the supervision of a registered nurse or physician, in areas demanding less judgment and knowledge than is required of the registered nurse; in the NCSBN model act, this is referred to as "a directed scope of nursing practice" (NCSBN, 1994, p.4). Practical nurse standards usually focus on the assessment and intervention portions of the nursing process. Some states provide a list of specific functions appropriate to the practical nurse, or list specific functions not permitted.

A variety of nursing assistants are employed in health care facilities; they may have titles such as mental health technician, nursing assistant, or medication technician. The preparation for and scope of practice for these individuals is a matter of serious concern to the public. With the current pressure to contain costs, these individuals may be assigned tasks and responsibilities requiring more than their educational preparation and competence. Laws regarding educational requirements and legal definitions of scope of practice have been used to control nursing assistant practice. For example, through the OBRA '87 regulations for long-term care facilities, a nationwide standard was established for the training and certification of nursing assistants for employment in these facilities. Each state administers the regulations and is free to raise the standards, but may not lower them.

QUALIFICATIONS FOR LICENSURE APPLICANTS

The qualifications for licensure may be described in detail in the law, or only general guidelines may be given, leaving the details up to the State Board of Nursing. The most common basic requirements are graduation from an approved educational program and proficiency in the English language. Some states make the educational requirements more specific—requiring, for example, high school graduation and either an associate or baccalaureate degree, or a diploma in nursing, for the registered nurse applicant.

All states require a passing score on a comprehensive examination, but do not specify which examination in the law; the current licensing examinations are discussed later in this chapter. Many states require that an applicant be of "good moral character," and some require "good physical and mental health."

TITLING

This section of the law reserves the right to use specific titles for those who have met the appropriate requirements. In some states, only the titles registered nurse and licensed practical nurse are regulated. Other states also regulate the use of titles for advanced practice, such as nurse practitioner and nurse midwife.

GRANDFATHERING

Whenever a new law is written, it usually contains a statement specifying that anyone currently holding a license may continue to hold that license if and when requirements for the license change. Without this provision, the enactment of a new law would require individuals who are currently licensed to reapply and to show that they meet the new standards.

However, not all changes in the law are grandfathered. When new requirements are instituted that the legislature believes are important for the safety of the public, all currently licensed individuals may be required to meet the new standards within a given period of time. For example, in 1987 the Washington state legislature in Washington State passed a bill requiring all licensed health professionals to have 7 hours of education regarding certain topics related to the acquired immunodeficiency syndrome. New applicants had to provide evidence of meeting this requirement before their licenses were granted; current license holders were required to meet this requirement before their licenses were renewed. Individuals seeking licensure by endorsement were also required to verify that they had completed the equivalent of seven hours of AIDS education.

LICENSE RENEWAL AND CONTINUING EDUCATION REQUIREMENTS

The length of time for which a license is valid and any requirements for the renewal of that license are specified in the law. In some states, license renewal requires only the payment of a fee. Many jurisdictions require evidence of continuing education for renewal. The documentation of continuing education may require the submission of records, or it may be attested to by signing a form. For example, California requires that the person seeking to renew an RN license list all continuing education courses taken, along with the number of continuing education units earned and the provider number of the agency offering the courses. In many states where the applicant is not required to submit records at the time of renewal, a procedure for random checking ensures compliance with the law. Continuing education requirements vary greatly—from as few as 15 hours every 2 years to as many as 24 hours every year.

FINANCIAL CONCERNS

Although the nurse practice act itself does not usually specify the fees to be charged for obtaining or renewing a license, general restrictions on the method of calculating fees and on how the fees may be used are often included in the act. The act may specify how the expenses of the Board of Nursing are to be met and who has legal authority to make decisions regarding the use of funds.

All states charge a fee for processing an application for licensure. At the time of initial licensure there are also fees for taking a licensing examination, and a fee must be paid to the company that prepares and scores an examination. The total cost for an initial examination and license is usually more than $100. In addition, there is a fee each time a license is renewed. For specific information on current licensure fees, temporary permits, and continuing education requirements, write to the Board of Nursing in the state in which you will practice.

NURSING EDUCATION PROGRAMS

Some state laws describe the requirements of nursing education programs in only the most general terms, leaving the details up to the Board of Nursing; in other states, the laws are specific. The law may specify the number of years of education required, the courses or content that must be included, and the approval process for particular programs. If the law is general, then the board sets more specific standards. All nursing education programs in a state must fulfill the requirements of the state law.

DISCIPLINARY ACTION

Disciplinary action refers to all penalties that may be imposed against an individual who has violated provisions of a licensing law. Disciplinary actions include restrictions on practice (such as working only under supervision), suspension of a license for a specified period, or revocation of a license. Disciplinary action can only be taken based on criteria stated in the law (Fig 7-3). In the past, most state acts contained general rules with regard to such matters as immoral and unprofessional conduct; because of their vagueness, however, these rules have been difficult to enforce in court. In addition, most courts have only supported revocation of a license when the offense was in some way related to practice issues that affected the public. Thus, most modern laws contain specific concerns such as the following:

- Fraud in obtaining a license
- Conviction of a felony

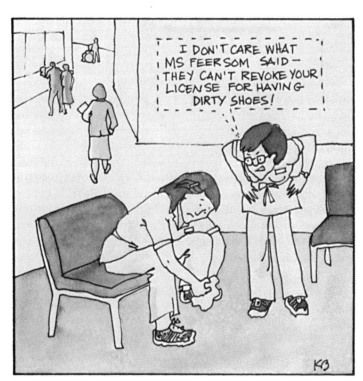

FIGURE 7-3
A nursing license may be revoked by the State Board of Nursing for reasons clearly spelled out in the law. These reasons may include fraud in obtaining a license, conviction of a felony, and conduct likely to harm the public.

- Substance abuse
- Harming the public

Some states now have clauses that call for license revocation for individuals who default on government sponsored educational loans, or on agreements regarding service in return for scholarship aid (New Legislation . . . , 1996).

VIOLATIONS AND PENALTIES

Specific power is provided to the nursing board to prosecute those who violate the provisions of the law. The board may be authorized to ask a court to halt a specific practice that it believes is contrary to the law until a full hearing can be held. This is called ''injunctive relief.'' This term refers to the court order called an injunction that requires an individual or organization to stop a particular activity.

EXCEPTIONS

Certain provisions may allow those who are not licensed to act as nurses in specific situations. Performing as a student while in an educational program is usually the primary exception. Those who are caring for family members or friends without pay are also exempted from license regulations. Those who are practicing nursing in a federal agency, such as a military hospital, are exempted from the local state law as long as they maintain a current license in another state.

ADMINISTRATIVE PROVISIONS

Each law requires administrative specifications detailing when the law will become effective and when a previous act will no longer be in force. Such provisions are of particular interest to nurses when a law is first passed, because nurses want to know when changes affecting them will take place.

Expanded Nursing Roles

Some nurse practice acts provide for the practice of nurses in expanded roles, including nurse midwives, nurse anesthetists, and nurse practitioners. Often the law requires that a person be certified for advanced practice by the ANCC or a nursing specialty organization (see section on certification later in the chapter). In some states no specific mention is made of expanded roles, but the Board of Nursing has approved specialty practice based on the provisions in the basic act. In still other states, practice in advanced practice roles is not legally sanctioned. Contact the Board of Nursing in the state in which you are interested for information about specialty practice.

As part of *Nursing's Agenda for Health Care Reform* (ANA, 1991), nurses have been working actively to support advanced practice roles for nurses. The ANA does not believe that the inclusion of expanded practice in the licensure law is the best method of ensuring safety in expanded practice. Some of the laws regulating specialty practice have provided for physician review of nursing's scope of practice; the ANA is concerned that these laws will take autonomy away from nursing and allow medicine to control some aspects of the nursing profession. The ANA is also concerned about the rigidity of these laws, which may not allow for evolving nursing roles. The ANA holds the position that the licensure law should regulate minimum safe practice, and that the profession should regulate advanced practice. This is the procedure in medicine, in which there is only basic licensure because a physician in specialty practice is regulated by specialty boards within the profession.

The National Council of State Boards of Nursing has taken the position that regulation of advanced nursing practice, to ensure public health and safety, should be the responsibility of the state board. In 1996, the NCSBN began a study process that could lead to a state-run testing program, and standardization of licensing for advanced nursing practice, if the NCSBN determines that this is the appropriate regulatory avenue for advanced practice nursing.

The Role of the Board of Nursing

The Board of Nursing (or its equivalent) is legally empowered to carry out the provisions of the law. The membership of the board, the procedures for appointment and removal, and the qualifications of board members are determined by the Nurse Practice Act. The board has the power to write the rules and regulations that will be used in daily operations.

The members of the State Board of Nursing usually are appointed by the governor. The law specifies the occupational background of the candidates; nominations are often made by nurses, but the final membership is appointed. North Carolina is the only state in which the registered nurse members of the state board are elected by the registered nurses in the state.

Boards of nursing range in size from 7 to 17 members. Prerequisites regarding the educational background of nurses who serve as board members vary from state to state. Some states require that the board include nurses from different occupational areas, such as education and nursing service. Most states have at least one public member of the board. A few have at least one physician on the nursing board.

Most states have a single board for registered nurses and licensed practical nurses. In some states, two separate boards exist. Each state board has a paid staff that usually is headed by a registered nurse who is employed as the executive director of the State Board of Nursing. The executive director is responsible for administering the work of the board and seeing that rules and regulations are followed. Some duties related to professional licensure may be performed by a centralized state agency acting in that capacity for all licensed occupations. The responsibilities of these centralized agencies may range from administrative matters, such as collecting fees, managing routine license renewals, and providing secretarial services, to decision making, relegating individual boards like the Board of Nursing, to an advisory status (Fig 7-4).

Each state board must operate within the framework of its own state law regarding the practice of nursing, but all cooperate with one another through the NCSBN. They also cooperate with the ANA and the National League for Nursing (NLN) in some matters, but maintain the separation that is required of a governmental body; for example, state boards acting together through the NCSBN contract with the company that prepares the licensing examinations for registered nurses and practical nurses that are used throughout the United States.

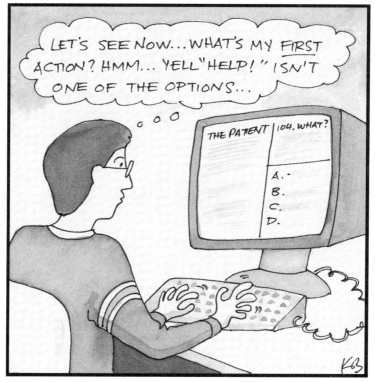

FIGURE 7-4
Questions on the NCLEX exam are designed to test ability to function safely as a nurse. Setting correct priorities is one aspect of safe practice.

The Board of Nursing typically must perform the following functions:

- Establish standards for licensure
- Examine and license applicants
- Provide for interstate endorsement
- Renew licenses, grant temporary licenses, and provide for inactive status for those already licensed who request it
- Enforce disciplinary codes
- Provide rules for revocation of license
- Regulate specialty practice
- Establish standards and curricula for nursing programs
- Approve nursing education programs

OBTAINING A NURSING LICENSE

There are two different procedures for obtaining a nursing license; one is used for obtaining an initial license and the other for obtaining a license when one is already licensed in another jurisdiction. The initial licensure process is called "licensure by examination." Obtaining a license in a second jurisdiction is called "licensure by endorsement." In both instances, the applicant for licensure must meet all provisions of the law (such as educational preparation, language proficiency, and legal residency status) in the state where he or she is seeking licensure. In the initial licensure process, the applicant must take and pass the standard licensing examination (NCLEX). When seeking licensure by endorsement, the applicant is not required to take another examination; the licensing examination results from the initial state are accepted as proof of minimum safe practice, but other requirements must be met. This process is discussed later in the chapter.

The Nursing Licensing Examination

The establishment of a licensing examination was an important part of early efforts to achieve a professional standard for the registered nurse. When each state adopted a licensing law, it also established a mechanism for examining license applicants. A major achievement in the history of licensure was the formation of the Bureau of State Boards of Nurse Examiners, which eventually led to the use of an identical examination in all states in 1950. The original examination, called the State Board Test Pool Examination, was prepared by the testing department of the NLN, under a contract with the state boards. Although each state initially determined its own passing score, most states agreed on an acceptable test score; eventually all states adopted a common passing score for the State Board Test Pool Examination. The current examination, called the NCLEX-RN for registered nursing and the NCLEX-PN for practical nursing, and used in all states and territories of the United States, is prepared and administered by the Educational Testing Service of Princeton, New Jersey, under a contract with National Council of State Boards of Nursing.

CONTENT OF THE EXAMINATION

Historically, the content of the nursing examination was divided into the categories of medical, surgical, obstetric, pediatric, and psychiatric nursing. Because nursing had changed in nature and these categories no longer adequately reflected nursing practice, the NCSBN adopted a different examination plan, which was implemented in July 1982. For this new examination, the National Council supported a research study, called the "RN Job Analysis," that identified nursing behaviors critical to maintaining a safe and effective standard of care (Display 7-2). This research has been repeated periodically to ensure that the test plan remains relevant to current nursing practice.

In all of these studies, newly licensed, practicing registered nurses are studied to determine both the frequency and the criticality of various behaviors. *Frequency* refers to how often the behaviors are required of the newly practicing registered nurse. *Criticality* refers to those actions that if performed incorrectly or omitted could cause serious harm to the client. These studies are reflected in the "Test Plan for the National Council Licensure Examination" (NCSBN, 1992b).

The NCLEX-RN examination questions are organized into categories based on the interaction of client needs and the steps of the nursing process. The client needs are (NCSBN, 1992b):

DISPLAY 7-2
Critical Requirements for Practice

I. **Exercises Professional Prerogatives Based on Clinical Judgment**
   A. Adapts care to individual patient needs.
   B. Fulfills responsibility to patient and others despite difficulty
   C. Challenges inappropriate orders and decisions by medical and other professional staff
   D. Acts as patient advocate in obtaining appropriate medical, psychiatric, or other help
   E. Recognizes own limitations and errors
   F. Analyzes and adjusts own or staff reactions in order to maintain therapeutic relationship with patient

II. **Promotes Patient's Ability to Cope with Immediate, Long-range, or Potential Health-Related Change**
   A. Provides health care instruction or information to patient, family, or significant others
   B. Encourages patient or family to make decision about accepting care or adhering to treatment regimen
   C. Helps patient recognize and deal with psychological stress
   D. Avoids creating or increasing anxiety or stress
   E. Conveys and invites acceptance, respect, and trust
   F. Facilitates relationship of family, staff, or significant others with patient
   G. Stimulates, remotivates patient, or enables patient to achieve self-care independence

III. **Helps Maintain Patient Comfort and Normal Body Functions**
   A. Keeps patient clean and comfortable
   B. Helps patient maintain or regain normal body functions

IV. **Takes Precautionary and Preventive Measures in Giving Patient Care**
   A. Prevents infection
   B. Protects skin and mucous membranes from injurious materials
   C. Uses positioning or exercise to prevent injury or the complications of immobility
   D. Avoids using injurious techniques in administering and managing intrusive or other potentially traumatic treatments
   E. Protects patient from falls or other contact injuries
   F. Maintains surveilolance of patient's activities
   G. Reduces or removes environmental hazards

V. **Checks, Compares, Verifies, Monitors, and Follows up Medication and Treatment Processes**
   A. Checks correctness, condition, and safety of medication being prepared
   B. Ensures that correct medication is given to the right patient and that patient takes or receives it
   C. Adheres to schedule in giving medication, treatment, or test
   D. Administers medication by correct route, rate, or mode
   E. Checks patient's readiness for medication, treatment, surgery, or other care
   F. Checks to ensure that tests or measurements are done correctly
   G. Monitors ongoing infusions and inhalations
   H. Checks for and interprets effect of medication, treatment, or care, and takes corrective action if necessary

(continued)

DISPLAY 7-2
Critical Requirements for Practice (continued)

VI. **Interprets Symptom Complex and Intervenes Appropriately**
   A. Checks patient's condition or status
   B. Remains objective, further investigates, or verifies patient's complaint or problem
   C. Uses alarms and signals on automatic equipment as adjunct to personal assessment
   D. Observes and correctly assesses signs of anxiety or behavioral stress
   E. Observes and correctly assesses physical signs, symptoms, or findings, and intervenes appropriately
   F. Correctly assesses severity or priority of patient's condition, and gives or obtains necessary care

VII. **Responds to Emergency**
   A. Anticipates need for crisis care
   B. Takes instant, correct action in emergency situations
   C. Maintains calm and efficient approach under pressure
   D. Assumes leadership role in crisis situation when necessary

VIII. **Obtains, Records, and Exchanges Information on Behalf of the Patient**
   A. Checks data sources for order and other information about patient
   B. Obtains information from patient and family
   C. Transcribes or records information on chart, Kardex, or other information system
   D. Exchanges information with nursing staff and other departments
   E. Exchanges information with medical staff

IX. **Utilizes Patient Care Planning**
   A. Develops and modifies patient care plan
   B. Implements patient care plan

X. **Teaches and Supervises Other Staff**
   A. Teaches correct principles, procedures, and techniques of patient care
   B. Supervises and checks the work of staff for whom she or he is responsible

- A safe, effective care environment
- Physiologic integrity
- Psychosocial integrity
- Health promotion–health maintenance

The nursing process is divided into the following five steps, each of which is tested in a designated percentage of the questions:

1. Assessing
2. Analyzing
3. Planning
4. Implementing
5. Evaluating

These two sets of concepts form a matrix for questions (Table 7-1). The multiple choice questions in the examination are typically based on situations that require a nursing response.

TABLE 7-1. Content Distribution of the NCLEX-RN Examination

Phases of the Nursing Process (% of Questions)	Client Needs—% of Questions			
	Safe, Effective Care Environment	Physiologic Integrity	Psychosocial Integrity	Health Promotion— Health Maintenance
Assess 15%–25%	25%–31%	42%–48%	9%–15%	12%–18%
Analyze 15%–25%	25%–31%	42%–48%	9%–15%	12%–18%
Plan 15%–25%	25%–31%	42%–48%	9%–15%	12%–18%
Implement 15%–25%	25%–31%	42%–48%	9%–15%	12%–18%
Evaluate 15%–25%	25%–31%	42%–48%	9%–15%	12%–18%

15% to 25% of the total number of test questions will be about assessment. Of these assessment questions 25%–31% will focus on assessment relative to a safe effective care environment. Using this matrix you can determine the distribution of questions for any test.

They are designed to test judgment and decision making, not simply knowledge of facts (NCSBN, 1992b).

Within these categories, safe practice behaviors are tested. For example, one question might determine an applicant's ability to assess a safe care environment, while another question might determine whether an applicant would implement the correct action to maintain safety. In the category of physiologic integrity, a question might focus on the appropriate assessment of a client with an illness that threatens physiologic integrity and another might focus on evaluating the outcomes of actions taken to preserve physiologic integrity. In this way questions address two aspects of the matrix plan.

In addition to assuming responsibility for test preparation, Educational Testing Services administers the computerized tests through contracted testing centers, scores the examinations, and reports scores to the state boards. The testing service is authorized to sell statistical information related to the examinations to the states and to individual schools.

Preparing questions for the examination is a complex process. Individuals who teach in nursing programs across the country are brought together as item writers. Together these individuals write questions based on the test plan. Questions are then reviewed by content experts, who are nurses currently working with new graduates. Another panel of individuals reviews the questions for bias. Each question is then verified for accuracy by using current nursing references; test construction experts also review the structure of all of the questions. The final versions of all questions are then tested by inclusion in a nongraded part of the license examinations being given to new graduates; the questions are then evaluated for their appropriateness as part of a future scored examination.

Computerized Adaptive Testing (CAT)

All NLCEX examinations (both RN and PN) are now administered through computerized adaptive testing (CAT). The CAT consists of a bank of examination questions administered through a computerized system. CAT had its first field trials in 1990, was tested across the country in 1993, and was adopted for all testing beginning in April 1994.

In this computerized test, the multiple choice questions are on a computer screen. The computer contains a large bank of questions; different individuals may be presented with different questions. The development of questions and the design of the computer program ensures that all tests are equivalent even when not identical. The computer program evaluates each response, and then selects an appropriate question to present next, choosing a slightly harder question if the previous question was answered correctly, or an easier question if the response was incorrect. The computer program ensures that all essential areas are tested, and that the balance of hard and easy questions and different aspects of the test matrix plan are all part of every examination. The minimum number of questions that might be administered is 75 and the maximum is 265. The maximum length of time for the examination is 5 hours, but a candidate performing especially well or very poorly might complete the exam in just 1 hour. One break is required after 2 hours of testing and others may be taken at the discretion of the applicant.

Each candidate for licensure makes an individual appointment at a testing site. At the testing site, the computers are located in a quiet room without distractions. Pencil and paper are provided for notes or calculations (calculators are not permitted). Security is tightly monitored.

Each question, along with its possible answers, is presented on a separate screen; if there is a brief situation, it appears on the same screen as the question and answers. Only two keys are used throughout the examination: the space bar moves between the alternative answers, and the ''enter'' key must be pressed twice to make a selection. A selection must be made to move to the next question. It is not possible to go back to a question previously answered. Some practice questions are provided to assure that the individual understands the process. When the individual has completed enough questions for the computer program to determine either a ''pass'' or a ''fail,'' the testing session is ended.

Scoring the Examination

The computer computes the score as the applicant answers questions. Based on the computation made as the applicant progresses, additional questions are presented to clearly determine whether the applicant meets the standards for safe, effective practice in all areas of the test plan. The score used to determine a pass or a failure is not a raw score (that is the number correct), but one derived from a complex statistical process that takes into consideration both the difficulty of a question and whether the response was correct. The test was not designed for the purpose of differentiating levels of excellence, only for demonstrating basic safe practice, and this is what the pass or fail communicates.

Every 3 years the National Council of State Boards convenes to consider the appropriateness of the passing score. In October 1995, the passing score for the NCLEX-RN was raised based on the increased expectations placed upon nurses in their work environments.

Although the computer immediately determines a score (upon the completion of the examination), the individual is not notified of the result at that time. The scoring information is communicated to the Educational Testing Service, which then notifies the appropriate board. The individual is notified of ''pass'' or ''fail'' status by the Board of Nursing in the state in which they are seeking licensure.

Preparing for the NCLEX-RN

Each individual must determine how best to prepare for the licensure examination. This is determined based on background and preferred study style. A review of the knowledge basic to nursing is important for most individuals. This may be done using course notes and texts, an NCLEX-RN review book, or a manual of nursing practice. Those who become very anxious in testing situations may want to focus on anxiety-reducing exercises to decrease anxiety during the examination. Those who find the process of test taking difficult can gain greater self-confidence by practicing test-taking techniques. This can be done through printed tests in books or computerized test preparation programs.

To prepare applicants to take the examination, the NCSBN has authorized the preparation of a study book that explains the examination, how it was written, and the scoring system, and that provides sample questions to familiarize applicants with the way the test is written. Many companies also prepare review books, sample examination questions, and computerized practice examinations that are used to prepare for the licensing examinations. Manuals that outline standard nursing practice relative to many different health care problems may be useful for reviewing nursing content. Live and videotaped review courses are available to those who want assistance with preparation.

The Licensure Examination for Practical Nursing

The licensure examination for the practical nurse, the NCLEX-PN, was designed in a manner similar to the NCLEX-RN. Client needs and the nursing process form the basis of this examination also. Based on a 1994 LPN/VN Job Analysis, the NCLEX-PN was modified (National Council, 1994). The new test, with slightly different categories in client needs, different test weights assigned to each category, and a higher passing score, was effective in October, 1996.

The practical nurse is expected to assume a dependent role in planning and evaluation, and a more independent role in data collection and implementation. The new test recognizes that many licensed practical nurses are employed in long-term care settings, with clients older than 65 years of age. The percentage of questions in each category are shown in Table 7-2. The testing and scoring processes are similar to those used for the NCLEX-RN examination, and a ''pass'' or ''fail'' is reported.

Future Trends in Examination

The NCSBN is investigating the potential for computerized Clinical Simulation Testing (CST), a more complex form of computerized testing of nursing licensure applicants (Bersky & Yocom, 1994). In this type of test, a client situation is presented on the computer screen. The applicant is asked to determine the appropriate action and type the answer into the keyboard. The applicant receives points for correct actions, and for the order or priority in which actions are chosen. Points are subtracted for inappropriate actions. Special note is made of actions that might harm a client. Consideration is being given to putting the situations on a videodisc to provide visual cues as well as written information (Bersky & Brady, 1993). This type of testing is much more expensive to develop and administer than a multiple choice question examination. CST was first field tested in 1991. Further testing in

TABLE 7-2. Content Distribution of the NCLEX-PN Examination

Phases of the Nursing Process —% of Questions	Client Needs—% of Questions			
	Safe, Effective Care Environment	Physiologic Integrity	Psychosocial Integrity	Health Promotion— Health Maintenance
Collect Data 30%	24%–30%	42%–48%	7%–13%	15%–21%
Plan 20%	24%–30%	42%–48%	7%–13%	15%–21%
Implement 30%	24%–30%	42%–48%	7%–13%	15%–21%
Evaluate 20%	24%–30%	42%–48%	7%–13%	15%–21%

30% of the questions on the practical nursing examination refer to collecting data. Of these 24% to 30% will be about collecting data in relationship to a safe, effective care environment. Using this plan the number of questions in each category can be calculated.

schools of nursing is scheduled for the 1997-1998 academic year. When the analysis of this testing is completed, the NCSBN, in its Delegate Assembly of 1999, will determine whether the CST will become a part of the licensing examination or be used for other educational and assessment purposes. The earliest implementation of this process, if approved, would be in 2001 (Overview . . . , 1996).

LICENSURE BY ENDORSEMENT

The process of obtaining a nursing license in a new state (when already licensed in one state) is called licensure by endorsement. There are no reciprocal agreements among states that provide for automatically moving licensure from one state to another. Sometimes people incorrectly assume a *reciprocity* among states for nursing licenses. Technically, reciprocity is the type of recognition provided for such items as a driver's license; you can drive in any state as long as your license from your home state is valid. At the time of this writing, there is no reciprocity in regard to nursing licenses. You cannot practice in a state, territory, or Canadian province in which you do not have that jurisdiction's license.

In licensure by endorsement, each case is considered independently, based on the rules and regulations of the state. However, owing to the uniformity of licensing laws throughout most of the United States and its territories, nurses have enjoyed easy mobility between geographical areas.

Because the same licensure examination is used nationwide, no state requires that the examination be retaken. Basic educational and legal requirements must be met. Sometimes a nurse moving to a new state must meet the current criteria for new licensure. In other states, a nurse must fulfill only the requirements that were in effect at the time of the original licensure. A state may require a nurse to meet other criteria, such as those for continuing education, before granting licensure by endorsement. In all cases, appropriate paperwork must be completed, necessary fees paid, and a license obtained before a nurse may begin employment.

If a nurse wishes to maintain licensure in more than one state, this may be done by paying the renewal fees and meeting other requirements for continued licensure, such as continuing education, in each state. Some nurses hold licenses in several different states in order to be able to work as a traveling nurse or to choose work in different locations.

A temporary license, which allows the applicant for licensure by endorsement to be employed while credentials are being verified and processed, is available in some states. Other states require that a permanent license be obtained before any employment is legal in those jurisdictions.

At the present time, North Dakota does not offer straight-forward licensure by endorsement to all nurses licensed in other states. In North Dakota, an associate degree is required for initial licensure as a practical nurse, and a baccalaureate degree is required for initial licensure as a registered nurse. All nurses registered in North Dakota were grandfathered into their licenses when this change in licensure regulations occurred. A registered nurse or licensed practical nurse from another state, who does not have the required degree and who seeks licensure by endorsement in North Dakota, must meet specific conditions and standards identified by the North Dakota Board; the conditions may include enrollment in an educational program to obtain the required degree. Based on individual evaluation, a temporary license may be granted while the individual fulfills the conditions specified for a regular license. North Dakota represents an exception to the general pattern of easy mobility for all registered nurses.

LICENSURE OF GRADUATES OF FOREIGN NURSING SCHOOLS

Graduates of foreign nursing schools who want to practice nursing in the United States must satisfy the Board of Nursing in their state that their education meets state requirements, and they must take the NCLEX-RN examination. To prevent the exploitation of foreign graduates who come to the United States to practice nursing and fail to pass the licensing examination, and to help ensure safety in health care for the U.S. public, the ANA and the NLN have sponsored an independent organization called the Commission on Graduates of Foreign Nursing Schools (CGFNS). This organization administers an examination to foreign-educated nurses that covers proficiency in both nursing and English, and helps the foreign-educated nurse to determine his or her chance of passing the actual licensing examination. Nurses may take the CGFNS examination in their own country, or in selected cities in the United States and Canada.

When there was a nursing shortage during the 1980s in the United States, recruitment of foreign-educated nurses was prevalent. A special regulation allowed these nurses to obtain a H-1A nonimmigrant preference visa from the U.S. Immigration and Naturalization Service, or a work permit from the U.S. Labor Department. The foreign-educated nurse had to pass the CGFNS examination to obtain this visa. Currently there is not a shortage of registered nurses in the United States. Therefore, the ANA and other labor organizations lobbied against renewal of the regulation allowing H-1A nonimmigrant preference work visas for nurses. Because it was not renewed, the general regulation was automatically rescinded, or ''sunsetted'' in September, 1995 (see section on Sunset Laws later in this chapter). H-1B nonimmigrant visas are still available for foreign-educated nurses with a bachelor's degree and experience. There is considerable debate as to what will be the fate of the many foreign-educated nurses in the United States when their work permits expire (Foreign Nurses . . . , 1995).

Many states require that foreign-educated nurses take the CGFNS examination before they are permitted to take the NCLEX examination for licensure. If foreign-educated nurses have not taken the test before emigrating, they must travel to one of the centers in the United States where this test is given. The nursing community has expressed concern about the exploitation of foreign-educated nurses who do not pass the licensing examination and then are employed as unlicensed assistive personnel (Foreign RNs . . . , 1995).

In addition to preparing and administering the CGFNS examination, the CGFNS organization also investigates and validates credentials held by graduates of foreign nursing schools for boards of nursing and other appropriate organizations. Nursing education throughout the world is varied and offers different titles and types of education. Those who are not familiar with a foreign nursing education and licensure system, and who lack foreign language proficiency, may have difficulty interpreting transcripts, diplomas, and other documents, and determining whether the credentials are equivalent to those of the licensed practical nurse or registered nurse in this country. CGFNS maintains current data on nursing around the world and has staff who are involved full time with this process; this enables CGFNS to provide an accurate evaluation of credentials from foreign nursing schools (Schaefer, 1990).

REVOCATION OR LIMITATION OF A LICENSE

A license to practice any occupation becomes a property right of the individual once the state has awarded it. As long as the individual renews a license by paying the appropriate fees and meeting any requirements, such as continuing education, a license cannot be revoked without cause. The possible reasons for revoking or limiting a license are spelled out in the law. (The common reasons were listed earlier, in the discussion of disciplinary action.)

The procedure for revoking a license includes a fact-finding process and a hearing, which functions in many ways like a court proceeding. The state board or a specially designated hearing board is responsible for conducting the hearing and making a decision. The board may provide a license with conditions, suspend a license until certain conditions are met, or revoke a license completely. For example, a nurse faced with charges of chemical dependency might be directed to enter a treatment program, to refuse employment involving direct responsibility for clients or access to drugs, and to be monitored for compliance. If these conditions are met, the individual may then be reinstated to full rights and privileges of licensure when treatment is completed. The board's decision may be appealed in a court of law in most states. The individual being threatened with revocation of a license should have an attorney for legal counsel throughout the proceeding. If a board of nursing finds that the individual's actions constitute a felony, the board is obligated to report that to the criminal authorities for prosecution.

As a licensed professional, you should be aware that you are responsible to your clients and to the state for your practice. You can act to protect your license through maintaining current knowledge and appropriate standards of practice. You should also understand and abide by the scope of practice as described in your individual nurse practice act (Green and others, 1995).

SUNSET LAWS

Most laws remain in effect until the legislature votes to rescind or replace them. Because this has resulted in archaic laws remaining in effect for many years, some states have passed what are known as "sunset laws." Sunset laws provide that any regulatory act, such as the Nurse Practice Act, will automatically be rescinded if not reauthorized. In states with sunset laws, nurses cannot wait for an opportune time to support changes in the Nurse Practice Act. Instead they must identify when sunsetting will occur and work in advance to sustain the current law or make changes. The advantage of sunset laws is that they guarantee that the legislature will review and evaluate agencies and programs.

INTERNATIONAL NURSING LICENSURE

Nursing education and nursing licensure differ greatly throughout the world. In Australia, nursing education has been moved into university settings, and future applicants for licensure in that country will be required to have a university education. In Italy, nursing education is now consolidated under broad programs administered by university nursing departments. The nations of Eastern Europe are facing many drastic changes in their health care systems as they change internally and form different relationships with the West. Nursing education was restricted during Soviet domination and many nurses had limited educational opportunities, with basic nursing education sometimes occurring at the high school level. These nurses are now seeking ways to broaden nursing education in their own countries and to interface with the international nursing community.

Because of these great differences, nursing credentials are not easily transferred internationally. The International Congress of Nurses (ICN) has supported the development of effective licensure legislation worldwide. In 1988, the ICN launched a project called "Nursing Regulation: Moving Ahead," which was funded by the W. K. Kellogg Foundation. This ongoing project has involved nurses and officials from 77 countries in seminars and studies. The publications produced by the project have been used by countries examining regulations involving nursing (Affara & Styles, 1990).

Individuals who are interested in international nursing need to consider their language proficiency and their educational backgrounds. Not all countries welcome nurses educated elsewhere. They may have a surplus of nurses and wish to avoid displacing local nurses. Others are concerned that nurses educated in affluent societies such as the United States and Canada may understand little about the health care needs and nursing practices in a developing country. Organizations actively working in the international health field will usually provide information on opportunities and licensure requirements in various countries. The ICN in Geneva can provide addresses of appropriate governmental authorities to contact regarding licensure in certain countries.

CERTIFICATION IN NURSING

Certification in nursing is primarily a professional, and not a legal, credential. The definition of certification adopted by the Interdivisional Council on Certification of the ANA (1978) states: "Certification is the documented validation of specific qualifications demonstrated by the individual registered nurse in the provision of professional nursing care in a defined area of practice." Certification is available from a variety of professional nursing and health care organizations.

Nurse anesthetists were the first nurses to be certified beyond the basic level. According to the American Association of Nurse Anesthetists (AANA), certified registered nurse anesthetists administer more than half of all anesthetics. Now there are many different kinds of nursing certification.

ANCC Certification

In 1988, the ANA established a credentialing center called the American Nurses' Credentialing Center, which assumed all of the ANA credentialing activities. The ANA invited all other organizations providing credentialing for nurses to join; some organizations joined, but many retained their individual programs.

ANCC certification is a method of recognizing nurses who have special expertise. Applicants must demonstrate current practice and knowledge beyond that required for licensure as a registered nurse. Effective in 1998, as approved by the House of Delegates in 1991, individuals seeking certification as generalists in all specialties will be required to have a baccalaureate in nursing; those seeking certification as specialists or advanced practice nurses will need a master's degree in nursing. These requirements are already in place in many certification programs. After submitting evidence of completing all requirements, a nurse may take the national examination for a specific certification. Certification is granted for a period of 5 years, after which the certification can be renewed by submitting new evidence of current practice and ability. Display 7-3 lists the various certification credentials available from the ANCC.

American Board of Nursing Specialties

In 1991, eight national nursing certification programs joined to establish the American Board of Nursing Specialties. These organizations were: the American Nurses' Credentialing Center of the ANA, the American Board for Occupational Health Nursing, the American Board of Neuroscience Nursing, the Association of Rehabilitation Nurses, the Council on Certification of Nurse Anesthetists, the National Board of Nutritional Support Certification, the Nephrology Nursing Certification Board, and the Orthopaedic Nurses Certification Board. According to their report, these eight organizations represent more than 65% of the total number of registered nurses certified in specialty practice (Specialty Certification . . . , 1991). The goals of this board are to ensure quality in specialty nursing, to improve the public's perception of specialty nurses, and to provide specialty nurses who bring a consistent standard of education and experience to their practice. This is a major breakthrough in the entire certification process for nursing.

Other Certification Programs

Other specialty organizations in nursing also have certification programs (Table 7-3). Most of these are administered by a separately titled and funded certification organization that is

DISPLAY 7-3
Certification Available Through the ANCC

GENERALIST CERTIFICATION

Cardiac Rehabilitation Nurse
College Health Nurse
Community Health Nurse
General Nursing Practice
Gerontological Nurse
Home Health Nurse
Informatics Nurse
Medical-Surgical Nurse
Nursing Continuing Education/Staff Development
Pediatric Nurse
Perinatal Nurse
Psychiatric and Mental Health Nurse
School Nurse

CLINICAL SPECIALIST CERTIFICATION

Adult Psychiatric and Mental Health Nursing
Child and Adolescent Psychiatrc and Mental Health Nursing
Community Health Nursing
Gerontological Nursing
Home Health Nursing
Medical-Surgical Nursing

NURSE PRACTITIONER CERTIFICATION

Acute Care Nurse Practitioner
Adult Nurse Practitioner
Family Nurse Practitioner
Gerontological Nurse Practitioner
Pediatric Nurse Practitioner
School Nurse Practitioner

NURSING ADMINISTRATION CERTIFICATION

Nursing Administration
Nursing Administration, Advanced

American Nurses Credentialing Center, 1996 Certification Catalog, Washington, DC: American Nurses Association, 1996.

TABLE 7-3 Certification Available Through Specialty Organizations*

Certification	Organization
Addictions Nursing (CARN)	CARN Certification, National League for Nursing
Critical Care Nursing (CCRN)	American Association of Critical Care Nurses Certification Corporation
Diabetes Educator (CDE)	National Certification Board for Diabetes Educators
Emergency Nursing (CEN) Flight Nursing (CFRN)	Board of Certification for Emergency Nursing
Enterostomal Therapy (CETN)	Enterostomal Therapy Nursing Certification Board
Gastroenterology (CGC)	Certifying Board of Gastroenterology Nurses and Associates
Hemodialysis Nurse (CHN) Peritoneal Dialysis Nurse (CPDN)	Board of Nephrology Examiners Nursing and Technology
Infection Control (CIC)	Certification Board of Infection Control
Intravenous Nursing (CRNI)	Intravenous Nurses Certification Corporation
Lactation Consultant (IBCLC)	International Board of Lactation Consultants Examiners

Maternal/Child Specialities
   Ambulatory Women's Health Care Nurses (RNC)
   High-risk Obstetric Nurse (RNC)
   Inpatient Obstetric Nurse (RNC)
   Low-Risk Neonatal Nurse (RNC)
   Maternal Newborn Nurse (RNC)
   Neonatal Intensive Care Nurse (RNC)
   OB/GYN Nurse Practitioner (RNC)
   Reproductive Endocrinology/Infertility Nurse (RNC)
	National Certification Corporation for the Obstetric, Gynecologic, and Neonatal Nursing Specialities

Neuroscience Nurse (CNRN)	American Board of Neuroscience Nursing Professional Examination Service
Nurse Administrator—Long-Term Care (RN, C)	Center for Credentialing Services NADONA/LTC Professional Exam Review System
Nurse Anesthetist (CRNA)	Council on Certification of Nurse Anesthetists
Nurse Midwife (CNM)	Association of Certified Nurse Midwives Certification Council
Nutrition Support Nurse (CNSN)	National Board of Nutrition Support Certification
Occupational Health Nursing (COHN)	American Board for Occupational Health Nurses
Oncology Nursing (OCN)	Oncology Nursing Certification Corporation
Ophthalmic Nursing (CRNO)	National Certifying Board for Ophthalmic Registered Nurses
Orthopedic Nursing (ONC)	Orthopaedic Nurse Certification Board
Pain Management (CNOR)	American Academy of Pain Management

Pediatric Specialties
   General Pediatric Nurse (CPN)
   Pediatric Nurse Practitioner (CPNP)
	National Certification Board of Pediatric Nurse Practitioners & Nurses

Perioperative Nurse (CNOR)	National Certification Board of Perioperative Nursing
Plastic and Reconstructive Surgical Nurse (CPSN)	Plastic Surgical Nursing Certification Board
Post-Anesthesia Nurse (CPAN)	American Board of Post-Anesthesia Nursing Certification Professional Examination Service
Rehabilitation Nurse (CRRN)	Rehabilitation Nursing Certification Board
School Nurse (CSN)	National Board for Certification of School Nurses
Urology Nurse (CURN)	American Board of Urologic Allied Health Professionals

*See Appendix B for addresses of organizations.

closely related to the specialty organization. This administrative structure is set up to protect the sponsoring organization from economic liability, to preserve tax-exempt status, and to provide a more objective approach to the credentialing process. Information on any of these specialty certification programs can be obtained by writing directly to the organization (see Appendix B).

The National Association of Pediatric Nurse Associates/Practitioners (NAPNAP) supports independent certification for the pediatric nurse practitioner. This has resulted in two certificates being awarded in the same area by two organizations. NAPNAP and the ANCC have had joint conferences regarding certification, with the hope of developing one jointly sponsored certification; however, fundamental differences still exist between the two organizations on how authority for determining standards should be established.

The Association for Women's Health, Obstetric, and Neonatal Nursing (AWHONN), formerly called the Nurses' Association of the American College of Obstetricians and Gynecologists (NAACOG), sponsors certification for nurses working in women's health care, obstetrics, and neonatal nursing.

The American Association of Critical Care Nurses (AACCN) sponsors certification of nurses in the critical care arena. Their certification confers the title Critical Care Registered Nurse (CCRN). Although this certification is not required to work in critical care, it attests to ongoing practice in critical care, along with continuing education directly related to the critical care field.

The American College of Nurse Midwives sponsors a certification program for nurses specializing in nurse midwifery. Nurses graduating from approved midwifery programs apply for certification through this organization. Approved programs may be at a basic level or at a master's degree level. The license to practice as a midwife depends, however, on the state licensure laws; some states do not allow the practice of nurse midwives. Some state laws recognize the certification as an appropriate credential for practice, and in other states no decision has been made.

Some organizations of health care workers offer credentialing to individuals in specific occupations that may include nurses. For example, the Society of Gastroenterostomal Assistants offers certification to individuals employed in gastroenterology laboratories. This certification is available to both registered nurses and licensed practical nurses. The Association for Practitioners in Infection Control certifies individuals who are professionals in infection control, including physicians, public health officers, and nurses.

Certification and Legal Recognition of Advanced Practice

Some states are using certification as a means of identifying competence in an expanded or specialized role for the registered nurse, and thus are giving legal recognition to the nurse possessing certification. The requirements and methods for obtaining certification remain under the control of the organization granting the certification, but the nurse receives a license from the state to practice in the expanded role. This is true of certified nurse anesthetists, who are all certified through the Council on Certification of Nurse Anesthetists, but who receive legal status to practice in anesthesia by the appropriate authority in their state (which may be the Board of Nursing—however, in some states nurse anesthetists practice under the Board of Medicine).

Titles being used in these expanded roles vary from state to state. Some current titles are advanced practice nurse (APN), advanced registered nurse (ARN), specialized registered nurse (SRN), nurse practitioner (NP), independent nurse practitioner (INP), advanced nurse practitioner (ANP), advanced registered nurse practitioner (ARNP), and certified registered nurse (CRN). In some states, the specialized nurse uses the title of a specific certification, such as family nurse practitioner (FNP) and pediatric nurse practitioner (PNP).

The National Council of State Boards of Nursing (NCSBN) is now working to develop more standardized titling across the states. The NCSBN has also adopted the position that the testing and licensing of nurses in advanced practice is the responsibility of the legal jurisdiction. Therefore, the NCSBN is moving toward the development of a testing program for advanced nursing practice. Those who now certify advanced practice nurses have voiced their opposition to this plan (Boards will weigh . . . , 1996).

Problems Related to Nursing Certification for Advanced Practice

There remain problems and inconsistencies in regard to certification in nursing. These relate to the areas of educational preparation and legal recognition. Programs that prepare nurses in various specialties have lacked uniformity. This is gradually changing as the requirements for certification are becoming more standardized. The situation is reminiscent of the early years of nursing education. In the past, not all specialty certifications have required the same educational, testing, or practice requirements. To remedy this, the American Nurses' Credentialing Center has established the master's degree as the requirement for initial certification of clinical specialists or nurse practitioners (advanced practice nurses), and the baccalaureate degree for initial certification in other specialty practice areas. Those who already are certified will retain certification as long as they continue to meet the practice and continuing education requirements. Increasing numbers of programs that prepare nurses for advanced practice are at the master's degree level. However, some programs that prepare nurses for advanced practice still accept any registered nurse, and are completed in 6 to 9 months. Thus, the same title may not always mean the same thing in terms of educational preparation.

Another problem is the disparity among states credentialing nurses in specialty areas; this hampers mobility and interferes with meeting the health care needs in areas of the United States where nursing specialists are not recognized. Some believe that the recognition of certification programs will help set national standards; when different states adopt the same certification as an appropriate way of credentialing, movement between those states is facilitated.

Also of concern is the proliferation of different titles in different states; many different titles may confuse the public and even those in health care. As legal regulation of advanced practice occurs, systemization of titles is likely to occur through the NCSBN.

THE FUTURE OF CREDENTIALING IN HEALTH CARE

The public, nurses, and other health care professionals, have been confused by credentialing in nursing because it involves so many different aspects of education, licensure, and certification. Because the ideal credential clearly communicates qualifications and competence, it is important for nursing to have a credentialing system that can be understood by others. Current changes are moving nursing closer to having an effective credentialing system.

One area of current study by the NCSBN concerns *multistate licensure* (Boards call. . . , 1996). As the health care system grows more complex, it is not uncommon for a health care-providing organization to operate across state boundaries. *Telenursing* includes the use of telecommunications technology (including the telephone, the facsimile, computers, teleconferencing, interactive television, and the video phone) to provide nursing services to individuals and groups. A telenurse may be in one state, with a client in a distant state; thus, questions regarding licensure requirements for a nurse who serves clients in more than one state have been raised. Does the nurse who provides telephone monitoring and advice for the client in another state need to be licensed in that client's state? This is a complex issue, because state licensing agencies are charged with protecting the public and have legitimate concerns regarding such areas as disciplinary action. Two major approaches to telenursing are being discussed by the NCSBN: rapid endorsement and mutual recognition. A computerized databank is being developed to facilitate rapid processing of endorsement applications and might be the basis for facilitating multistate licensure (Majek, 1996). Mutual recognition would require that states share disciplinary information and also could affect state revenue. The exact nature of multistate licensure must still be worked out by the various states (National Council Begins . . . , 1996).

Many *new health care occupations* related to new procedures and processes in medical care are developing. Those who believe the state should take positive action to protect the public continue to exert pressure to license additional health care providers. Those who oppose credentialing of additional individual groups of health care workers believe that modern-day employers are able to assess workers and to differentiate among them on the basis of competence. Some who oppose credentialing of individual health occupations believe that licensing the institution that hires the employees would be an adequate safeguard for the public.

Another approach to credentialing in health care is *certifying specific competencies* rather than an entire field of practice. Those advocating this approach believe that it would facilitate the development of individuals with a broad range of competencies suited to a particular setting. For example, in a rural area one individual might be certified as competent to perform certain basic x-ray examinations (such as for simple fractures), basic laboratory studies (such as complete blood count and urinalysis) and some basic client care procedures (such as bathing, toileting, feeding, and positioning). Because more complex procedures are sent to a larger center and there is no need for a full-time person in any of these positions, basic care would be made available in a convenient and low-cost manner. Certification of specific competencies by the employing agency is sometimes referred to as *site-based examination* and *site-based certification*. One concern about this method of certifying competencies is the focus on technical skills, without adequate recognition of the knowledge base needed for decision making and judgment. Other concerns are the complexity of keeping track of the many specific competencies, and the difficulty with job mobility when competencies are not standardized.

A *comprehensive reform* of all health care workforce regulation has been proposed by the Center for the Health Professions (Finocchio and others, 1995). Based on a study that was supported by the Pew Charitable Trust, the report titled ''Reforming Health Care Workforce Regulation'' (commonly referred to as one of the ''Pew Reports on Health Care Workforce Regulation''), made ten recommendations for change in regulations. These are found in Display 7-4. These recommendations are based on what is termed a S.A.F.E. focus

DISPLAY 7-4
Recommendations for Reforming Health Care Workforce Regulation

1. Standardize regulatory terms
2. Standardize entry-to-practice requirements
3. Remove barriers to the full use of competent health professionals
4. Redesign health professional board structures and functions
5. Educate the public
6. Collect data on the health professions
7. Develop, implement, and evaluate continuing competency requirements
8. Reform the professional disciplinary process
9. Develop tools to evaluate regulatory effectiveness
10. Understand the organizational context of health professions regulation; develop partnerships to streamline regulatory structures and processes

The Center for the Health Professions. "What's the fuss?" Front & Center, San Francisco: University of California, Summer, 1996.

(*S*tandardized where appropriate, *A*ccountable to the public, *F*lexible to support optimal access, and *E*ffective and *E*fficient in protecting and promoting the public's health, safety, and welfare.) Many of these recommendations, such as educating the public in regard to health professional regulation and collecting data on the health professions, are supported by almost everyone. Others such as developing, implementing, and evaluating continuing competency requirements raise many questions in the minds of both health professionals and regulatory boards.

The National Council of State Boards of Nursing provided leadership in a national meeting in December of 1995 to discuss the Center for Health Professions' recommendations and their implications for nursing regulation. The response of those in attendance was that nursing has been supporting the broad goals of these recommendations and has achieved goals in many areas. However, there was concern that the stated goals are unfocused and go beyond what can be accomplished through regulation alone. Although some of the policy suggestions in the report are controversial, there appeared to be a willingness to engage in constructive dialogue and encourage the participation of legislators, consumers, and health professionals in decision making. In August, 1996 the NCSBN published a detailed response to the Pew Report as a special section in its Issues Newsletter. For each recommendation, a discussion and specific policy option were provided (Lund and others, 1996).

KEY CONCEPTS

- Credentials are written proof of qualifications and may include diplomas conferred by educational programs, certification or registration by professional groups, and legal licenses conferred by governmental agencies.

- Permissive licensure allows for those meeting certain standards to be licensed, whereas mandatory licensure requires that all individuals who wish to practice in the field be licensed to practice.
- Nursing leaders began efforts to obtain legal licensure in 1896. The first permissive licensure law was passed in 1903 by North Carolina, and the first mandatory licensure law was passed in New York in 1947.
- Legal rules governing nursing practice are found in the licensure law passed by a legislative body. Further provisions governing nursing are found in the rules and regulations established by the administrative agency in whom the legislation vests authority.
- The nursing practice act usually contains a definition of nursing, and addresses qualifications for licensure applicants, use of titles, renewal and continuing education requirements, grandfathering, financial concerns, nursing education programs, disciplinary action, violations and penalties, administrative provisions, and expanded nursing roles.
- The Board of Nursing (or its equivalent) is the administrative agency with the authority to carry out the provisions of the Nurse Practice Act.
- A license to practice nursing must be obtained from the state or province in which you wish to work. An initial license is termed licensure by examination and subsequent licenses may be obtained in other jurisdictions through licensure by endorsement.
- The NCLEX-RN examination is administered through a computerized plan that covers the five steps of the nursing process and four areas of client needs, and that identifies competence for entry-level safe nursing care.
- Graduates of foreign nursing schools must have their credentials reviewed and may be required to take the CGFNS examination, which reviews both nursing content and English language ability, before being admitted to take the NCLEX examination.
- A license may be revoked by the State Board of Nursing, a designated disciplinary board, or a court of law based on specific reasons stated in the Nurse Practice Act.
- Certification provides evidence of specialized clinical knowledge and ability beyond the basic level. Certification as a nurse practitioner may be used as a basis for legal approval to practice in an expanded role.
- Concerns about the future of health care worker credentialing include issues of public accountability,

Critical Thinking Activities

1. A student about to graduate from a registered nursing program in New York wishes to practice nursing in New Jersey. Investigate the steps she should take to ensure that she may legally practice nursing in New Jersey as soon (after graduation) as possible.
2. A registered nurse who has been working in Indianapolis, Indiana for 10 years decides to relocate to Orlando, Florida. What are the steps that the nurse should take to ensure that she is able to work as a registered nurse in Florida?
3. A registered nurse with 5 years of general medical-surgical acute care experience is interested in working in the critical care unit of a hospital in your community. Seek information regarding how this nurse could obtain a critical care position in your community. Compare that process with what would be required of you as a new graduate to move into such a position.

text continued

Critical Thinking Activities   (continued)

4. A nurse in your state receives a notification from the Board of Nursing that a complaint has been lodged with the board in regard to her practice. Find out what the process would be in your state for this nurse to respond to the complaint. What resources will this nurse need? What are the possible consequences if the complaint is sustained?

5. Choose an allied health occupation found in a health care facility in which you have clinical practice. Investigate the credentials needed for that occupation and how the credentials would be obtained in your state. Analyze a way in which you could work collaboratively with an individual in this health occupation.

REFERENCES

Affara F, Styles M. Nursing regulation moves ahead. Int Nurs Rev 37(4):307–311, 1990

American Nurses Association. Nursing's Agenda for Healthcare Reform. Washington, DC: American Nurses Publishing Co., 1991

American Nurses Association Congress for Nursing Practice. Suggested State Legislation: Nursing Practice Act, Disciplinary Diversion Act, Prescriptive Authority Act. Kansas City, MO: American Nurses Association, 1990

American Nurses Association. Nursing: A Social Policy Statement. Kansas City, MO: American Nurses Association, 1980

American Nurses Association. The Study of Credentialing in Nursing: A New Approach, vol 1. The Report of the Committee. Kansas City, MO: American Nurses Association, 1978

Bersky A, Brady D. A new generation of competence assessment in nursing: Computerized clinical simulation testing (CST). Issues 14(1):1–8, 1993

Bersky AK, Yocom CJ. Computerized clinical simulation testing: Its use for competence assessment in nursing. Nurs Health Care 15(3):120–127, 1994

Boards will weigh plan to test NPs. Am J Nurs 96(6):69, 73, 1996

Boards call for work to continue on a multistate license for nurses. Am J Nurs 96(10):78, 18, 1996

Finocchio LJ, Dower CM, McMahon T, Gragnola CM, and the Taskforce of Health Care Workforce Regulation. Reforming Health Care Workforce Regulation: Policy Considerations for the 21st Century. San Francisco: Pew Health Professions Commission, 1995

Foreign RNs' fate unclear as visa program ends. Am J Nurs 95(10):77, 80–81, 1995

Green A, Crismon C, Waddill L, Fitzpatrick O. Are you at risk for disciplinary action? Am J Nurs 95(7):36–42, 1995

Lund E, Bouchard J, Graves C, Osman C, VanWingerden C, Bosma J, Creal D, Hutcherson C, Sheets V. National Council of State Boards of Nursing's Response to the Pew Taskforce on Health Care Workforce Regulation. Issues 17(3):Special Section 1–6, 1996

Majek M. Licensure verification process under construction by Boards of Nursing. Issues 17(3):5, 1996

National Council begins revising models for nursing regulation. Issues 17(3):3, 1996

National Council of State Boards of Nursing. Test Plan for the National Council Licensure Examination for Practical Nurses. Chicago: National Council of State Boards of Nursing, 1994a

National Council of State Boards of Nursing. Job Analysis of Newly Licensed Practical/Vocational Nurses. Chicago: National Council of State Boards of Nursing, 1994b

National Council of State Boards of Nursing. Model Nursing Practice Act. Chicago: National Council of State Boards of Nursing, 1994c

National Council of State Boards of Nursing. Model Nursing Administrative Rules. Chicago: National Council of State Boards of Nursing, 1994d

National Council of State Boards of Nursing. Job Analysis of Newly Licensed Registered Nurses. Chicago: National Council of State Boards of Nursing, 1992a

National Council of State Boards of Nursing. Test Plan for the National Council Licensure Examination for Registered Nurses. Chicago: National Council of State Boards of Nursing, 1992b

National Council of State Boards of Nursing. Model Nursing Practice Act. Chicago: National Council of State Boards of Nursing, 1982

New Legislation. The Nursing Commission Newsletter 2(1):2, Olympia, WA: Washington State Department of Health, 1996

Overview of the computerized clinical simulation test (CST) project. Issues 17(1):7-9, 1996

Practice questions: A framework for thinking. Issues 10(3):3-5, 1989

Schaefer B. International credentials review: Crucial and complex. Nurs Health Care 11(8):431–432, 1990

Snyder ME, LaBar C. Issues in Professional Practice, Vol. 1, Nursing: Legal Authority for Practice. Washington, DC: American Nurses Publishing Co., 1984

Specialty certification groups form organization. Am Nurse 23(4):20, 1991

FURTHER READING

American Association of Colleges of Nursing. Position statement: Certification and regulation of advanced practice nurses. Washington, DC: AACN, 1994

Cronenwett LR. Molding the future of advanced practice nursing. Nurs Outlook 43(3):112–118, 1995

Fiesta J. Why nurses lose their licenses, Part I. Nurs Management 24(10):12,14, 1993

Fiesta J. Why nurses lose their licenses, Part II. Nurs Management 24(11):14–15, 1993

Fiesta J. Why nurses lose their licenses, Part III. Nurs Management 24(12):16, 1993

Henry PF. Your due process rights in a disciplinary action. Nurse Pract Forum 2(4):210–211, 1991

Konradi D, Stockert P. Preparing for the NCLEX-RN. Imprint 40(1):6–9, 1993

Parker J. Development of the American Board of Nursing Specialties. Nurs Management 25(1): 33–35, 1994

Spencer-Cisek P, Sveningson L. Regulation of advanced nursing practice: Part two—certification. Oncology Nursing Forum 22(8):39–42, 1995

Wall DM, Miller DE, Widerquist JG. Predictors of success on the newest NCLEX-RN. West J Nurs Res 15(5):628–643, 1993

Legal Responsibilities for Practice

We must be willing to identify the unnecessary, ineffective, and burdensome parts of our (licensing) system and strive to correct the problems. (Schowalter, 1995).

Objectives

After completing this chapter, you should be able to:

1. Identify two general sources of law and describe their differences.
2. Explain the role of institutional policies and protocols in legal decision making.
3. Describe some situations in which nurses may be involved in criminal law.
4. Define liability, identifying situations in which liability is shared by employers or supervisors.
5. State points to be considered in the purchase of professional liability insurance.
6. Explain the most commonly recurring legal issues in nursing.
7. Explain how informed consent, advance directives, and the Patient Self-Determination Act support the patient's rights.
8. Discuss the nurse's responsibility in the specific issues that can constitute malpractice.
9. Identify factors that contribute to a suit being instituted against a health care professional, and explain how an individual nurse might prevent legal suits.
10. Explain the various aspects of testifying for a legal proceeding.

KEY TERMS

Administrative law
Advance directive
Claims brought insurance
Claims occurred insurance

Common law
Court
Criminal law
Deposition

Discovery

Durable power of attorney

Durable power of attorney for health care

Guardian

Informed consent

Liability

Liability insurance

Malpractice

Minor

Negligence

Patient Self-Determination Act

Privileged communication

Regulatory law

Res ipsa loquitor

Statutory law

Suit

Testimony

Tort

L egal issues are those that are decided by law. *Law* includes those rules of conduct or action recognized as binding, or enforced by a controlling authority such as the local, state, or national government. *Ethics* are the principles of conduct governing one's relationships with others—basic beliefs about right and wrong. Legal and ethical issues are often discussed together because of their interrelationships. Ethics and the law go hand in hand, with one supporting the other. Ethics may address questions entirely different from those addressed by the law. In some situations people will find that the law and their own ethical beliefs are divergent; these are the most difficult circumstances in which to make decisions. In this chapter we will focus on how the law affects nursing practice. Ethics are discussed more completely in Chapters 8 and 9.

Examples and situations relating to legal issues are given throughout this chapter to help you understand the specific concepts discussed. Many more factors would be considered in arriving at an actual legal decision than can be presented in a brief paragraph. It is the interaction of multiple factors that makes absolute predictions regarding legal outcomes in specific situations impossible. Specific factual data may contribute to different decisions in cases that appear similar on the surface. Different judges and juries may also interpret facts and law in various ways, resulting in dissimilar outcomes for cases that appear to be alike.

If you have a question about a specific personal situation, you would be well advised to consult an attorney who is experienced in medicolegal matters. The facility where you are employed may have a legal counselor who is available to you. Another source of legal aid is your nurses' association attorney. If you desire private counsel, suitable names may be recommended by your local bar association.

SOURCES OF LAW

There are two general sources of law: statutory law and common law (Fig. 8-1).

Statutory Law

Statutory law is composed of enacted law and regulatory law. *Enacted law* includes laws enacted by a legislative body such as a county or city council, a state or provincial legislature, the U.S. Congress or Parliament; these laws carry the greatest weight in court. The Constitution of the United States is considered statutory law. States, provinces, and other governmental bodies license nurses through statutory nursing practice acts in order to protect

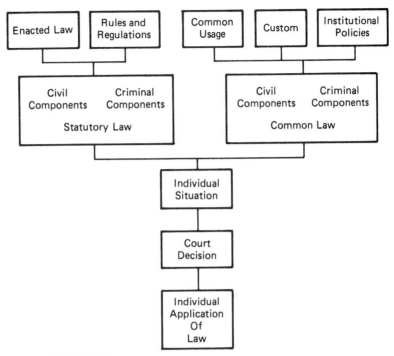

FIGURE 8-1
Civil law and criminal law both may affect a nursing situation.

the public. Through these acts, nurses become legally accountable to patients and to the state for the quality of care provided. See Chapter 7 regarding nursing licensure.

Regulatory law includes the rules and regulations established by governmental agencies to carry out their duties assigned in statutory law. These rules and regulations are sometimes referred to as *administrative law.* Rules and regulations formulated by the State Board of Nursing, and other legally established bodies that regulate nursing practice, are in this category. These agencies are authorized through enacted laws to establish rules and regulations. These rules and regulations must be within the areas addressed in the statutory law. If a board enacted a rule believed to be contrary to an underlying statutory law, an individual affected by the rule could appeal to a court. The court could overturn the rule if the court found it to be outside the scope of, or contrary to, the intent of the enacted law. Unless it is contrary to statutory law, regulatory law has the same force as enacted law.

Common Law

Common law derives from common usage, custom, and judicial decisions or court rulings. Previous judicial decisions or rulings in court cases are used to establish precedents for interpretations of both statutory and common law. Rulings are binding within the jurisdiction of the particular court that determines them, but are used in a more general way (as guidelines) in other jurisdictions. Common law is fluid and cannot be defined with precision. In general, statutory law carries more weight in court than does common law.

The issue of abandonment of a patient illustrates how common law applies to nursing. No statutory laws dictate that a nurse cannot leave a seriously ill patient without ensuring that someone else will provide care, but common practice and custom (which could be supported through the testimony of nurses and other health care workers) require that nurses do not abandon their patients. Failure to meet this standard might be deemed a violation of common law.

Rulings

A *ruling* or *advisory opinion* made by a state board or by an attorney general is an attempt to provide a guideline based on an interpretation of the statutory and common law relative to a specific situation, and is not a final legal decision. Different boards and attorneys general might vary in their opinions. The validity of an opinion only stands until the issue is brought before a court and the court rules on the situation. The final decision in any legal issue rests with a court.

Rights and Responsibilities in Health Care

Rights and responsibilities have both legal and ethical aspects. In the United States, basic rights are specified in the first fourteen amendments to the Constitution; this section of the Constitution is called the Bill of Rights. These rights protect the individual from governmental interference in basic areas of life. From these primary rights, other rights are deduced. For example, although the right to privacy of medical records is not specifically discussed in the Bill of Rights, the right to be secure in one's own home against unreasonable search and seizure is guaranteed; this basic right has led to court decisions supporting the right to privacy regarding one's own affairs, including medical records.

In the United States, because the Constitution is supreme over any other source of law, no statutory or regulatory law may interfere with the rights enumerated in the Bill of Rights. In other countries, rights may be more limited, or may be part of the statutory law enacted by a legislative body that carries less weight than the U.S. Constitution. Some countries have no counterpart to the rights found in the United States.

Some of the rights we speak of are not legally supported, but are based on ethical beliefs. For example, we often speak of a "right to health care." There is no legal basis for this right in the United States, but there are many who believe there is an ethical basis for this right. In some countries, such as Canada and Great Britain, health care is a right supported by the law. In these countries, health care for all has been established through legislation and administrative rules and regulations.

Responsibilities often accompany rights. If a right is guaranteed, the government and designated others have legally mandated responsibilities to ensure that those rights are upheld. In the matter of the right to privacy of medical records, all health care workers have legally mandated responsibilities to ensure that privacy is upheld.

The individual who holds a right may also have responsibilities. These responsibilities are sometimes a matter of ethics, rather than mandated by law. An individual with a right to health care may have the responsibility to use that resource wisely and to cooperate effectively in achieving the desired health outcomes.

The Role of Institutional Policies and Protocols

Institutional policies provide guidance in the proper actions to be taken in specific situations, and identify the individuals responsible for taking action. Established hospital policies may be considered common usage (common law) by the court, and therefore may become important as a basis for legal decisions. Policies may protect the institution itself, and the employees of an institution, from legal difficulties if they are based on current practice and sound legal advice.

Most often policies are developed by members of the hospital staff who have expertise in the practice area under consideration. An attorney may also be consulted to ensure that policies conform to legal requirements. Final approval of policies often rests with the board of trustees, directors, or commissioners who have ultimate responsibility for the financial and legal management of the organization.

Institutional policies are changed in response to new situations and new expectations in society. Usually there is an established institutional route for the change or expansion of a hospital policy. Nurses may be in a position to recognize the need for such a change as they use a policy and compare it with the latest professional information.

A *protocol* or *procedure* provides specific guidelines on performing a task. The purpose of protocols and procedures is to ensure that there is consistent, sound practice in an institution. Just as policies must be updated, so should protocols and procedures.

CLASSIFICATION OF LAWS

Law can be divided into civil and criminal components. Both statutory law and common law may be subdivided in this way.

Criminal Law

Criminal law applies to law that affects the general welfare of the public. A violation of criminal law is called a *crime* and is prosecuted by the government. On conviction, a crime may be punished by imprisonment, parole conditions, a loss of privilege (such as a license), a fine, or any combination of these. The punishment is intended to deter others from committing the crime and to punish the violator.

Civil Law

Civil law applies to laws that regulate conduct between private individuals or businesses. A *tort* is a violation of a civil law in which another person is wronged. Private individuals or groups may bring a legal action to court for breach (or breaking) of civil law. The judgment of the court results in a plan to correct the wrong and may include a monetary payment to the wronged party. Nurses may find themselves involved with both civil and criminal laws, either separately or within the same situation.

CRIMINAL LAW AND NURSING

Because a violation of any law governing the practice of any licensed profession may be a crime, you must be aware of the extent of the Nurse Practice Act. Where the Nurse Practice Act requires that actions (such as administering drugs) be performed only under the direction of a physician, that explicit authorization must exist. Standing orders that refer to specific situations, as well as the usual orders written for an individual patient, may be adequate authorization. However, custom or usual practice will not substitute for the specific authorization required by law. A violation of a professional practice act may be prosecuted as a crime even if no actual harm occurred to the patient.

SITUATION   ## Situation: Violation of a Practice Act

A registered nurse working nights in a nursing home has an elderly resident awake complaining of indigestion. The nurse assesses the resident carefully and determines that this, indeed, appears to be simple indigestion and heartburn. After checking the medication record, the nurse determines that there is no prn order for any type of antacid or other medication that might relieve the resident's distress. She notes that the physician is one who dislikes being called at night and that further, this physician is considered a very approachable individual when she visits residents. The nurse decides to go ahead and give a dose of an antacid and ask the day nurse to call the physician and request a telephone order for the medication.

The Nurse Practice Act does not give the nurse the authority to diagnose disease and prescribe medication, regardless of the situation. The Medical Practice Act and the Nurse Practice Act on Advanced Nursing Practice contain this authorization. This, then, is a violation of the law and is a crime, even though the resident was not harmed.

Violation of laws related to the care and distribution of controlled substances is also a crime.

SITUATION   ## Situation: Violation of Narcotic Laws

In making the routine check of the narcotic record before going off duty, the night nurse notes that the record does not match the actual count of morphine in the supply. She is tired and does not wish to spend the time searching the record and correcting the mistake. Instead, she makes a false entry for a patient who did not receive a narcotic so that the record appears correct.

Because the laws regulating controlled substances are rigid, this would be a violation of the law.

It is costly to the state to undertake criminal prosecution; therefore, even when they are discovered, some violations of criminal law are not prosecuted in court. Knowing this, some nurses make the error of believing that "minor" violations are acceptable. Even when not prosecuted in court, criminal action could result in the loss of a job and in the loss of a license to practice nursing.

Nurses have also been charged with committing such serious crimes as murder and assault while in the role of caregiver. These serious crimes are investigated, prosecuted, and tried by the criminal courts. A license to practice nursing may be temporarily withdrawn while such charges are investigated and tried. If the individual is found innocent, the license may then be restored. If the individual is convicted of the crime, the nursing license may be revoked in addition to sentencing and other penalties.

CIVIL LAW AND NURSING

Civil law relates to legal disputes between private parties. Malpractice actions brought in health care situations involve civil law.

Torts

Torts are civil wrongs committed by one person against another (Bernzweig, 1996). The wrong may be physical harm, psychological harm, or harm to reputation, livelihood, or some other less tangible value. The action that causes a civil wrong may be either intentional or unintentional. An intentional tort is one in which the outcome was planned, although the person involved may not have believed that the intended outcome would be harmful to the other person.

SITUATION   Situation: Intentional Tort

An elderly, somewhat forgetful, but competent resident in a long-term care facility decides not to take an ordered antidepressant medication, although he clearly shows signs of depression. The nurse believes that the patient needs the medication. Therefore, she dissolves it in juice and does not tell the resident. She later informs the resident's son of her action, thinking it will be praised. She is surprised to find the son very angry, and he threatens legal action.

The nurse purposely made the resident take the medication, even though he had refused it. This was her planned intent. Even though she thought it was in the resident's best interests, the resident was wronged in losing his right to informed consent. A court would generally agree that loss of informed consent is a wrong. If legal action is taken, the nurse may be found to have committed an intentional tort (that is, a planned wrong to another person).

An unintentional tort is a wrong committed against another person or property that was not intended to happen. The most common cause of an unintentional tort is negligence.

Negligence

Negligence is the failure to act as a reasonably prudent person would have acted in a specific situation (Guido, 1992). If harm is caused by negligence, it is termed an *unintentional tort*, and damages may be recovered. *Negligence* is a broad term that has many applications in society. All negligence has the following four essential characteristics (Fiesta, 1994):

1. Harm must have occurred to an individual.
2. The negligent person must have been in a situation where he or she had a duty toward the person harmed.
3. The person must be found to have failed to fulfill his or her duty. This is called "breach of duty." This might include either doing what should not have been done (commission of an inappropriate action) or failing to do what should have been done (omission of a necessary or appropriate action).
4. The harm must be shown to have been caused by the breach of duty.

SITUATION **Situation: Negligence**

A homeowner fails to repair a broken step at the entrance to his home. He fails to warn a guest of the broken step, and the guest trips on the broken step in the dark and is injured.

Negligence could be charged: the injury is the harm; the homeowner had a duty toward the guest to safeguard that guest from foreseeable harm; a reasonably prudent person would have repaired the step or at least warned the guest; and the injury can be shown to have been a direct result of the homeowner's failure to act prudently.

Each of these points must be addressed in any legal action. The presence of harm is often clear. For example, if a person fractured a hip, no one would dispute that this was harm. When the harm is so clear, and the responsibility for the harm so straightforward, that anyone would agree on it, the expression *res ipsa loquitur* is used. This is Latin for "the thing speaks for itself." In this case the harm does not need to be "proved" to the court, because all would agree that harm occurred. However, all harm is not so straightforward. For example, when a person claims emotional suffering, the court must determine whether harm actually occurred.

SITUATION **Situation: Res Ipsa Loquitor**

An individual was undergoing surgery. During the surgery, an emergency occurred that demanded a great deal of attention by all of the care providers. During this emergency situation, the failure to complete a count of the sponges used in the open abdomen was overlooked. The wound was closed and the patient transferred to post-anesthesia recovery, and from there to a unit. The wound did not begin to heal but rather showed signs of infection. When this did not clear with treatment, an x-ray of the abdomen was performed and the radiopaque thread in the sponge revealed its position. The patient was returned to surgery and the sponge was removed. If this case were taken to court, the court might well determine that the doctrine of res ipsa loquitor applied. There was a sponge in the abdomen; it was the cause of infection; the sponge could not have gotten in the abdomen except during surgery; and the surgical team was responsible in the operating room for all that occurred to the patient while there. The thing quite literally would speak for itself.

Malpractice

Malpractice is a term used for a specific type of negligence. It refers to the negligence of a specially trained or educated person in the performance of his or her job. Therefore, *malpractice* is the term used to describe negligence by nurses in the performance of their duties.

The definition of malpractice is almost the same as the definition of negligence, with one modification: the professional person must have had a *professional duty* toward the person injured. For example, the nurse was acting as a nurse for the person injured (in either a paid or volunteer capacity). Additionally, the harm that occurred to the injured person or to the property must be based on a failure to act as a reasonably prudent *professional* would have acted in the situation. This is a higher standard than is required of the general public (Bernzweig, 1996). (See Display 8-1).

Just as all parts of the situation are clear in some general negligence situations and not in others, the professional duty is similarly clear in some instances and not in others. The nurse who is assigned to care for a patient in a hospital clearly has a duty to that patient. In some situations, duties overlap and more than one nurse might have a duty toward the same patient; whether a supervisor, another nurse on the unit, or a nurse visitor has a professional duty to a patient might be in dispute. Again, the court would decide whether a duty was present.

A breach of duty, as mentioned earlier, is a failure to act according to the standards of the profession in a particular situation (Fiesta, 1994). To determine that a breach of duty was present, a court must determine what constitutes a professional standard of practice for that situation.

The final question becomes one of identifying the cause of the harm that occurred. Malpractice is only present if a breach of duty was the cause of the harm. In the case of the sponge left in the abdomen: if the nurses failed to complete a sponge count, the failure to safeguard the patient (breach of duty) could be shown to be a direct cause of the infection (the harm). The cause of harm is not always so clear and may be part of the dispute in a legal action. Remember that, as discussed earlier in the chapter, a breach of duty may be either the ommission of a correct action or the commission of an incorrect action (Fig. 8-2).

DISPLAY 8-1
Essential Elements of Malpractice

- Harm to an individual
- Duty of a professional toward an individual
- Breach of duty by the professional
- Breach of duty as the cause of harm

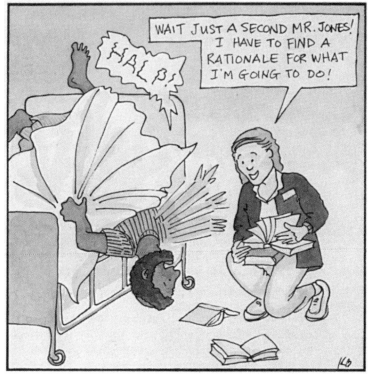

FIGURE 8-2
A reasonably prudent nurse uses common sense as well as nursing theory.

SITUATION **Situation: Omission of Correct Action**
An elderly, disoriented person is admitted to an acute care facility. The nurse fails to establish a plan for monitoring and maintaining safety for this person. The patient falls out of bed during the night, sustaining a fractured hip.

This could be found to be malpractice. The nurse was working in a professional capacity and had a duty to this patient. The patient can be shown to have sustained an injury. It may be demonstrated through testimony by nurses and reference to standard nursing texts that a reasonably prudent registered nurse would have been expected to take action to protect this patient from falls. It was the nurse's failure to act that caused the fall and fracture. This failure to act could constitute malpractice.

SITUATION **Situation: Commission of Inappropriate Action**
A postoperative patient has an order to ambulate. The nurse assigned to this patient finds that the patient's condition has changed drastically since the order was written. The patient has a

fever and a rapid pulse and is complaining of severe abdominal pain. The nurse proceeds to have the patient ambulate. The patient faints, sustaining a head injury in the fall. This necessitates additional hospitalization, x-ray films, and diagnostic procedures.

Again, this could be found to be malpractice. The nurse was working as a professional with a duty to this patient. The patient can be shown to have sustained an injury. It may be demonstrated that a reasonably prudent nurse would have recognized that the change in the patient's condition called for altering the plan of care and not ambulating at this time. This was the breach of duty. Ambulating the patient in that condition was the cause of the fall and the head injury. Therefore, malpractice could be found, owing to inappropriate action on the part of the nurse.

LIABILITY

A *liability* is an obligation or debt that can be enforced by law. In the case of malpractice, a person found guilty of any tort (whether intentional or unintentional) is considered legally *liable*, or legally responsible, for the outcome. The person legally liable usually is required to pay for damages to the other person. These may include actual costs of care, legal services, loss of earnings (present and future), and compensation for emotional and physical stress suffered. Although liability is legally determined by a court, an individual who believes that he or she would be held legally liable if a court were consulted, may agree to pay damages (or that individual's insurance company may agree to pay) without actually going to court. This may be done even when the person denies true negligence or malpractice, but chooses to settle the issue because a court case would be more costly than the damages to be paid.

LIABILITY INSURANCE

Liability insurance transfers from the individual to a large group the legal costs and any settlement related to a suit. The expectation is that most individuals will not be sued, and that the pool of premiums will therefore adequately cover the costs of those who are sued, the administrative costs of managing the policies, and the profit for the insurance company. The individual benefits by transferring risk from himself or herself to the insurance company for the cost of the insurance policy.

A liability insurance crisis exists in the United States. The cost of liability insurance for some health care providers has escalated at an extraordinary rate. Some of the factors that have caused this to happen are the large judgments that have been made, the number of suits that have been brought, the large fees that attorneys receive, and the high profits of insurance companies. Nurses in independent advanced practice have been especially affected by the increase in premiums, because their incomes have traditionally been moderate and they cannot charge fees sufficient to cover insurance costs that may equal those of physicians. Nurses who are employed in more traditional settings are able to obtain malpractice insurance for a modest cost.

The American Nurses Association (ANA) has initiated a data bank related to legal claims against nurses. The organization is asking all registered nurses to provide information to it regarding legal action in which they have been named as a defendant. The ANA's purpose is to have adequate records to support its contention that the low level of suits against nurses in all areas of practice should translate into low-cost liability insurance.

Some states have initiated legislation that allows for awards to cover actual losses and costs of care, while limiting awards for pain and suffering and other nontangible factors. Sometimes this legislation has been accompanied by restrictions on insurance company rates. Some laws are also being amended to restrict the monetary liability of any party according to the percentage of responsibility. For example, if damages were set at $10,000 and each of two defendants were determined to be responsible for 50% of the problem, one party could not be made to pay more than $5,000, even if the other party had no assets and could not pay. Liability laws continue to be a major concern for nurses because nurses are being named in an increasing number of suits.

Institutional and Individual Insurance

Many hospitals and other institutional employers carry liability insurance that covers both the institution and its employees. Some hospitals may limit the coverage that their policies provide for individual employees in an effort to hold down costs.

Even if an employer carries liability insurance, it is often advisable for the individual professional to carry an independent policy. An independent policy may cover the person in voluntary activities as well as on the job. It also will follow the person who moves from one employer to another. If a legal action is instituted against the professional, the individual liability insurance policy may provide independent legal counsel.

Some nurses state that they do not carry insurance because it might encourage people to bring suit against them. They are under the mistaken assumption that persons will not sue if it means financial hardship for the person being sued; most individuals who sue do not know whether a nurse carries individual insurance. In addition, insurance is not the only source of payment for a judgment. Judgments may be levied against most tangible assets, including houses, cars, and savings; judgments also may be levied against future earnings. Married nurses who reside in community property states should realize that one half of the assets of a family may be vulnerable to a judgment. Community property states at this time include Arizona, California, Idaho, Louisiana, Nevada, New Mexico, Texas, and Washington. These factors combine to support the need for the individual professional to carry liability insurance that will provide legal counsel and protection in the case of any judgment.

Analyzing Insurance Coverage

Individual liability insurance for registered nurses is available from a variety of insurance companies (directly through their agents) and through professional organizations that offer coverage as a service to members. When investigating individual liability insurance, ask the agent or company the following questions:

1. In what situations would I, as an individual, be covered?
2. In what situations would I not be covered?

3. How is my coverage affected by my actions? For example, if I failed to follow hospital policy, would I still be covered?
4. What are the monetary limits of the policy?
5. Does the policy provide me with an attorney?
6. Is the policy renewable at my option? What factors affect renewability?
7. Does the insurance cover incidents that occurred while the policy was in force, regardless of when the claim is brought (*claims occurred insurance coverage*), or does it cover incidents only if I am currently insured (*claims brought insurance coverage*)?
8. What is the cost compared with other policies?

Asking these questions will help you to compare policies from different insurance carriers. When coverage appears equal, you might ask how long a company has been in business and how long it has been providing nursing liability insurance. You will want to be insured with a reliable, stable company.

Liability insurance coverage that is carried by the hospital should be just as carefully investigated by the nurse employee. Questions 1 through 4 above apply to institutional insurance policies as well as to individual insurance policies. In addition, you should ask the following questions about an institutional policy:

1. Does the policy provide me with a personal attorney, or will the same attorney be working for the hospital?
2. At what point would the hospital no longer be responsible and would I become personally responsible?
3. How would my job be affected if a lawsuit were filed or payment awarded based on an action against me? (Check institutional policy as well as the insurance company policy.)
4. Does the insurance company have the right to seek restitution from me if it pays a claim based on my actions?

It is important that you have accurate answers to these questions so that you can make an informed decision regarding your need for an individual policy.

Insurance Cost and Coverage

The ANA has a group policy providing $500,000 per claim and $1 million total in 1 year as basic coverage for the registered nurse. Optional higher limits are available. The cost for basic coverage in 1996 was approximately $89 per year. Inflation can be expected to increase this cost. Since the 1970s, the cost of the basic coverage provided by the ANA policy rose from approximately $12 per year to its current amount. Several commercial companies offer liability insurance policies with comparable rates. These are often advertised in nursing journals.

As previously stated, liability insurance coverage for specialty practice as a nurse practitioner, nurse anesthetist, or nurse midwife is much more expensive. Group policies are available for some of these individuals through professional organizations. Some individuals are covered by institutional policies and do not try to maintain individual policies.

National Data Bank

In the United States the federal government is now maintaining a "National Data Bank" on licensed health care providers. This is separate from and has a purpose different from the data being collected by the ANA. By law, all judgments, settlements paid, or convictions for malpractice, and all situations in which a health care provider's privileges to practice are curtailed or withdrawn, must be reported to this data bank. All institutions must consult this data bank for information before giving any health care provider privilege to practice in the institution. The purpose of the National Data Bank is to protect the public from incompetent professionals who continue to practice by moving from one place to another.

LEGAL ISSUES IN NURSING

Some legal issues recur frequently in nursing practice. It is wise for the nurse to try to understand these particular issues as they relate to individual practice.

Personal Liability

As an educated professional, you are always legally responsible or liable for your actions (Bernzweig, 1995). Thus, if a physician or supervisor asks you to do something that is contrary to your best professional judgment and says, "I'll take responsibility," that person is acting unwisely. The physician or supervisor giving the directions may be liable if harm results, but that would not remove your personal liability.

SITUATION   **Situation: Personal Liability**

The registered nurse giving medications on a large medical unit notes that an order for digoxin (a heart medication) is considerably larger than the usual dose. She looks up the medication in a reference book and finds that she is correct about the dosage. The ordered dose is several times the usual dose. The nurse then calls the supervisor and explains the situation.

The supervisor double checks the order with the registered nurse and then states: "Dr. Jones is an outstanding physician. I am sure he has a good reason for ordering this dose. Go ahead and give the medication as ordered. I'll take responsibility." The nurse then gives the medication, and the patient suffers a toxic reaction.

The registered nurse could be held liable for giving the incorrect amount of medication. She had the knowledge and judgment to recognize that the dose was much larger than usual, and she failed to check with the physician. A statement by the supervisor does not remove the nurse's personal responsibility for her own actions. Because even a competent physician might make an error, the nurse had a responsibility to clarify the order. The supervisor and the physician could be held liable in addition to the nurse, but not instead of her.

Although each person is legally responsible for his or her own actions, the example above illustrates that there are also situations in which a person or organization may be held liable for actions taken by others.

Employer Liability

The most common situation in which a person or organization is held responsible for the actions of another is in the employer–employee relationship. In many instances, an employer can be held responsible for torts committed by an employee. This is called the doctrine of *respondeat superior* (let the master respond). The law holds the employer responsible for hiring qualified persons, for establishing an appropriate environment for correct functioning, and for providing supervision or direction as needed to avoid errors or harm. Therefore, if a nurse, as an employee of a hospital, is guilty of malpractice, the hospital may also be named in the suit. The employer's liability may exist even if the employer appears to have taken precautions to prevent error.

It is important to understand that this doctrine does not remove any responsibility from the individual nurse, but it extends responsibility to the employer in addition to the nurse. If, for example, a hospital has a procedure that does not conform to good nursing practice as you know it, and you follow that procedure, you will still be liable for any resulting harm. You are expected to use your education and experience to make sound judgments regarding your work.

SITUATION **Situation: Employer Responsibility for a Staff Nurse**

A nurse working in a long-term care facility is responsible for planning and coordinating the care of a severely debilitated resident. This elderly man is totally dependent for all activities of daily living due to a recent stroke. He is not eating and drinking adequately. He faints and is discovered to have very low blood pressure and a rapid weak pulse. He is sent to the local hospital, where he is admitted for dehydration secondary to inadequate fluid intake. Investigation reveals that no assessment of his fluid or nutritional status has been recorded, nor was there any plan to ensure that nutritional and fluid needs were met.

Both the nurse and the long-term care facility in this situation might be found liable for harm that resulted. The nurse had a personal, professional responsibility to accurately assess the resident and to institute care to meet his basic needs. The facility also had a responsibility to make sure that policies, procedures, and protocols were in place to ensure appropriate assessment and care, and that employees followed through on them.

Charitable Immunity

In some states, nonprofit hospitals have "charitable immunity." This means that the non-profit hospital cannot be held legally liable for harm done to a patient by its employees. The employees of that nonprofit hospital are still legally liable for their own actions. The trend in legislation is toward the repeal of laws providing for charitable immunity. Those active in the consumer movement have argued that no institution should be relieved of responsibility in such a blanket fashion. If you are employed by a nonprofit institution, it is important that you know whether the law in your state provides charitable immunity for the institution.

Supervisory Liability

When a nurse is in the role of charge nurse, head nurse, supervisor, or any other role which involves supervision or direction of other people, the nurse is potentially liable for the actions of others. The supervising nurse is responsible for exercising good judgment in a supervisory role. This includes making appropriate decisions about assignments and delegation of tasks. If an error occurs and the supervising nurse is shown to have exercised sound judgment in all decisions made in that capacity, the supervising nurse may not be held liable for the error of a subordinate. If poor judgment was used in assigning an inadequately prepared person to an important task, the supervisory nurse might be liable for resulting harm. The extent of the subordinate's responsibility would depend on his or her level of education and training. Persons with insufficient education or training might not be liable for some errors; the more education subordinates have, the more likely they will be liable.

SITUATION   **Situation: Supervisory Responsibility for an Educated Staff Member**

Two sudden admissions to the coronary care unit create a situation in which additional help is needed to care for the patients in the unit.

The staff supervisor calls the person whose name appears first on the list of temporary placement registered nurses. This nurse agrees to come in immediately. The nurse is not asked whether she has education or experience in coronary care, nor does she volunteer this information. She has no background or experience in coronary care; however, she is assigned to this unit because of the need for additional help.

While working in the coronary care unit, the temporary nurse is assigned the complete care of two patients. Because of her inability to read the monitors, a potentially life-threatening problem is not identified until the patient "arrests." Resuscitation efforts are successful, but the patient suffers some brain damage.

Both the staffing supervisor who placed the inadequately prepared nurse in the unit, and the temporary nurse herself, could be found liable—the supervisor for incorrectly assigning the nurse, and the nurse for not recognizing her own limitations. The educational preparation of the temporary nurse gave her the background to understand that expertise was needed in this situation, and that she did not possess that expertise. If the situation were changed so that the temporary nurse was reviewed for expertise in coronary care and found to have that expertise, then the supervisor might not be liable for the error of the temporary nurse. The supervisory function of ascertaining level of preparation and ability to meet the standards of the job would have been carried out.

Situation: Supervisory Responsibility for Staff Member With Limited Education

The evening nursing supervisor is responsible for adjusting personnel assignments when employees are absent. She decides to send an extra nursing assistant to the emergency department to assist. This nursing assistant has never been assigned to the emergency department before and has no education or training other than the orientation to basic patient care given by the hospital. The supervisor instructs the nursing assistant to take care of the desk and answer the phone while others are busy.

While the nursing assistant is alone at the desk, a family enters the emergency department with an infant in acute distress. The nursing assistant instructs the family to sit down and wait until a nurse comes out of one of the rooms.

It is a long time before a nurse appears and care for the infant is instituted. The infant has a complicated recovery that is later shown to be due to the delay in initial treatment.

The supervisor might be found negligent in this case for assigning the nursing assistant to emergency department duties without proper direction or supervision. The nursing assistant might not be found negligent because she had no basis for recognizing the seriousness of the situation or for recognizing her own lack of ability to meet the responsibilities involved in being at the desk in an emergency department.

Duty to Report or Seek Medical Care for a Patient

A nurse who is caring for a patient has a legal duty to ensure that the patient receives safe and competent care. This duty requires that the nurse maintain an appropriate standard of care and also that the nurse take action to obtain an appropriate standard of care from other professionals when that is necessary. For example, if a nurse identifies that a patient needs the attention of a physician, and fails to make every effort to obtain that attention, the nurse has breached a duty to the patient.

Situation: Failure to Seek Medical Care for Patient

The registered nurse is caring for a postoperative patient during the night. The patient's blood pressure begins to drop and the pulse begins to rise. The nurse's assessment indicates that the patient may be bleeding internally. The nurse institutes a plan for close nursing monitoring and calls the surgeon to describe the situation. The surgeon gives a telephone order to increase the intravenous fluid rate and states that he will see the patient in the morning. The patient's condition continues to deteriorate, but the nurse does nothing further to ensure that a physician examines the patient.

If the outcome is unfavorable, the nurse can be found to have breached a duty to the patient. The patient relies on the nurse to provide appropriate care and to identify when a physician is needed. The nurse could have made other telephone calls to the surgeon and failing the success of that, could have followed the facility's procedure for asking another physician (such as the emergency department physician) to see the patient.

The nurse has a duty to continue all efforts to obtain appropriate medical care for the patient. If the nurse had followed all procedures, sought another physician, and continued efforts when initial attempts were unsuccessful, the nurse would not have breached a duty. The nurse cannot guarantee a physician's care but can guarantee that the patient will not be left without an advocate.

Confidentiality and Right to Privacy

Confidentiality and the right to privacy with respect to one's personal life are basic concerns in our society. All information regarding a patient belongs to that patient. This right has been inferred from interpretation of the federal constitution, but is explicitly stated in some state laws.

In theory, this right should protect a patient's privacy. However, third party payers (such as insurance companies and HMOs) will not reimburse for care if they do not receive the records they request. The result is that patients must frequently sign statements giving blanket approval for all information to be sent to the third party payer. They may be unaware of exactly what information is sent or who may see it.

When computerized records are transmitted to insurance companies, they no longer contain only a brief statement of diagnosis and treatment; they may contain detailed accounts of interactions between a patient and a mental health professional, health information of a sensitive nature, and genetic information that could be used inappropriately. Because increased use of computerized records can result in easier retrieval and cross-referencing of records from a variety of sources, the general public, health care providers, and government officials are becoming more concerned about potential invasions of privacy.

A nurse who gives out information without authorization from the patient or from the legally responsible guardian can be held liable for harm that results. If you have any question about who the legally responsible guardian of a patient is, be sure to consult with your administrative authority. There may be a court-appointed legal guardian, or the situation may be governed by specific state laws regarding who becomes the responsible guardian when the person is unable to give personal consent. The hospital administration should be able to ascertain the correct guardian.

Only those professional persons involved in the patient's care who have a need to know about the patient can be allowed routine access to the record. A physician who is not involved in the patient's care or who does not have an administrative responsibility relative to that care is not allowed routine access. Persons not involved in care can only be allowed access to the record by specific written authorization or by court order. You should be cautious about what information you share verbally and with whom.

A directory information policy has been adopted by many acute care hospitals. This policy gives specific guidelines regarding what may be revealed according to freedom of information laws, and does not violate confidentiality; usually a patient's name and sex, and a general statement of condition (satisfactory, serious, and so on) may be revealed. This is a wise standard for general hospitals and nursing homes with no written policy to follow. In some instances, especially those involving treatment for alcoholism, drug abuse, and acquired immunodeficiency syndrome, even revealing the information that an individual is hospitalized is considered a legal violation of confidentiality.

Medical records professionals state that it is not uncommon for attorneys, family members, media representatives, or law enforcement officials to request access to patient records or specific patient information without having express consent of the patient or a legal court order to view the records or be given information. Those unfamiliar with laws regarding privacy sometimes reveal information inappropriately. If you are ever approached for patient information by someone who purports to have authority, your best course of action is to refer that individual to appropriate administrative personnel who can determine the validity of the request.

A new concern is that more health care agencies are using fax machines to send patient information to one another. Faxes have a legitimate purpose in that continuity of care is enhanced when information is shared. When you send a document by fax machine, however, you may not assure that confidentiality is maintained. Some facilities have a policy requiring that you call ahead and designate a specific person who is to be present to receive the fax. The cover page often states that this is confidential material and should not be read by anyone other than the designated recipient. If your facility or agency has no policy regarding the safeguarding of faxed information, you would be wise to raise the concern.

Other new areas of concern are the Internet and e-mail. Through these avenues, a health care provider may consult with other professionals to provide the best diagnostic and treatment services to the patient. However, on-line computer communications are not private. Those with the necessary skill may intercept and read any e-mail or Internet message. Therefore, the identity of patients must be protected in any such communication.

SITUATION   ## Situation: Breach of Confidentiality

A nurse in a small community hospital discusses with a friend the admission of a woman community member for treatment of cancer. The nurse's friend then talks to others, who talk to still others, until there is widespread knowledge of the patient's cancer in the community. The woman's daughter hears about her mother's cancer diagnosis at school and is very upset.

The nurse could be held liable for revealing this information in a suit charging breach of privacy and confidentiality. The harm is the emotional distress to the woman and her family. If the breach of confidentiality could be traced to the nurse's conversation, the nurse's action would be considered the direct cause of harm.

Defamation of Character

Any time that shared information is detrimental to a person's reputation, the person sharing the information may be liable for defamation of character. Written defamation is called libel. Oral defamation is called slander. Defamation of character involves communication that is malicious and false. Sometimes such comments are made in the heat of anger. Occasionally statements written in a patient's chart are libelous. Severely critical opinions may be stated as fact. An example of such a statement might be ''The patient is lying,'' or ''The patient is rude and domineering.'' Patients may charge that comments in the chart adversely affected their care by prejudicing other staff against them. The prudent nurse will chart only objective information regarding patients and give opinion in professional terms, well documented with fact. A chart might read: ''The patient states. . . Observation reveals . . .''; this provides factual information for the reader without making potentially libelous accusations. In conversations, the prudent nurse avoids discussing patients.

SITUATION   ## Situation: Slander

Two registered nurses are leaving the floor for their coffee break. They are discussing the patients in their care as they wait for the elevator. They enter the elevator with a number of other people and continue their conversation. The first nurse says: "That Mrs. Johnson in room 201. I don't know whether I can take another day of her! She's impossible!" The other nurse replies: "I know just what you mean. I had her last week and she was just on the bell all the time. If you ask me, there's nothing wrong with her that a good swift kick wouldn't cure!" First nurse: "Do you really think she's faking?" Second nurse: "I'm sure of it. Have you ever watched her when her husband comes to visit?"

A relative of the patient is one of the people in the elevator and overhears the conversation. The relative reports the conversation to the patient.

If the patient brings suit, the nurses involved might be found guilty of slander. The nurses were discussing the patient in a place where others could hear the conversation. The comments clearly identified the patient, reflected opinions that were not supported with fact, and potentially could jeopardize the patient's reputation and standing in the community.

Defamation of character also may be charged by a health care provider who believes that statements made by another professional are false, malicious, and have caused harm. There are accepted mechanisms for confidentially reporting inappropriate care or errors; these should be used, and critical statements to uninvolved third parties should not be made. In many states, licensed professionals are required to report poor practice or illegal acts on the part of other professionals. Criticism reported without malice and in good faith, through the appropriate channels, is protected from legal action for defamation.

Privileged Information

Privileged communication refers to information shared with certain professionals that does not need to be revealed even in a court of law. All states consider certain types of communication (between client and attorney, between patient and doctor, or between an individual and a member of the clergy) privileged. Not all states recognize the nurse–patient relationship as one in which privileged communication takes place; even those states that recognize nurse–patient communication as potentially privileged do not consider *all* communication between patients and nurses privileged. It is important that you understand that privilege is a limited concept. Only a court can determine if privilege exists in any specific case. If a court does not determine information to be privileged, then you are legally obligated to testify about the communication.

Informed Consent

Every person has the right to either consent to or refuse medical treatment.

LEGAL REQUIREMENT

The law requires that a person give voluntary and informed consent to treatment. *Voluntary* means that no coercion exists; *informed* means that a person clearly understands the choices being offered. Included in the discussion must be the alternatives for treatment, the risks of any treatment proposed, the relative value of any treatment proposed, and the risks of not having treatment. This consent may be either verbal or written. Written consent usually is preferred in health care to ensure that a record of consent exists, although a signature alone does not prove that the consent was informed. A blanket consent for "any procedures deemed necessary" is not usually considered adequate consent for specific procedures. The form should state the specific proposed medical procedure or test.

The patient's medical condition usually is not accepted by the courts as a valid reason for not giving the patient complete and accurate information. Currently, there are no clear guidelines as to what constitutes complete information. Courts have generally supported the idea that usual risks need to be disclosed, but that rare or unexpected risks do not have to be discussed.

The law places the responsibility for obtaining consent for medical treatment on the physician. It is the physician's responsibility to provide appropriate information, and he or she is liable if the patient charges that appropriate information was not given.

A nurse may present a form for a patient to sign, and the nurse may sign the form as a witness to the signature. This does not transfer the legal responsibility for informed consent for medical care to the nurse. If the patient does not seem well informed, the nurse should notify the physician so that further information can be provided to the patient; although the nurse would not legally be liable for the lack of informed consent, the nurse has ethical obligations to assist the patient in exercising his or her rights and to assist the physician in providing appropriate care.

ADVANCE DIRECTIVES

Advance directives are legal documents attesting to the wishes of an individual in regard to health care in situations in which he or she is no longer capable of giving personal informed consent. They are completed in "advance" of the situation in which they might be needed, and "direct" the actions of others. There are several types of advance directives. A living will provides information on general preferences regarding end-of-life issues.

A *durable power of attorney for health care* is a document that legally designates a decision-maker should the person be incapacitated. This document may also contain specific advance directives such as whether tube feedings, intravenous fluids and nutrition, ventilator support, and other such treatments should be instituted if the individual is found to be terminally ill or in a persistent vegetative state.

In 1990, the Patient Self-Determination Act (PSDA) was passed by the U.S. Congress. It took effect in 1992, and required that on admission to any health care service (hospital, long-term care center, or home care agency) patients be given an opportunity to determine what lifesaving or life-prolonging actions they want to be carried out. The agency must provide adequate information for the individual to make an informed decision regarding these important matters. As a result of this legislation, agencies reviewed and revised policies and protocols regarding consent. In many agencies, a nurse has the responsibility to provide the education and obtain a signature on a document indicating preferences.

Information regarding the results of the PSDA is being analyzed by several government agencies to determine whether there has been a change in practice. Some have suggested that the manner in which self-determination and the possible alternatives are explained greatly influences patient choices; one suggestion has been that these matters first be discussed in the health care provider's office, before admission. When this is possible, it allows for more time to consider alternatives and consult significant others. The final decision is then made away from the pressure of the health care environment. (See Chapter 10 for a further discussion of planning for end-of-life issues.)

CONSENT FOR NURSING MEASURES

Nurses must obtain a patient's consent for nursing measures undertaken. This does not mean that exhaustive explanations need to be given in each situation, because courts have held that patients can be expected to have some understanding of usual care. Consent for nursing measures may be verbal or implied. The nurse may ask, "Are you ready to ambulate now?" The patient answers, "Certainly," providing verbal consent. Alternatively, the nurse may state, "I have the injection the doctor ordered for you. Will you please turn over?" If the patient turns over, this is implied consent.

The nurse should remember that the patient is free to refuse any aspect of care offered. However, like the physician, the nurse is responsible for making sure that the patient is informed before making a decision. Good nursing care requires that you use all means at your disposal to help the patient comprehend the value of proposed care. For example, the postoperative patient needs to understand that getting into a chair is part of the plan of care, not a convenience for the nurse or simply a change to prevent boredom. Thus, a patient's refusal of care is accepted only after the patient has been given complete information.

COMPETENCE TO GIVE CONSENT

A person's ability to make judgments based on rational understanding is termed *competence*. Dementia, developmental disabilities, head injuries, strokes, and illnesses creating loss of consciousness are common causes of an inability to make judgments. Determining competence is a complex issue. Illness, age, or condition alone do not determine competence. Legal competence is ultimately determined by the courts. The general tendency of the courts has been to encourage whatever decision making an individual is capable of, and to restrict personal decision making as little as possible.

When a person is legally determined to be incompetent, consent is obtained from a legal guardian. A legal guardian is constrained from making some types of decisions. For example, if the health care action could be identified as injurious to the individual involved, a court may need to be consulted regarding consent. An example of this would be the discontinuation of dialysis for an incompetent individual; when such an individual leaves no clear advance directive regarding such a situation, the health care providers might insist on getting a court decision before accepting the consent of the guardian to terminate the dialysis.

Health care providers often encounter those for whom no legal determination of competence has been made, but who do not seem able to make an informed decision; examples include the very confused elderly person, the inebriated person, and the unconscious person. The law in each state specifies who is allowed to give consent in such situations. There are also guidelines to follow in determining that a person cannot give his or her own consent. Your facility policy should contain directions to guide you in obtaining legal consent; if it does not, you should consult an administrative person for a decision. Determining who is able to give legal consent in such a situation is not a nurse's responsibility.

If a person truly is not capable of making decisions, the nurse should attempt to present necessary nursing actions in a way that elicits cooperation and avoids confrontation over decisions. Competence may change from day to day, as a person's physical illness changes; an individual may be competent to make some decisions, such as ''I don't like rice and I won't eat it!,'' but incompetent to make other decisions—for example, decisions regarding financial matters. These changes in competence require care providers to adjust their own planning to incorporate patient self-determination whenever possible, even when the person is legally incompetent.

WITHDRAWING CONSENT

Consent may be withdrawn after it is given. People have the right to change their minds. Therefore, if after one intravenous infusion a patient decides not to have a second one started, that is his or her right. As a nurse, you have an obligation to notify the physician if the patient refuses a medical procedure or treatment.

CONSENT AND MINORS

The consent of a minor usually is given by a parent or legal guardian. You should also obtain the minor's consent when he or she is able to give it. Increasingly, courts are emphasizing that minors be allowed a voice when it concerns matters that they are capable of understanding. This is especially true for the adolescent, but this consideration should be given to any child who is 7 years of age or older. When a minor refuses care and the legal guardian has authorized that care, you should not proceed until legal clarification is given. Your nursing supervisor should be consulted.

Minors who live apart from their parents and are financially independent, or who are married, are termed *emancipated minors*. In most (but not all) states an emancipated minor can give consent to his or her own treatment. Some states have specific laws allowing minors to give personal consent (without also obtaining parental consent) for treatment of sexually transmitted disease, or for obtaining birth control information and supplies. You should be sure of the law in your own state if you practice in an area where this is a concern. Most institutions have developed policies to guide employees in making correct decisions in this and other areas dealing with consent.

Emergency Care

Care in emergencies has many legal repercussions, therefore, the judgment that an emergency exists is important. Certain actions may be legal in emergencies and not legal in non-emergency situations. In emergencies, the standard procedures for obtaining consent may be impossible to follow. Further, in emergencies, personnel must sometimes take on responsibilities that they would not undertake in a non-emergency situation. Critical thinking on the part of all health care professionals is essential when differentiating an emergency from a nonemergency.

Most facilities that provide emergency care have policies and procedures designed to ensure that there is adequate support for claiming that an emergency exists. Thus, the policy will often state that at least two physicians in the emergency department must examine the patient and concur that the emergency requires immediate action, without waiting for consent. This ensures maximum legal protection for the physician and the institution.

CONSENT IN EMERGENCIES

If a true emergency exists, consent for care is considered to be implied. The law holds that if a reasonable person were aware that the situation was life threatening, he or she would give consent for care. An exception to this is made if the person has explicitly rejected such care in advance; an example is a Jehovah's Witness carrying a card stating his personal religion, and that he does not wish to receive blood or blood products. This is one reason emergency department nurses should check a patient's wallet for identification and information related to care; if this is done with another person, and a careful inventory of contents is made and signed by both, there should be little concern about liability in taking emergency action.

STANDARDS OF PRACTICE AND EMERGENCIES

Standards of practice in emergencies also differ from those in non-emergency situations. In hospital emergencies, the nurse sometimes may be in the position of identifying an emergency and whether a needed action is one that only a physician usually performs; the hospital is expected to have a policy and procedure, which the nurse would follow, to verify and document the situation fully. This usually involves consultation with a supervisory nurse and verification of the emergency situation, as well as attempts to obtain medical assistance. Again, critical thinking by the nurse is essential to determine whether a true emergency exists.

When ''life or limb'' is truly in danger, the courts have held that a nurse can do those things immediately necessary, even if they usually are considered medical functions, provided the nurse has the essential expertise to perform the actions safely and correctly. The matter of having essential expertise is crucial; this is why all members of an emergency response team must learn all aspects of the ''code'' procedure. If, for any reason, the physician were unable to respond to the code, the role of the leader would be assumed by a nurse who was prepared with this essential expertise.

SITUATION   Situation: Nursing Action in a Hospital Emergency

In an orthopedic unit, it is common to care for patients with new casts. A young man with a newly applied long-leg cast is admitted via the emergency department at 6 pm. The nurse assigned to this patient's care carefully makes all the appropriate observations throughout the evening and documents his findings. The nurse notes that the leg is beginning to swell and that the edges of the cast are beginning to cut into the skin. At that time, the nurse notifies the supervisor that a problem is developing, and that he thinks the physician should be notified. The supervisor agrees and the nurse begins to try to contact the physician. The nurse continues to make observations, noting increasing swelling, color changes in the exposed toes, and loss of sensation. The physician cannot be reached and no other physician is immediately available.

The nurse follows the hospital procedure for seeking medical attention and for determining when an emergency exists. After consultation with the supervisor, the nurse decides that an emergency exists and that the cast needs to be cut open to relieve the pressure. Cutting a cast open is considered a medical procedure in this hospital.

The nurse has been taught how to use a cast cutter in emergency situations. Thus, the nurse possesses the essential expertise. The nurse, with the supervisor's approval, cuts open the cast and secures it in place with an elastic bandage. All observations made, consultations carried out, attempts to notify the physician, and the final action taken are carefully documented in the chart. Hospital policy was followed throughout the situation to ensure that all necessary steps had been taken.

Although this action went beyond usual nursing practice, it would not be considered a violation of either the nursing or the medical practice acts, because an emergency existed and the results of inaction would have been serious. Additionally, the nurse had the expertise and was prepared to carry out the necessary action safely. This emergency care is usually limited to specific technical procedures that the nurse has learned. It does not include diagnosing disease or prescribing medication, unless there are specific standing orders relative to the situation.

NONINSTITUTIONAL EMERGENCY CARE

Emergencies encountered outside the health care environment present other problems. Anyone rendering aid in an emergency is expected to behave as a reasonably prudent person would in such a situation. The nurse rendering aid in an emergency must behave as a reasonably prudent nurse in that situation. Thus, the standard is higher than for the nonprofessional person, although the nurse is not expected to perform as if he or she were in an institutional setting. The physical situation and the psychological situation are both considered when determining what is reasonably prudent nursing action.

All states and Canadian provinces have "Good Samaritan" statutes that encourage health care professionals to give aid in emergency situations. The first of these statutes was enacted in California in 1959 (Bernzweig, 1995). These statutes vary in content and comprehensiveness but relieve a professional of some liability when reasonable care is used. These laws often make people feel more secure when rendering aid.

Each nurse must make an individual decision about rendering emergency aid in a specific situation. The decision involves ethical as well as legal considerations. If the profession of nursing is a public trust and nurses are truly involved in the business of caring, then failure to come to the aid of an individual who is in serious danger is an ethical violation of that trust. To date there has been no instance of a nurse being sued for coming to the aid of someone in an emergency situation (Bernzweig, 1995; Fiesta, 1994). Professional liability insurance does provide coverage when the nurse assists in this way—which may make you feel more comfortable about rendering emergency aid.

In many states, emergency personnel must render all possible aid, including all resuscitative measures, when they are called to an emergency situation. This has sometimes resulted in the resuscitation of a terminally ill person who had previously stated that resuscitation was not desired; as more individuals receive terminal care in their homes, this will become an increasing concern.

Legislation allowing for patient self-determination in regard to emergency responders has now been passed in some states. The law usually stipulates the precise circumstances under which an individual may provide an advance directive in regard to emergency procedures, and how that directive must be documented so that emergency personnel can honor it. All emergency responders must be aware of their responsibilities in regard to advance directives.

Fraud

Fraud is deliberate deception for the purpose of personal gain and is usually prosecuted as a crime. However, it may also serve as the basis of a civil suit. Situations of fraud in nursing are not common. One example would be trying to obtain a better position by giving incorrect information to a prospective employer. By deliberately stating (falsely) that you had completed a nurse practitioner program to obtain a position for which you would otherwise be ineligible, you are defrauding the employer. This may be prosecuted as a crime, because you are also placing members of the community in danger of receiving substandard care. You may also commit fraud by trying to cover up a nursing error to avoid legal action. Courts tend to be more harsh in decisions regarding fraud than in cases involving simple malpractice, because fraud represents a deliberate attempt to mislead others for your own gain and could result in harm to those assigned to your care.

SITUATION   **Situation: Fraud**

A registered nurse is giving medications to the patients to whom she is assigned. When she presents a patient with his pills, he states that he was sure the doctor had discontinued the red pill because he had had a reaction to it the evening before. The nurse states that she is sure these are the correct medications. The patient takes the pills and the nurse charts the medications. The patient subsequently has a reaction. The nurse becomes frightened, goes back, and alters the medication record to make it appear that the medication was not given.

This situation could be considered fraud. The deception was the changing of the record, and the personal gain was freedom from responsibility for the error.

Assault and Battery

Assault is saying or doing something to make a person genuinely afraid that he or she will be touched without consent. Battery is unconsented or unlawful touching of a person. Neither of these terms implies that harm was done; harm may or may not occur. For an assault to occur, the person must be afraid of what might happen, even if the threatening person would not or could not carry out the threat. "If you don't take this medication, I will have to put you in restraints" is an example of an assault. For battery to occur, the touching must occur without consent. Remember that consent may be implied rather than specifically stated. Therefore, if the patient extends an arm for an injection, he cannot later charge battery, saying that he was not asked. But if the patient agreed because of a threat (assault), the touching would still be considered battery because the consent was not freely given.

Assault and battery are crimes under the law. However, most of these cases in health care are instituted as civil suits by the injured party, rather than as criminal cases by the governmental authorities. An example of a case that is most likely to be prosecuted as a civil case is given in the following situation.

SITUATION   **Assault and Battery**

A patient admitted to a psychiatric hospital refused to take any antipsychotic medications. The staff decided that her need for the medications was great, and therefore, planned to restrain her and give her injectable antipsychotic medications.

A court might consider this to be assault and battery. Although the patient was mentally ill, there is no indication that a court ever found her incompetent to make her own decisions. Mental illness alone does not constitute incompetence and this woman had the right to refuse treatment.

Assault and battery are most commonly treated as criminal cases when they involve suspected abuse of a patient. Most of us in health care are shocked and dismayed to learn of instances where care providers were abusive. Individuals who have difficulty with impulse control and anger may become frustrated with a patient and threaten, push, shove, or otherwise harm the individual. Most jurisdictions have laws requiring that anyone who knows of abuse to a dependent patient, whether a child, a developmentally delayed adult, or an elderly person, report that abuse to the proper authorities. Within an institution, there should be policies and procedures for this type of reporting. Appropriate authorities must conduct a careful investigation in order to ensure protection of the rights of the person accused.

False Imprisonment

Making a person stay in a place against his wishes is false imprisonment. The person may be forced to stay either by physical means or verbal means. It is easy to understand why restraining a patient or confining a patient to a locked room could constitute false imprisonment, if proper procedures were not first carried out. Again, false imprisonment is a crime,

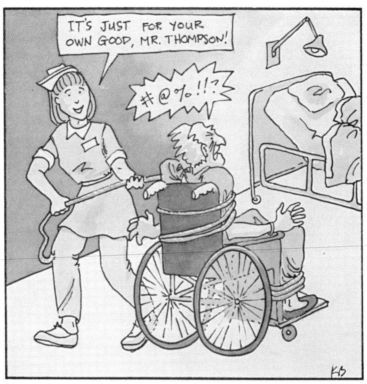

FIGURE 8-3
The improper use of restraints may constitute "false imprisonment."

but when it occurs in health care it is most often the basis of a civil suit rather than a criminal case (Fig. 8-3).

The law is less clear about keeping a patient confined by nonphysical means. If you remove a patient's clothes for the express purpose of preventing his leaving, you could be liable for false imprisonment. Threatening to keep a person confined with statements such as "If you don't stay in your bed, I'll sedate you," can also constitute false imprisonment.

Any time a patient needs to be confined for his or her own safety or well-being, it is best to help the person understand and agree to that course of action. If the patient is not responsible, the guardian or legal representative may give permission (this is a return to the issue of who may give consent). The third alternative is to objectively document the need in the patient's record and obtain a physician's order as soon as possible. Be sure to follow the policies of the facility.

In a conventional care setting you cannot restrain or confine responsible adults against their wishes. All persons have the right to make decisions for themselves, regardless of the consequences. The patient with a severe heart condition who defies orders and walks to the bathroom has that right. You protect yourself by recording your efforts to teach the patient the need for restrictions and by reporting the patient's behavior to your supervisor and the physician.

In the same context, the patient cannot be forced to remain in a hospital. If a patient wants to leave against medical advice, that is the patient's right. Again, you document your efforts in the record and follow applicable policies to protect the facility, the physician, and yourself from liability. The example of an intentional tort given earlier in this chapter involved false imprisonment.

A hospital may not detain a patient for nonpayment of a bill. The hospital is free to take legal action against the person who does not pay, but refusing discharge also constitutes false imprisonment.

False imprisonment suits are a special concern in the care of the psychiatric patient. Particular laws relate to this situation. In the psychiatric setting, you may have patients who have voluntarily sought admission. The same restrictions on restraint or confinement that apply to the patients in the general care setting apply to these patients. Other patients in the psychiatric setting may have been committed involuntarily according to the laws of the state. Specific measures may be used to confine the involuntarily committed patient. These are usually defined by law in terms of situation, type of restraint allowed, and length of time restraining may be used. If you work in a psychiatric setting, you should review specific policies regarding restraint to protect patients and to assist staff in functioning within the legal limits.

FACTORS THAT CONTRIBUTE TO MALPRACTICE CLAIMS

Poor results or harm that occur in the course of nursing practice usually are not followed by a suit. An understanding of some of the factors that enter into whether a suit is instituted may help you.

Social Factors

Much is being written about changes in the public's attitudes toward health care personnel. Health care is big business, and patients complain increasingly of not being known as individuals. Patients are more willing to bring suit against someone who is part of a large, impersonal system.

Health costs are high, and some people think hospitals and physicians have the ability to pay large settlements, whether directly or through insurance. If a patient's own income is lessened or disrupted by an illness, he or she might bring suit as a solution to economic difficulties. Increased public awareness of the size of monetary judgments that have been awarded may also be an economic incentive to initiating a suit.

Suit-Prone Patients

Some people are more likely to bring suit, for real or imagined errors. If these people are recognized as being suit-prone patients, it is possible for you to protect yourself through increased vigilance in regard to care and thorough record-keeping. Although we would warn you to guard against stereotyping, the following general descriptions may help you to avoid problems. Suit-prone patients usually are identified by overt behavior in which they are persistent fault finders and critics of personnel and of all aspects of care. They may be uncooperative in following a plan of care and sensitive to any perceived slight.

Persons who exhibit hostile attitudes may extend their hostile feelings to the nurses and other health care persons with whom they have contact. The nurse who becomes defensive when faced with hostility only widens the breach in the nurse–patient relationship. It is necessary to pay careful attention to those principles of care learned in psychosocial nursing that deal with how to help the hostile patient. Assisting patients in solving their own problems and offering support are the best forms of protection for the nurse.

Another type of patient who appears more suit-prone is the very dependent person who uses projection to deal with anxiety and fear. These individuals tend to ascribe fault or blame for all events to others and are unable to accept personal responsibility for their own welfare. Again, meeting these patients' needs with a carefully considered plan of care is the answer.

A common error is to withdraw and become defensive when confronting a suit-prone patient; this reaction occurs partly because a situation is unpleasant and partly because a staff member feels personally threatened by the patient's behavior. This reaction increases the likelihood of a suit if a poor result occurs.

Another incorrect nursing response to the suit-prone patient is to become more directive and authoritarian. This tends to increase the patient's feeling of separation and distance from the staff and again increases the likelihood of suit.

When the staff is helped to view the patient as a troubled person who manifests his or her problems in this manner, sometimes they find it easier to be objective. The patient is in need of all the skill that the prepared nurse can bring to the emotional problems. The suit-prone patient does not always end up suing; much depends on the response of health care personnel.

Suit-Prone Nurses

Nurses may also be suit-prone. Nurses who are insensitive to the patient's complaints, who do not identify and meet the patient's emotional needs, or who fail to identify the limits of their own practice may contribute to suits instituted not only against the nurse but also against the employer and the physician. The nurse's self-awareness is critical in preventing suits.

Staff members may contribute to a patient's distrust of care through complaining about working conditions, telling patients about problems occurring on the unit, and disparaging other health care providers. There is a distinction between informing a patient that you must meet someone else's needs, and therefore will not return for a specified period of time, and giving the patient the impression that you do not have time to attend to his or her needs (Fig. 8-4).

PREVENTING MALPRACTICE CLAIMS

The most significant thing you can do to prevent malpractice claims is to maintain a high standard of care. To do this, you may work at improving your own nursing practice and also the general climate for nursing practice where you work. You can do this in a variety of ways.

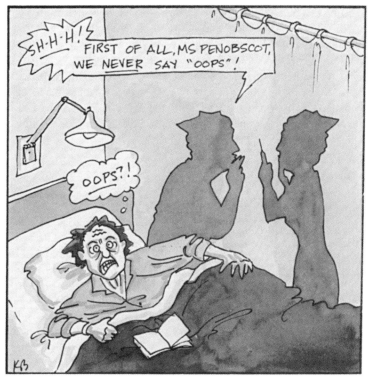

FIGURE 8-4
Certain things can be done to prevent malpractice suits.

Self-Awareness

Identify your own strengths and weaknesses in practice. When you have identified a weakness, seek a means of growth. This may include education, directed experience, or discussion with colleagues.

Be ready to acknowledge areas of weakness to supervisors, and do not accept responsibilities for which you are not prepared. For example, the nurse who has not worked in pediatrics for 10 years and accepts an assignment to a pediatric unit without orientation and education is setting the stage for an error to occur. Lack of current familiarity with the area is not a defense against liability. As a professional you should not accept a position if you cannot meet the criterion of being a reasonably prudent nurse in that setting. In instances of true emergency (eg, disaster, flood), courts may be more lenient, but ''we need you here today'' is not an emergency.

Adapting Proposed Assignments

As discussed previously, nurses may find themselves assigned to units where they have little or no experience with the types of patient problems they will encounter. It is reasonable to be assigned to assist an overworked nurse in a special area if you can assume duties that are within your own competence, and allow the specialized nurse to assume the specialized duties. It is not reasonable or safe for you to be expected to assume the specialized duties. Thus, if you were not prepared for coronary care, you might go to that unit, monitor the intravenous lines, take vital signs, and make observations to report to the experienced coronary care nurse; the experienced nurse would then be able to check the monitors, administer the specialized medications, and make decisions. Note that this does fragment the patient's care, and would not be appropriate as a permanent solution—but could alleviate a temporary problem in a safe manner.

Following Policies and Procedures

It is your responsibility to be aware of the policies and procedures of the institution that employs you. If they are sound, they can be an adequate defense against a claim, providing they were carefully followed.

For example, the medication procedure may involve checking all medications against a central medication Kardex; if you do this and there is an error in the Kardex, you might not be liable for the resulting medication error because you followed all appropriate procedures and acted responsibly. The liability would rest with the person who made the error in transcribing the medication from the physician's orders to the Kardex. If, however, you had not followed procedure in checking, you might also be liable because you did not do your part in preventing error. As discussed previously, policies are often designed to provide legal direction.

Changing Policies and Procedures

As nursing evolves, changes are needed in policies, procedures, and protocols. Part of your responsibility as a professional is to work toward keeping all of these up to date. Are there written policies to deal with emergency situations? Statements such as ''Oh, we've always done it this way'' are not adequate substitutes for clearly written, officially accepted policies. Often facilities that are reluctant to make changes based on the suggestions of individual nurses are much more receptive to new ideas when the legal implications of outmoded practice are noted. References such as the guidelines produced by the Agency for Health Care Policy and Research (AHCPR) may provide strong support for needed changes in practice.

Documentation

Nurses' records are unique in the health care setting. They cover the entire period of hospitalization, 24 hours a day, in a sequential pattern. Your record can be the crucial factor in avoiding litigation. Documentation in the record of observations made, decisions reached, actions taken, and the evaluation of the patient's response are considered much more solid evidence than verbal testimony, which depends on one's memory.

Because each case is determined by the facts as well as by the applicable law, clear documentation of all relevant data is important. For legal purposes, observations and actions that are not recorded may be assumed not to have occurred. Documentation needs to be factual, legible, and clearly understandable. Only approved abbreviations should be used. Narrative notes should have clear statements, and errors should be corrected according to the policy of the facility. Liquid erasing fluid, erasures, and heavy crossing out may be interpreted as attempted fraud in record keeping. You should avoid any statement that implies negligence on the part of any health care provider. Properly kept records may also protect you from becoming liable for the error of another, by demonstrating that you did everything in your power to prevent harm, including consulting with others. These records might include a complete log of telephone calls to a physician, and consultation with any relevant supervisor. Documentation should support that you followed all relevant policies and procedures when an emergency occurred. Although it is easy to become impatient with the time required by ''paper work,'' complete and clear documentation is often the basis of a successful defense against a claim of malpractice.

One concern about problem-oriented records and charting ''by exception'' is that these formats may provide less detailed information and may be less helpful in defense against litigation. This does not have to be the case. You can use any system of charting and record-keeping to provide appropriate and adequate documentation of care. If you identify something that needs to be recorded and cannot find a provision within your system to make that recording, you can be sure that others have experienced the same difficulty. You might begin inquiries toward establishing a clear mechanism for the record-keeping that concerns you. When nurses serve on committees to review and plan charting procedures, it is wise for them to seek consultation with the attorney for the facility; this helps to ensure that the plan for record-keeping is legally sound as well as professionally useful.

THE NURSE AS WITNESS

In the course of your practice as a registered nurse, a time may come when you will be asked to serve as a witness in a legal proceeding. There are several kinds of cases that involve the nurse as a witness.

The first type is a personal injury action in which a person has been injured (for example, in an automobile accident) and you or your organization has been involved in the care of that person. Your testimony in such a case might be on behalf of the injured person, to help describe the injuries and the care received for those injuries. For example, you may be asked to testify regarding the care given in a burn center to a victim of an electrical accident who received considerable nursing care during the recovery period.

The second type of lawsuit that involves the nurse as a witness is one in which a patient brings a lawsuit against persons or organizations who have provided health care that the patient believes was below the standard of the community. Medical malpractice is alleged in such a situation. The nurse may be included among those who are charged with malpractice. For example, the nurse may have to give evidence regarding medical record notes, or care given to the patient in the days before the alleged malpractice occurred. In both of these situations, the nurse's concern is with the specific factual details of a particular case.

A nurse may also be involved in a lawsuit as an expert witness. An expert witness, under Rule 702 of the Federal Rules of Evidence, accepted in the federal courts and many state courts, is defined as ''a witness qualified as an expert by knowledge, skill, experience, training, or education'' who may testify in the form of an opinion or otherwise. The purpose of testimony as an expert witness is to provide information and opinion that can be used by the court in making a decision. When you appear as an expert nursing witness, your testimony provides an opinion that will assist the judge or jury to understand complex areas of nursing care. You provide a professional opinion, that relates to your area of expertise, on the appropriate care for a given situation. For example, if you are an operating room nurse, you may be given medical records from another hospital and asked to render an opinion, on the basis of your expertise, as to whether the standard of nursing care given at the first hospital was within the standards of the community. Your role as an expert may not be accepted without question in a legal action. You may have to clearly state the qualifications, including your education and experience, that enable you to make a judgment.

When you become involved in any legal action, you should be sure that you understand both your rights and your obligations in regard to legal action.

Discovery

In a civil lawsuit (one between parties for the recovery of damages) a lengthy discovery process leads up to the trial. Discovery involves gathering information through documents (such as previous medical records and results of mental and physical examinations), interrogatories (written questions answered under oath), and depositions. A deposition is a formal proceeding in which each attorney has an opportunity to question a witness, and a sworn verbatim record is made by a court reporter (Guido, 1992). Depositions are often held in attorneys' offices or in a health care facility for the convenience of the health care providers. Sometimes depositions are taken to preserve the testimony of a witness for trial and are used in place of live testimony at trial. Most depositions in which you would participate, however, would be depositions for discovery purposes.

Often cases are settled before trial because of information obtained in the discovery process. The person bringing suit may be persuaded that no malpractice occurred or that it cannot be proved, and may drop the suit. On the other hand, the persons or institutions being sued (or their insurance companies) may determine that it is in their best interests to avoid a trial and agree to pay damages; this is often done without admitting that malpractice occurred. A settlement may require that no party to the settlement reveal its terms to others.

Testimony as a Witness in Deposition or at Trial

When you are asked to consult as an expert witness, your role is based on your knowledge of nursing practice. When you are asked to testify as a witness to *fact*, you will be testifying to the exact situation and circumstances of the event or events in question. You should always consult an attorney before talking to anyone about a matter in which you have been asked to testify, especially a malpractice action (Display 8-2).

The attorney who asks you to testify as an expert witness should be able to provide you with the information you need about your testimony. Feel free to ask that attorney what your role is in the case, and in which areas you are expected to testify. The attorney is likely to discuss in detail what questions will be asked of you and to ask what your answer would be to those questions.

DISPLAY 8-2
Guidelines for Testifying

- Answer only the questions asked.
- Do not volunteer additional information.
- Admit if you do not remember.
- Refer to your written documentation to support your answers.
- Be brief and direct.
- Do not use medical or technical terminology unless essential—then explain your terms.
- Explain when a simple yes or no would be misleading.
- Note differences between hypothetical cases presented and the one under consideration.

When nurses are asked to testify as to the facts of a situation, they sometimes believe that because they have done nothing wrong they do not need legal counsel. The law is complex, and you could jeopardize the position of an institution for which you work, or even jeopardize yourself and your professional future, with unwise statements. The person who is bringing suit may alter or amend the original complaint to involve new defendants including you. If you have liability insurance, you should advise your insurance company of your role as a witness, and an attorney will be assigned to talk with you. If you are covered by an employer's policy, you should consult with the appropriate administrative representative immediately to obtain legal counsel. This attorney should assist you in understanding the questions in the case, your role, and how you can protect yourself in the situation (Fig. 8-5).

As a witness, you will be required to swear or affirm to tell the entire truth. Failure to tell the entire truth is perjury. You are expected to answer the questions asked of you to the best of your ability; however, you do not have to provide an answer that would incriminate yourself—nor do you have to answer a question for which you do not remember or know the answer. It is perfectly permissible to state ''I do not remember'' or ''I do not know'' if you do not.

It is helpful to use words and terms that can be understood by those who are not familiar with medical terminology, or to explain medical terminology when its use is essential. If hypothetical situations or cases are presented for your response, be sure to note the differences between the hypothetical case and the one currently under consideration before you respond.

Be brief and direct when answering questions. Do not volunteer additional information that has not been asked for by the attorney. You may open up entire areas of inquiry that would not be considered without your comments. It is the attorney's job to ask the question to bring out the facts to which he or she wants you to testify. The opposing attorney will have an opportunity during cross-examination to ask you additional questions that the attorney believes are necessary for the facts of the case. However, be cautious about simply answering ''yes'' or ''no.'' In some instances an explanation is essential; a simple answer may sound as if you did not perform appropriately (Aiken, 1994).

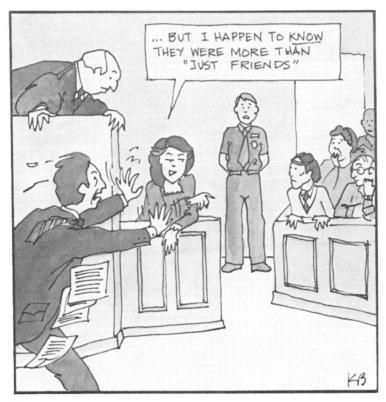

FIGURE 8-5
When testifying in court you should answer only the questions asked. Do not introduce other information.

KEY CONCEPTS

- Law includes those rules of conduct or action recognized as binding or enforced by government.
- Statutory law is enacted by legislative bodies, whereas regulatory law includes those rules and regulations established by administrative bodies within the government.
- Civil law encompasses those laws regulating private conduct between individuals. Criminal law regulates actions having to do with the safety of the community as a whole. Violations of criminal law are considered crimes, whereas violations of civil law are considered torts.
- Legal rights are derived from constitutional guarantees, and carry with them responsibilities. Other rights are ethically determined, and while not supportable by law, do govern the behavior of health care professionals.
- Malpractice actions brought against health care workers involve civil law. Nurses may be involved in cases related to intentional torts, negligence, or malpractice.
- The individual who is negligent or has committed malpractice is legally liable for the effects of that action. This means there is an obligation to the individual wronged.

- Liability may be focused on the individual, the supervisor, or the employer.
- Liability insurance may be purchased that transfers the cost of being sued and the cost of any settlement from the individual to a large group.
- A number of legal issues recur in nursing. Among these are the duty to report or seek medical care for a patient, protection of the patient's confidentiality and the right to privacy, defamation of character, privileged information, the various issues related to informed consent, and issues related to different types of emergency care.
- Nurses can also be involved in criminal cases related to fraud, assault and battery, and false imprisonment. In some cases, however, a civil suit may be brought against a nurse, in which case the nurse may not be prosecuted for criminal behavior.
- A number of factors contribute to malpractice claims. These include social factors, characteristics of suit-prone patients, and characteristics of suit-prone nurses.
- A nurse can do many things to prevent malpractice claims. Being aware of your own practice, accepting only those assignments for which you are prepared, following policies and procedures, and properly documenting care are among the most important.
- Nurses may be called as witnesses in trials because of their expertise in a particular area, or because of personal involvement in the case being tried. You must understand both your rights and your obligations in regard to legal action before giving a deposition or testimony.

Critical Thinking Activities

1. You are accepting a position in a clinic. When might you ask about professional liability insurance coverage? Formulate specific questions. Identify the person who would be the best source of this information. How will you proceed if this person does not have the information you seek? If the interviewer tells you that the clinic is very well covered by liability insurance, will you purchase personal malpractice insurance? Why or why not?
2. You have taken a position as a night nurse in a long term-care facility. One of the nursing assistants speaks of residents in very negative terms. You have observed her assisting a resident to the bathroom and she seemed abrupt and somewhat rough. A resident says to you "You have to be really nice to her (gesturing toward the door where the nursing assistant just exited) or she'll take it out on you next time." What should be your response to the resident? What action if any should you take? What is your legal liability if you do nothing? What is your legal liability if you initiate action against this nursing assistant?
3. You have taken a new position as a home health nurse. One of your patients is an elderly woman with a long history of diabetes who has a leg ulcer. Your role is to assess the patient in relationship to her diabetic management and wound care, and teach as needed. While you are in the home, her husband tells you that he has been having pain in his knee and asks if you would examine it and tell him whether it is all right to use a heating pad on it, and whether he should take ibuprofen or some Tylenol. Do you have a duty to help him? Why or why not? What will your response be? What legal issues

text continued

Critical Thinking Activities   (continued)

are involved in this situation? If you advise him and your advice turns out to be incorrect, what legal action could he take?

4. You have been called as a witness of fact to testify in a malpractice case against a local orthopedic surgeon regarding a patient for whom you cared. You are anxious about testifying. How can you best prepare for this? From whom should you seek assistance and guidance?

5. A good neighbor and friend experiences an unfortunate episode of extremely poor care in a local hospital where you are employed. She discusses this with you and asks your advice regarding initiating a suit. What are your obligations in this situation, both as a friend and as a professional? What are your obligations as an employee of the institution? If you need help reaching a decision, to whom can you turn?

REFERENCES

Aiken TD. Legal, Ethical, and Political Issues in Nursing. Philadelphia: FA Davis, 1994

Bernzweig EP. The Nurse's Liability for Malpractice, 6th ed. St. Louis: Mosby-Year Book, 1996

Fiesta J. The Law and Liability, 2nd ed. New York: John Wiley & Sons, 1994

Guido GW. Legal Issues in Nursing: A Source Book for Practice. Norwalk, CT: Appleton-Lange, 1992

FURTHER READING

Aiken TD. Depositions: What you need to know. J Legal Nurs Consult 6(4):9–10, 1995

Carson W. Nursing and professional boundaries: Legal barriers to practice. Am Nurse 25(2):24, 1993

Fiesta J. Law for the nurse manager: Legal issues in long-term care—part I, Nurs Manage 27(1): 18–19, 1996;—part II, Nurs Manage 27(2):18–9, 1996

How to read and understand your professional liability insurance policy. Am Nurse 27(8):24–25, 1995

The legal side. Am J Nurs (regular feature)

The legal side: Bedside computers and confidentiality. Am J Nurs 95(10):75–76, 1995

Regan Reports on Hospital Law. Providence: Medica Press (quarterly publication)

Regan Reports on Medical Law. Providence: Medica Press (quarterly publication)

Regan Reports on Nursing Law. Providence: Medica Press (quarterly publication)

Regan WA. OR nursing law. AORN J (regular column)

Schirm V, Gray M, Peoples M. Nursing personnel's perceptions of physical restraint use in long term care. Clin Nurs Res 2(1):98–110, 1993

Sullivan GH. Legally speaking. RN (regular column)

Grant AE, Ashman AA. Legal issues: Fax machines can land you in court. Regist Nurs J 8(1):16, 1996

Tammelleo AD. Court upholds nurse's refusal to float. Case in point: Winkleman v. Beloit Memorial Hospital (483 N.W. 2d 211—WI[1992]). Regan Reports on Nursing Law 33(2):2, 1992

Weiler K. Patient self-determination: Is anyone really listening? J Gerontol Nurs 19(10):42, 1993

9

Ethical Concerns in Nursing Practice

Only an ethics which is grounded in the breadth of being, not merely in the singularity or oddness of man, can have significance in the scheme of things.
(Salk, The Phenomena of Life)

Objectives

After completing this chapter, you should be able to:

1. Discuss the concept of ethics and its application in the health care field.

2. Describe four ethical theories that may be used when considering ethical problems.

3. Explain how personal religious and philosophical viewpoints, the Code for Nurses, and the Patient's Rights document are used as bases for ethical decision making.

4. Discuss how sociocultural and occupational factors affect ethical decision making for nurses.

5. Outline a framework for ethical decision making.

6. Discuss how ethics relates to commitment to the patient, commitment to personal excellence, and commitment to nursing as a profession.

7. Review the ethical and legal obligations related to the chemically impaired nursing colleague.

KEY TERMS

Authoritarian	Ethics	Social equity
Autonomy	Fidelity	Teleology
Beneficence	Ideal observer theory	Theory of obligation
Chemical dependency	Justice	Utilitarianism
Codes of ethics	Morality	Values
Cultural relativism	Mores	Values clarification
Deontology	Natural law	Values conflict
Duty	Nonmaleficence	Veracity
Ethical dilemma	Paternalistic	

A s a nurse you will participate in making judgments that involve human lives and the welfare of individuals, families, and communities. Many of these decisions will require a different background of knowledge than does the clinical judgment you have been developing. To a large extent, you will be dealing with ethical and moral concerns.

Morality refers to the rightness or wrongness of an action and is based upon a society's mores or customs. Ethics is a study of morality. Decisions that must be made regarding ethical and moral issues are primarily concerned with what is "right" or "good" for an individual. You have already had exposure to some of these decisions—including the decision not to resuscitate a patient, or the decision to withdraw treatment. You already understand that these are not easy decisions to make. Fortunately there are some guiding principles to assist us in the process.

In this chapter we will discuss some of the approaches to ethical decision making, and we will give examples of how it is applied in the health care arena. We will also provide some direct application to your performance as a nurse and to personal decision making. As you read about ethical issues and conflicts, and discuss them in your classroom or with a classmate, we urge you to respect others by carefully listening to them and honestly attempting to understand their positions and their accompanying values and beliefs. Only by considering all aspects of an issue can we seek and find understanding for ourselves.

UNDERSTANDING THE CONCEPT OF ETHICS

In the formal sense, ethics is a branch of philosophy referred to as moral philosophy. The word *ethics* is derived from the Greek term *ethos* which means customs, habitual usages, conduct and character. DeGeorge (1993) defines ethics as a "systematic attempt to make sense of our individual and social moral experience, in such a way as to determine the rules that ought to govern human conduct, the values worth pursuing, and the character traits deserving development in life." Since the time of Socrates and the Golden Age of Greece, philosophers have attempted to provide a logical approach to some of the questions of human conduct that arise in our lives. Some divide this discipline into three areas: *meta-ethics*, which deals with the extent to which moral judgments are reasonable or justifiable; *normative ethics*, which examines individual rights and obligations as well as the common good; and *descriptive ethics*, which focuses on what people actually do in given situations (Davis & Aroskar, 1991). Closely associated with the concept of ethics is that of *morals*. This word, derived from the Latin *mores,* means custom or habit. Morals are the basic standards for what we consider right and wrong. Morals or standards are usually based on religious beliefs and, to some extent, social influence and group norms. When we use the words ethics and morals together we are talking about conduct, character and motives for action. We typically describe the behavior we observe as good, right, desirable, honorable, fitting or proper; or, we might describe the behavior as bad, wrong, improper, irresponsible, or evil. You will quickly realize that such perceptions are based on *values,* and that each of us (and each society) has differing sets of values. Values are most commonly derived from societal norms, religion, and family orientation and provide the framework for making decisions about the actions we take everyday of our lives (Aiken, 1996). For example, if you were raised to believe in and support the teachings of the Roman Catholic Church, you value human life as beginning at the time of conception. Therefore, you probably would have difficulty accepting abortion as an alternative to unwanted pregnancy. We all have been in a situation in which we experienced a *values conflict*. This occurs when we must choose between two things, both of which are important to us. For example, if you are a new mother you probably would like to spend all of your time with your child; however, if you must also help provide support for the family, and that requires leaving the child to go to work, you have a values conflict.

Most of the time we don't think about our values—we just accept them. We are most apt to think about them when we have a difficult decision to make, when something goes wrong, or when we find ourselves in a conflict because of differing values. In nursing we work with a very diverse patient population and therefore are exposed to a wide variety of values and ethical standards. The need to give conscientious care to all patients often forces us to examine our own values. The process that fosters the identification of significant values is known as *values clarification* (Steele & Harmon, 1979). We examine what we believe is good, bad, beautiful, worthy, meaningful and so forth, and explore the process of determining our personal values. The process of values clarification assists us in making choices and facilitates decision making, because we have a better understanding of our own value systems and, therefore, a better understanding of ourselves.

It is important to have a good understanding of yourself when you are faced with an *ethical dilemma*. An ethical dilemma occurs when an individual must make a choice between two equally unfavorable alternatives. For example, assisted suicide provides an ethical dilemma for many. Although they are certainly opposed to seeing a loved one spend the last months of life in great pain and suffering, they are equally opposed to assisting with an earlier death. In ethical dilemmas there is usually no perfect solution, and those making decisions often find themselves in the position of having to defend their decisions. Although there are times when a difference in values and decisions can be accepted, there are other times when differences put people into direct conflict. Should you experience such a situation, we urge you to be constructive (rather than destructive) in the methods you choose to work toward resolving the differences.

BASIC ETHICAL CONCEPTS

Basic concepts that are involved in most ethical situations include rights, autonomy, beneficence, nonmaleficence, justice, fidelity, veracity, and the standard of best interest. Identifying how they apply to a particular situation and balancing their competing claims often present a challenge.

Rights

Typically we think of a *right* as a just claim or entitlement, or as something that is owed to an individual on a legal, moral or ethical basis. In common usage this is often extended to include privileges, concessions, and freedoms. Rights form the basis of most professional codes and legal judgments. (See Chapter 8 for more discussion of rights as used in the legal sense.) The discussion of the other ethical concepts is founded on the belief that people are entitled to certain rights. We deal with the issue of ''rights'' any time we are talking about the right of a person to self-determination. If a patient is admitted to a hospital and refuses treatment, and there is a strong indication that the patient could recover, should the physicians and nurses respect the patient's right to self-determination? The problems that occur when one individual's rights come in conflict with the values of another provide us with many challenges and dilemmas.

Federal legislation has been passed to ensure that individual rights are respected. The Patient Self-Determination Act, also known as the Danforth amendment, requires that agencies receiving Medicare money ask patients if they have advance directives, inform patients of their right to refuse treatment under state law, and educate staff and the community about those rights. This act was created because of our society's fundamental belief in the individual's right to decide. However, this act does little to recognize cultural diversity and sensibility to groups such as Chinese-Americans, who have a unique but different set of values and well-defined role relationships (Fung, 1994).

Although the concept of rights is almost taken for granted in our Western culture, there are some who suggest that there are no human rights and that we cannot talk about rights, the violation of rights, or moral judgments, because the validity of all moral judgments is culturally relative. In other words all rights and judgments must be able to be applied to all cultures. This concept is known as *cultural relativism.* Carried to the fullest extent, this concept would bar us from saying that human rights violations are occurring in the world, because those living in the cultures in which we believe violations are occurring may not recognize those actions as violations of rights. The concept of cultural relativism would limit us to determining when rights are being violated in our culture (Buchanan, 1996). Cultural relativism embraces the notion that groups and individuals hold different sets of values that must be respected. This is an interesting concept to consider in relationship to health care practices with which we have great difficulty, such as female circumcision. Although it is appalling to us, in some non-Western cultures concerns about virginity, marriageability, the husband's sexual pleasure, and religious beliefs dictate that female children be circumcised. Members of these cultures do not view this practice as mutilation; rather, it is thought to result in the improved appearance of female genitalia. To be referred to as uncircumcised is a terrible insult (Lane & Rubinstein, 1996). As our world becomes smaller, we will need to learn how to deal with such differences.

Autonomy

Autonomy involves the right of self-determination, independence and freedom (Aiken, 1994). It comes from the Latin *auto* meaning "self" and *nomy,* which means "control." Some refer to autonomy as respect for the individual and include the expectation that each individual will be treated as unique and as an equal to every other individual (Davis & Aroskar, 1991). Other words frequently associated with autonomy include dignity, inherent worth, self-reliance, and individualism. When we consider an individual's autonomy, the way we approach a problem may result in the decision-making process becoming more time consuming. Giving consideration to an individual's autonomy also requires that justification be provided for why the patient is not participating in decision making, if in fact the patient is not. In today's health care delivery system, it is important to respect patients' rights to make decisions about and for themselves, even when we do not agree with those decisions. For example, you may have difficulty supporting the decision of a new mother, who is a Jehovah's Witness and whose life is in danger because of blood loss, not to receive a blood transfusion.

As with most other rights, there may be restrictions on the right to choose. When one person's autonomy interferes with another's rights, health, or well-being, limitations may be imposed. Does a patient's right to self-determination allow that individual to choose a certain expensive treatment, if that choice would unjustly deny money to another person for another treatment? What if a patient demands a bone marrow transplant that wipes out the health department's entire budget for immunizations? Does the autonomy of a patient with a highly communicable disease take precedence over the right of the community not to be exposed to the disease? If there are to be limitations, what should those limitations be? In what instances should the legal system interfere with personal decision making?

For some individuals, autonomy may be less important than values related to the family. Is this acceptable? Who decides how much autonomy is "enough?" Once again, we must consider the idea that autonomy is predominantly a Western value. For example, tribal life occurs under more strenuous circumstances than we normally encounter; it requires more cooperation, less variation from the norm. The individual's freedom to do things is far more limited because it is directed toward the common good of the community.

Beneficence and Nonmaleficence

Beneficence refers to the obligation to do good, not harm, to other people. It also requires that we act in the best interests of others (Cohen, Cohen, & Thomasma, 1988). Thus, the concept of beneficence extends from promoting good to *nonmaleficence* (the prohibition of intentional harm). As far back as Hippocrates, physicians were entreated to do no harm. Florence Nightingale stated that the patient should be no worse for having been nursed. In health care we recognize that sometimes we unintentionally do harm to individuals. Nosocomial infections, adverse drug reactions, and the side effects of such treatments as irradiation and chemotherapy for cancer are certainly harmful to the individuals who experience them. In some cases, given the alternatives, a patient will opt not to have the treatment (eg, irradiation). The ethical mandate is that we refrain from intentionally inflicting harm. Sometimes it is difficult to accept that a side effect of a particular treatment might result in harm to a patient;

Good is a general term of approval or commendation, and may be defined as that which produces favorable results, is beneficial, effective, honorable, worthy, respectable, proper, valid, desirable, pleasant, or healthy (Webster's New World College Dictionary, 1996, p. 581). Thus, we tend to think of it as that which promotes life, development and fulfillment. We view it as "good" when a friend makes a quick recovery from surgery, when a child graduates from high school or college, or when aging parents are able to take that long-awaited trip they have been planning for years.

It is sometimes difficult to decide who will determine what is good for a specific person in a specific situation. In most instances we expect that people will make their own decisions about what is good for them. But who decides for the infant with regard to procedures such as immunizations that inflict some degree of pain, but have long-lasting and positive benefits? Who decides for the individual who is unconscious or is mentally incompetent?

Another problem centers around what is good. Is all life good, or are there situations in which not living is better than life? Is it better to sustain life in the face of disability, or is it better to allow a person to die and have suffering end? If giving good care to one patient means that lesser care will be given to another, how can we defend such an action?

What if giving good care means violating good nursing economics (cost containment)? There are no simple answers, and the answers will not be the same for everyone.

The issue of sanctity of life is of major concern in the health care arena. Some would argue that all life is good. Others would adamantly assert that life is not good when the quality of life is poor; this latter belief has led to serious discussions regarding euthanasia, supported the establishment of such groups as the Hemlock Society, and has resulted in at least three states initiating legislation supporting assisted suicide. Many people, particularly physicians, believe that the principles of respect for the patient and relief from suffering fail to do justice to the internal values, professional integrity, and norms of medicine (Miller and Brody, 1995). Quality-of-life issues also emerge in instances where parents are advised that a fetus has a life-compromising condition such as meningomyelocele. Surrounding all issues dealing with the sanctity of life are religious views, particularly those maintaining that all life is sacred. Certainly arguments regarding the ''right to life'' play a major role in discussions regarding abortion, whether supported by religious beliefs or personal value systems. The ''right to life'' also affects our personal beliefs about capital punishment.

Thus it can be said that although the topics of medical futility and the sanctity of life are popular, there exists little consensus about them. As a nurse you will often encounter difficult situations in the care of your patients in which opposing values play against one another. Understanding your own values, which may change over time, is important in these situations.

Justice

Justice refers to the obligation to be fair to all people. The concept is often expanded to what is called *distributive justice*—which requires that individuals be treated equally regardless of race, sex, marital status, medical diagnosis, social standing, economic level, or religious belief (Davis & Aroskar, 1991). We must ask, ''How is fairness defined?'' Does fairness mean that people should be treated the same? In terms of access to health care, is it just for one person to receive more resources than another? If so, what makes it ''just,'' and how does that relate to the distribution of scarce medical resources? Does age make a difference in what we consider just? Should it? Does justice imply that the government should provide the resources or services individuals cannot provide for themselves? Can we measure fairness in any objective sense? What should occur when one person's rights interfere with the rights of another? These issues will be discussed in greater detail in Chapter 10.

Fidelity

Fidelity refers to the obligation to be faithful to the agreements, commitments and responsibilities that one has made to oneself and others. Fidelity is the foundation of the concept of accountability that we hear about so frequently in nursing today. What are the responsibilities of health care personnel to individuals, employers, the government, society, and self? When these responsibilities conflict, which should take priority? In reality, which do take priority? Are nurses obligated to provide care to all patients? Under what circumstances if any might this be challenged? What if the health care provider and the patient disagree as to obligations and responsibilities? Who makes the decision as to what constitutes fidelity?

Veracity

Veracity refers to telling the truth or not intentionally deceiving or misleading patients. From childhood we are all admonished to tell the truth and to avoid lying. When we are children this seems straightforward. As we become adults, we see more and more instances where the choices are less clear. For example, do you tell the truth when you know it will cause harm to an individual (nonmaleficence)? Do you tell a lie when it would make someone less anxious and afraid? You might see this as beneficence (doing good), but then you have abandoned the principle of veracity.

Sissela Bok, an ethical philosopher, has written an extensive treatise entitled *Lying: Moral Choice in Public and Private Life* (Bok, 1978). In this book she explores the ethical principles that relate to lying and then relates these to specific areas of concern, one of which is lies to the sick and dying. She concludes that lying, by its very nature, is detrimental to the liar as well as to the person to whom the lie is told. She recognizes that justifications for lying do exist in situations where the truth will cause greater harm than the lie.

Bok concludes that lying to the sick and dying rarely is justified. The loss of trust in caregivers, the anxiety created by not knowing the truth, the loss of opportunity to deal with personal and family concerns, and other adverse consequences of not being told the truth far outweigh the perceived benefits of lying. She points out that the damage associated with sad news or risks is usually less severe than physicians or other caregivers think it will be. She states that lying should be seen as an unusual step and one that requires reasons to be set forth and debated, and alternatives to be weighed carefully.

The Standard of Best Interest

When a decision must be made about a patient's health care and the patient is unable to make an informed decision, it is done in the *standard of best interest*. As the name implies, it is based on what the health care providers or family believe is best for that individual. Such decisions are based on the individual's expressed wishes or on documents such as living wills. Health care professionals strive to avoid unilateral decisions made by a health care provider. Unilateral decisions often imply that the decision maker knows what is best for the patient. When this occurs it is referred to as *paternalism*.

ETHICAL THEORIES

It is not our intent to delve with any depth into the writings of early philosophers. However, because ethical theories are mentioned frequently in the literature that deals with bioethical issues, some background seems appropriate.

An ethical theory is a moral principle or a set of moral principles that can be used to assess what is morally right or morally wrong in a given situation. Over the years we have called on the theories of philosophers to guide us in our decision making.

The most widely used theories are presented in Table 9-1. You are encouraged to consider various ethical approaches and discuss with your classmates when each might be used appropriately. For example, an application of utilitarianism (or consequentialism) as seen in the health care industry would be the justification of capitation in the managed care organization (MCO). Because the MCO pays a certain amount of money per member per

TABLE 9-1. Major Ethical Theories and Theorists

Theory Title (Other Names)	Theorist Associated With Work	Basic Principles of Theory
Utilitarianism (often referred to as teleology, consequentialism, or situation ethics, although there are some differences)	Jeremy Bentham (1748–1832) & John Stuart Mill (1806–1873)	An act is right when it brings the greatest good for the greatest number. A second principle allows the end to justify the means. Fits well into Western society's values regarding work ethic and the behavioristic approach to education, philosophy, and life.
Deontology (formalistic system, the principal system of ethics, or duty-based ethics)	Immanuel Kant (1724–1804)	Ethical decision making is based on moral rules and unchanging principles (or motivations which are derived from universal values) considered separately from the consequences. The fundamental principle is called the categorical imperative.
Natural Law	St. Thomas Aquinas (1223–1274)	Actions are morally right when they are in accord with our nature and end as human beings. Good should be promoted, evil avoided, and ethics is grounded in our concern for human good.
Social Equity and Justice	J. Rawls	If people of reason were placed in a situation of ethical choice, they would choose the alternative that supported the most disadvantaged person. Supports justice and equal rights for everyone.
Ideal Observer	R. Firth	Requires that decisions be made from a disinterested, dispassionate, omniscient, consistent viewpoint with full information about the situation and the consequences available (difficult criteria to fulfill).

month to a contracted provider, the MCO would argue that it has provided the greatest good for the greatest number of members (Stahl, 1996). An example of deontology might be applied to the situation in which all persons involved in a research study have a complete understanding (informed consent) of the study and its purposes. The participant is not simply a means to an end.

FACTORS THAT INFLUENCE ETHICAL DECISION MAKING

All people must determine their own grounds for making ethical decisions. Some people rely on formal philosophical or religious beliefs that define matters in relation to what is believed to be the truth or good or evil. Others make decisions based on personal life experiences or on the experiences of those dear to them. Still others rely on professional codes of ethics to give guidance on ethical issues. In reality, ethical decision making often involves a combination of all of these factors.

Ethical decisions are not made in a vacuum. Many factors exert pressure and demand response as we search for appropriate answers to the dilemmas that we face. All facets of today's world are experiencing change, and nursing is no exception. The ''truths'' of yesterday are being challenged by the realities and new problems confronting us today.

In studying ethical issues it is important for you to understand the many forces that are operating simultaneously in our society. These forces are not independent or mutually exclusive, but act and react with one another in a constantly changing milieu, causing evolutionary changes in all segments of society (Fig. 9-1).

Personal Religious and Philosophical Viewpoints

Your personal viewpoint certainly will be a major factor influencing your ethical decision making. Achieving self-understanding in values is a lifelong learning task, and undoubtedly your position on various issues will change as you move through life. Values are the product of our life experiences and are influenced by family, friends, culture, environment, education, and many other factors. Because of this our values may change.

Religious beliefs form the basis for ethical decision making for some people. A person

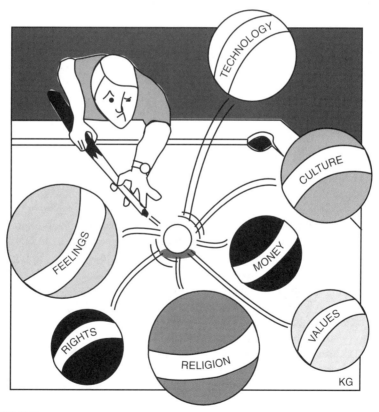

FIGURE 9-1
Decisions made in relation to one aspect of an ethical situation will affect all other aspects of the problem.

who is a member of a particular religious group may not ascribe to all of the beliefs of that group. However, individuals make their own decisions with regard to each situation, which in some cases may not parallel the doctrines of their religious group. For example, some Muslims maintain that women should be completely separated from men, and wear veils when in the presence of men. They would find any health care setting that did not respect this belief to be in conflict with their basic values. Other Muslims do not adhere to this strict interpretation of Islamic law, and women wear modest clothing but do not wear veils. They would be more comfortable in most Western health care settings because they would not feel a conflict with their personal values.

You will want to consider your personal values when seeking a nursing position after graduation. Nursing offers a wide variety of job opportunities to the new graduate. In choosing a job, you certainly cannot expect to avoid all conflict or problem situations, but you will want to avoid working in an area in which there is constant conflict. Before you accept a position, you may want to consider whether it has the potential to conflict with your basic beliefs. For example, if you are ethically opposed to abortion, it would be wise to avoid employment on an obstetric unit or in a community clinic where therapeutic abortions are performed routinely. In this situation, making your views known and refusing certain assignments after you begin employment might result in termination because the employer may justifiably assert that you agreed to fulfill all the responsibilities of the position when you accepted employment.

Similarly, you might choose to work in an area that supports your personal value system or strong ethical commitment. For example, the hospices for the dying in England were begun by religious groups who saw value in the life of the dying person. Their religious beliefs were and have continued to be part of their approach to care. If you strongly value your own ethnic or cultural approach to health care, you might choose to work in a health care setting where that approach is part of the philosophy.

Codes for Nurses

Through their professional organizations, nurses have developed some common guidelines to use in making ethical decisions. They are contained in the American Nurses Association's (ANA) Code for Nurses, and the International Council of Nurses' Code for Nurses. Each attempts to outline the nurse's responsibilities to the patient and to the profession of nursing.

The ANA code is somewhat unique among professional codes because it addresses fairly specific issues and does not confine itself to matters of etiquette or broad general statements. Warren T. Reich, editor-in-chief of the *Encyclopedia of Bioethics,* was quoted as stating, ''This is probably the most interesting and responsive code I have ever read'' (New encyclopedia. . . , 1977, p. 8). Tentative codes were presented by nurses in the 1920s, the 1930s, and the 1940s. Finally, in 1950, a code of ethics was adopted. It has been revised several times since then, most recently in 1976. Early versions stated that a nurse had an obligation to carry out a physician's orders; later versions, however, stress the nurse's obligation to the patient. This includes protecting the patient from incompetent, unethical, or illegal practice. An ad hoc committee of the ANA also developed interpretive statements which enlarge upon and explain the code in detail. The interpretive statements were last revised in 1985. The Code for Nurses is presented in Display 9-1.

The International Council of Nurses' Code was revised in 1973 and reaffirmed in 1989.

DISPLAY 9-1
American Nurses Association Code for Nurses

PREAMBLE

The Code for Nurses is based on belief about the nature of individuals, nursing, health, and society. Recipients and providers of nursing services are viewed as individuals and groups who possess basic rights and responsibilities, and whose values and circumstances command respect at all times. Nursing encompasses the promotion and restoration of health, the prevention of illness, and the alleviation of suffering. The statements of the Code and their interpretation provide guidance for conduct and relationships in carrying out nursing responsibilities consistent with the ethical obligations of the profession and quality in nursing care.

1. The nurse provides services with respect for human dignity and the uniqueness of the client unrestricted by considerations of social or economic status, personal attributes, or the nature of health problems.
2. The nurse safeguards the client's right to privacy by judiciously protecting information of a confidential nature.
3. The nurse acts to safeguard the client and the public when health care and safety are affected by the incompetent, unethical, or illegal practice of any person.
4. The nurse assumes responsibility and accountability for individual nursing judgments and actions.
5. The nurse maintains competence in nursing.
6. The nurse exercises informed judgment and uses individual competence and qualifications as criteria in seeking consultation, accepting responsibilities, and delegating nursing activities to others.
7. The nurse participates in activities that contribute to the ongoing development of the profession's body of knowledge.
8. The nurse participates in the profession's efforts to implement and improve standards of nursing.
9. The nurse participates in the profession's efforts to establish and maintain conditions of employment conducive to high quality nursing care.
10. The nurse participates in the profession's effort to protect the public from misinformation and misrepresentation and to maintain the integrity of nursing.
11. The nurse collaborates with members of the health professions and other citizens in promoting community and national efforts to meet the health needs of the public.

Source: Code for Nurses with Interpretive Statements. *Reprinted with permission of the American Nurses Association.*

The introductory section of this code addresses the general responsibilities of the nursing profession. Five sections follow, dealing with the more specific concerns of people, practice, society, coworkers, and the profession. In addition, the International Council of Nurses has written a Pledge for Nurses, which is a statement of affirmation and acceptance of the personal and ethical responsibilities of being a member of the nursing profession. Both of these documents can serve as guidelines for ethical conduct. The International Council of Nurses' Code is presented in Display 9-2.

DISPLAY 9-2
International Council of Nurses Code for Nurses Ethical Concepts Applied to Nursing (1972)

The fundamental responsibility of the nurse is fourfold: to promote health, to prevent illness, to restore health and to alleviate suffering.

The need for nursing is universal. Inherent in nursing is respect for life, dignity, and rights of man. It is unrestricted by considerations of nationality, race, creed, colour, age, sex, politics or social status.

Nurses render health services to the individual, the family and the community and coordinate their services with those of related groups.

NURSES AND PEOPLE

The nurse's primary responsibility is to those people who require nursing care.

The nurse, in providing care, promotes an environment in which the values, customs and spiritual beliefs of the individual are respected.

The nurse holds in confidence personal information and uses judgment in sharing this information.

NURSES AND PRACTICE

The nurse carries personal responsibility for nursing practice and for maintaining competence by continual learning.

The nurse maintains the highest standards of nursing care possible within the reality of a specific situation.

The nurse uses judgment in relation to individual competence when accepting and delegating responsibilities.

The nurse when acting in a professional capacity should at all times maintain standards of personal conduct that would reflect credit upon the profession.

NURSES AND SOCIETY

The nurse shares with other citizens the responsibility for initiating and supporting action to meet the health and social needs of the public.

NURSES AND CO-WORKERS

The nurse sustains a cooperative relationship with co-workers in nursing and other fields.

The nurse takes appropriate action to safeguard the individual when his care is endangered by a co-worker or any other person.

NURSES AND THE PROFESSION

The nurse plays the major role in determining and implementing desirable standards of nursing practice and nursing education.

The nurse is active in developing a core of professional knowledge.

The nurse, acting through the professional organization, participates in establishing and maintaining equitable social and economic working conditions in nursing.

Source: Reprinted with permission of the International Council of Nurses.

The Patient's Rights

The patient's rights are another consideration in decision making. Ideally, we have always recognized them in some way. As early as 1959, the National League for Nursing formulated a statement regarding patient's rights. For many years, however, health care professionals assumed that they knew what was best for patients and made many decisions without consulting or considering the rights of the patient. For example, a patient with a specific disease was not offered information about possible treatment alternatives, even when valid alternatives did exist. The patient's physician made the decision regarding which treatment method was preferable, and that was the only one presented to the patient. This is another example of paternalism, discussed earlier in this chapter.

As the health consumer movement became more active, greater attention was paid to the rights of the patient. Today patients may expect to be informed of all alternatives for treatment and often want to participate in choosing a type of treatment, weighing the possible benefits and risks of the treatment methods presented. The law has also supported the right to informed decision making.

In 1973, the American Hospital Association published A Patient's Bill of Rights (AHA, 1992), which outlines the rights of the hospital patient and serves as a basis for making decisions about hospitalized patients. Some have criticized this document, saying that it is rather innocuous because it simply reminds patients of their rights (such as privacy, confidentiality, and informed consent) but says nothing of hospitals that fail to act in accordance with these rights. The AHA revised this document in 1992. In the introduction, hospitals are encouraged to modify and adapt the AHA document to their individual situations and communities. The revised document speaks more forcefully regarding the hospital's responsibility for providing medically indicated care and services. In addition, it emphasizes the collaborative nature of health maintenance, which requires patient as well as provider responsibility. The Patient's Bill of Rights is presented in Display 9-3.

Some groups, nurses' associations among them, have also formulated statements regarding the rights of the health care consumer. In some states, the rights of the health care consumer are being formalized into legal statements.

Of particular interest currently is the development of legislation that would protect the confidentiality of medical records. As computer-based patient records have become the state-of-the-art system for managing patient records, and as more personal data are collected by the federal government, concerns about adequate protection of personal information have emerged. In light of the many conglomerates that manage care, and the tremendous amount of information handled by insurance companies, it is easy to imagine how privacy could become unmanageable. Although the Federal Privacy Act passed by Congress in 1974 established the right of citizens to know that certain information is available in a record system, no legislation exists that focuses specifically and deliberately on confidentiality rather than privacy. Many believe we need to ensure the confidentiality, security, accuracy, and integrity of personal health information. In 1995, the Institute of Medicine published a report titled *Health Data in the Information Age*, which recommended that Congress enact legislation to establish a uniform requirement for the assurance of confidentiality and protection of privacy rights for person-identifiable data (Detmer & Steen, 1996).

DISPLAY 9-3
The Patient's Bill of Rights

INTRODUCTION

Effective health care requires collaboration between patients and physicians and other health care professionals. Open and honest communication, respect for personal and professional values, and sensitivity to differences are integral to optimal patient care. As the setting for the provision of health services, hospitals must provide a foundation for understanding and respecting the rights and responsibilities of patients, their families, physicians, and other caregivers. Hospitals must ensure a health care ethic that respects the role of patients in decision making about treatment choices and other aspects of their care. Hospitals must be sensitive to cultural, racial, linguistic, religious, age, gender, and other differences as well as the needs of persons with disabilities.

The American Hospital Association presents *A Patient's Bill of Rights* with the expectation that it will contribute to more effective patient care and be supported by the hospital on behalf of the institution, its medical staff, employees, and patients. The American Hospital Association encourages health care institutions to tailor this bill of rights to their patient community by translating and/or simplifying the language of this bill of rights as may be necessary to ensure that patients and their families understand their rights and responsibilities.

BILL OF RIGHTS*

1. The patient has the right to considerate and respectful care.
2. The patient has the right to and is encouraged to obtain from physicians and other direct caregivers relevant, current, and understandable information concerning diagnosis, treatment, and prognosis.

    Except in emergencies when the patient lacks decision-making capacity and the need for treatment is urgent, the patient is entitled to the opportunity to discuss and request information related to the specific procedures and/or treatments, the risks involved, the possible length of recuperation, and the medically reasonable alternatives and their accompanying risks and benefits.

    Patients have the right to know the identity of physicians, nurses, and others involved in their care, as well as when those involved are students, residents, or other trainees. The patient also has the right to know the immediate and long-term financial implications of treatment choices, insofar as they are known.
3. The patient has the right to make decisions about the plan of care prior to and during the course of treatment and to refuse a recommended treatment or plan of care to the extent permitted by law and hospital policy and to be informed of the medical consequences of this action. In case of such refusal, the patient is entitled to other appropriate care and services that the hospital provides or transfer to another hospital. The hospital should notify patients of any policy that might affect patient choice within the institution.
4. The patient has the right to have an advance directive (such as a living will, health care proxy, or durable power of attorney for health care) concerning treatment or designating a surrogate decision maker with the expectation that the hospital will honor the intent of that directive to the extent permitted by law and hospital policy.

    Health care institutions must advise patients of their rights under state law and hospital policy to make informed medical choices, ask if the patient has an advance directive, and include that information in patient records. The patient has the right to timely information about hospital policy that may limit its ability to implement fully a legally valid advance directive.

(continued)

DISPLAY 9-3
The Patient's Bill of Rights (continued)

5. The patient has the right to every consideration of privacy. Case discussion, consultation, examination, and treatment should be conducted so as to protect each patient's privacy.

6. The patient has the right to expect that all communications and records pertaining to his/her care will be treated as confidential by the hospital, except in cases such as suspected abuse and public health hazards when reporting is permitted or required by law. The patient has the right to expect that the hospital will emphasize the confidentiality of this information when it releases it to any other parties entitled to review information in these records.

7. The patient has the right to review the records pertaining to his/her medical care and to have the information explained or interpreted as necessary, except when restricted by law.

8. The patient has the right to expect that, within its capacity and policies, a hospital will make reasonable response to the request of a patient for appropriate and medically indicated care and services. The hospital must provide evaluation, service, and/or referral as indicated by the urgency of the case. When medically appropriate and legally permissible, or when a patient has so requested, a patient may be transferred to another facility. The institution to which the patient is to be transferred must first have accepted the patient for transfer. The patient must also have the benefit of complete information and explanation concerning the need for, risks, benefits, and alternatives to such a transfer.

9. The patient has the right to ask and be informed of the existence of business relationships among the hospital, educational institutions, other health care providers, or payers that may influence the patient's treatment and care.

10. The patient has the right to consent to or decline to participate in proposed research studies or human experimentation affecting care and treatment or requiring direct patient involvement, and to have those studies fully explained prior to consent. A patient who declines to participate in research or experimentation is entitled to the most effective care that the hospital can otherwise provide.

11. The patient has the right to expect reasonable continuity of care when appropriate and to be informed by physicians and other caregivers of available and realistic patient care options when hospital care is no longer appropriate.

12. The patient has the right to be informed of hospital policies and practices that relate to patient care, treatment, and responsibilities. The patient has the right to be informed of available resources for resolving disputes, grievances, and conflicts, such as ethics committees, patient representatives, or other mechanisms available in the institution. The patient has the right to be informed of the hospital's charges for services and available payment methods.

The collaborative nature of health care requires that patients, or their families/surrogates, participate in their care. The effectiveness of care and patient satisfaction with the course of treatment depend, in part, on the patient fulfilling certain responsibilities. Patients are responsible for providing information about past illnesses, hospitalizations, medication, and other matters related to health status. To participate effectively in decision making, patients must be encouraged to take responsibility for requesting additional information and instructions. Patients are also responsible for ensuring that the health care institution has a copy of their written advance directive if they have one. Patients are responsible for informing their physicians and other caregivers if they anticipate problems in following prescribed treatment.

(continued)

DISPLAY 9-3
The Patient's Bill of Rights (continued)

Patients should also be aware of the hospital's obligation to be reasonably efficient and equitable in providing care to other patients and the community. The hospital's rules and regulations are designed to help the hospital meet this obligation. Patients and their families are responsible for making reasonable accommodations to the needs of the hospital, other patients, medical staff, and hospital employees. Patients are responsible for providing necessary information for insurance claims and for working with the hospital to make payment arrangements, when necessary.

A person's health depends on much more than health care services. Patients are responsible for recognizing the impact of their life-style on their personal health.

CONCLUSION

Hospitals have many functions to perform, including the enhancement of health status, health promotion, and the prevention and treatment of injury and disease; the immediate and ongoing care and rehabilitation of patients; the education of health professionals, patients, and the community; and research. All these activities must be conducted with an overriding concern for the values and dignity of patients.

* These rights can be exercised on the patient's behalf by a designated surrogate or proxy decision maker if the patient lacks decision-making capacity, is legally incompetent, or is a minor.

A patient's Bill of Rights was first adopted by the American Hospital Association in 1973. This revision was approved by the AHA Board of Trustees on October 21, 1992.

©1992 by the American Hospital Association, 840 North Lake Shore Drive, Chicago, Illinois 60611. Printed in the U.S.A. All rights reserved. Catalog no. 157759.

Social and Cultural Attitudes

Changes in the attitudes of society as a whole profoundly influence each of its segments. For example, the changing roles of women, the shifting attitudes toward marriage and the family, and the changing status of minorities have all required nurses to reexamine their personal feelings and alter their way of providing nursing care.

Ethical concerns are the by-products of a number of factors at work in our society today, including the role of the individual and the family. In the health care field this is most pointedly illustrated by the use of the terminology "health care" as opposed to "medical care." Health care suggests much greater involvement of others and places the patient in the center of the activity, whereas medical care places the physician in the key role. The meaning of "consumer unit" is shifting from an individual to a whole family or even a whole community. The focus of care also has changed from one that was primarily disease oriented to one that focuses on prevention and wellness.

The size of the group being affected by ethical decisions has a bearing on the decision-making process. The smaller the group, organization, or society that is involved in or affected by the decision making, the easier the process of arriving at an acceptable alternative.

For example, the Oregon Medicaid system limits care for HIV-infected people based on the reasoning that their average life expectancy is short (Hall, 1996). It is unlikely that this decision could have been made if the state had a large population of people who were HIV-infected. The larger the group affected by a decision, the more complex it becomes. Many of our ethical considerations now involve our society as a whole or, in some cases, the world; therefore, solutions are difficult.

The value a society places on the individual or the family directly influences the standard of care (Fig. 9-2). In Western society, we believe in each person's right to exercise choice based on individual beliefs and conscience. We also place high value on preserving individual life; therefore, we often use tremendous resources to try to achieve additional years, months, or even days of life. A society that placed greater emphasis on the community good than on the individual might not choose to use resources in that way. The standard of care might aim for comfort without the use of expensive treatment modalities.

A culture's religious values and belief in an afterlife directly affect ethical issues. The Hindu belief in rebirth after death and the immutability of fate affects decisions about using health care resources. Those who believe that an outcome is predetermined by fate will not choose to commit major resources and efforts toward altering that outcome.

The population, or, more accurately, the overpopulation of a country relative to its resources may also have a direct bearing on the value placed on life. The material resources to provide many health services may not be available. Decisions may be made to eliminate certain costly health care procedures even though they are known to be effective and desired by individuals.

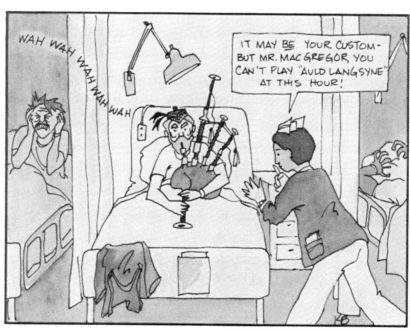

FIGURE 9-2
In providing care, the nurse respects the beliefs, values, and customs of the individual.

Science and Technology

Scientific advancement and technology have left us wrestling with concerns that would have been considered science fiction 50 years ago. Before the development of kidney dialysis, we accepted the fact that people with nonfunctioning kidneys would soon die. After machines that could filter body wastes became available, a genuine dilemma arose over who would have dialysis and who would not; the number of people needing treatment far exceeded the personnel, time, and equipment available to treat them. As the technology became available, the ethical questions refocused on decisions to end treatment rather than on issues related to initiating treatment.

Other technology has had similar effects. The advent of machines that could artificially breathe for someone challenged the medical and legal professions to examine their definitions of life, and brought into focus problems of whether and when to turn off a ventilator. Heart and lung machines that could adequately perfuse the body while the heart was stopped for surgical procedures enabled operations to be performed that were unheard of 50 years before. Fetal monitors, which can be attached to women while they are in labor, provide a continuous readout of the status of the fetus. Such monitoring has resulted in a greater number of infants delivered by cesarean section. The transplantation of organs from one individual to another has created untold ethical dilemmas. Individuals with acquired immunodeficiency syndrome have a limited life expectancy even with the best of health care. Should they be encouraged to participate in sometimes risky research to advance scientific knowledge and the possibility of future benefit to others? How far should experimentation go? Should it include the transfusion of bone marrow from a baboon? Thus, scientific and technological advances continue to present some ethical questions for which no answers are readily apparent.

Legislation

Social change and legislation are constantly interacting. Legislation may follow changes in society's attitudes, converting new ideas into law. For example, a greater acceptance of infants born to single mothers has resulted in legislation that changed the wording of birth certificates, and dropped the word "illegitimate." Similarly, attitudes are being challenged regarding parenting by lesbian and gay couples, either through artificial insemination or adoption.

When social change is desired, legislation may be actively sought to require people to behave in new ways. This was true for much of the civil rights legislation. A change in society was desired, and supporters of civil rights sought legislation as one step toward change. Recent legislative action that addresses the needs and opportunities available to the disabled has brought about changes in public policies, procedures, and even architecture.

Judicial Decisions

The judicial system provides a major avenue for debating and trying to solve ethical problems. We find that more issues are being taken to court, and that judicial decisions are used more often as the basis for determining appropriate action. As you continue to study this topic, note that we have often cited a landmark decision in regard to an ethical issue. The process does not stop there, however. Some people may disagree with a judicial decision and continue to oppose it. Judicial decisions may also be overturned by higher courts. Meanwhile, the questions regarding the individual person's role in carrying out a judicial decision remain. For example, although the law in the past forbade abortions, some physicians believed so strongly in the right of the individual to have the procedure done and were so upset by the results of nonprofessional abortions that they were willing to perform them despite the law prohibiting them. These physicians were, of course, liable to prosecution if they were caught, and some were prosecuted for performing illegal abortions. The issues of abortion and government funding of the procedure are still very controversial. It is not likely that these issues will be resolved in a way that is satisfactory to everyone.

Funding

The financing of health care represents a major area of conflict that has ethical dimensions. The government has become more involved in providing funds for health care. Some people are asking how much time, money, and energy we should allocate to health care, and how those resources should be divided. How obligated are we as a society to make some form of health care available to all? What is it that health care can and cannot provide? Which is more important, prevention or cure? Health care includes controversial procedures, such as abortions, sterilization, and transplantation; some taxpayers do not ethically sanction these procedures and do not want their tax dollars used to fund them. Thus, decisions about funding challenge basic values.

FACTORS IN THE WORK ENVIRONMENT THAT AFFECT ETHICAL DECISION MAKING

By virtue of the positions they hold in the health care system, nurses have special pressures influencing them as they try to make decisions. An awareness of these factors may help you as you struggle with personal problems in decision making.

Status as an Employee

Most nurses are not in independent practice, but are employed by hospitals, nursing homes, community agencies, or outpatient facilities. Pressures divide the nurse's loyalty among patient, employer, and self. You will notice that codes do not speak of responsibilities to the employer, yet, from an ethical standpoint, you have certain loyalties and obligations to the employer who pays your salary and makes decisions regarding your work. It is not unusual for an ethical decision to involve conflict between the best interests of the employer and the patient.

When discussing ethical decisions in the abstract, most people say that, of course, the patient's best interest should be the only priority. In real situations, however, the issues often are not so clearly defined. If a nurse's decision affects the employer adversely, the result may be job loss, poor references, and a severely curtailed economic and career future. For example, one physician was known to routinely require his patients to sign blank surgical permits on admission to the hospital; a staff nurse became upset with this procedure after learning that the patients often did not understand what was being planned. Eventually, she discussed the matter with the physician, pointing out that she did not believe it was ethical to require the patients to sign the blank documents, especially because they were not informed of alternative methods of treatment. The physician became angry and complained to the hospital administration, threatening to take his surgeries elsewhere. This might have created a considerable economic loss for the hospital and, depending on the action of the administrator, the nurse might have been labeled a troublemaker, and even discharged to placate the physician.

Collective Bargaining Contracts

Collective bargaining contracts can protect nurses in making ethical decisions. By formalizing reasons and procedures for termination of employment, and outlining grievance measures so that individual nurses have a mechanism for protecting themselves, a contract may provide greater freedom. (See Chapter 12 for more discussion of collective bargaining and grievance measures.)

Some people believe that contracts hamper individual freedom. The supervisor who believes that an employee does not deliver optimal care may feel unable to do anything about the situation, because the correction and termination processes under a contract are so complex. Often many steps related to notifying the employee of unsatisfactory work and providing assistance for employee improvement are required before a person can be discharged.

Collegial Relationships

Relationships among nurses who work together as effective colleagues and support one another, share in decision making, and present a unified approach to others can provide an excellent climate for ethical decision making. All too often such relationships are lacking in health care institutions. Nurses feel alone and are not experienced in seeking out and providing support to one another. Greater effort on the part of all nurses in this area might be rewarding and is certainly long overdue.

Authoritarian and Paternalistic Backgrounds

The historically authoritarian and paternalistic attitudes of physicians and hospitals often have relegated nurses, most of whom are women, to dependent and subservient roles. These role differentiations have discouraged nurses from taking independent stands on issues, and they continue to affect relationships in the health care field. In some settings, ethical decisions are made without the participation of nurses, yet nurses are expected to implement whatever decisions are made.

More nurses are speaking out against an approach that leaves them out of the decision-making process. Nurses today might expect a physician to discuss the possibly futile treatment of a critically ill patient with the patient, with the family, and with the nursing staff. The patient would be encouraged to express personal needs, the family's views would be included, and the nurses' input would be part of the decision-making process regarding the medical plan of care.

If a nurse makes an ethical decision on the basis of the patient's best interest, but contrary to the physician's or hospital's interest, public support may be forthcoming. The public increasingly sees health care as big business, and tends to support those who champion consumer interests that conflict with the institution's interests. This support may be short lived and therefore should not be relied on for protection against the adverse consequences of an ethical decision.

Ethics Committees in Health Care

Many hospitals have had ethics committees for years. Such committees were traditionally composed of physicians and existed for the purpose of monitoring the behavior of physicians. They acted when a physician's inappropriate behavior, such as arriving at the hospital intoxicated, was reported to them. Today the scope of ethics committees has enlarged considerably. Membership has grown, and, representatives of the hospital administration, the community, and a variety of health care disciplines are being included. An ethicist may serve as a consultant or as a member of the committee. If nurses participate, they have a formal mechanism to share in ethical decision making.

With their expertise and experience, the members of ethics committees help individuals who must make ethical decisions to identify whether they have all the relevant information, to determine other options they have not considered, and to compare the situation with basic ethical principles and theories. Often the committee acts in an advisory capacity to medical staff members and families struggling with difficult decision making. Ethics committees may also help institutions establish policies in regard to ethical concerns that tend to recur in that setting.

Consumer Involvement in Health Care

With consumers involved in decision making, nurses again may face situations in which they are expected to take action based on the conclusions of others. Many nurses may find this as problematic as action based on a physician's decision. For example, an elderly diabetic who is experiencing gangrene of the foot may refuse amputation saying, ''If I'm going to die, I'm going to die whole.'' The nurse, recognizing the life-saving benefit of the amputation, may have difficulty maintaining effective communication and rapport with the patient and family, because of her own convictions that an amputation is the best treatment. Mental health is another area in health care in which nurses may struggle. Patients may refuse to comply with the recommended treatment and as a result live in a homeless, psychiatrically unhealthy situation. This also is very difficult for family members.

A FRAMEWORK FOR ETHICAL DECISION MAKING

When faced with ethical decisions, most of us hope to find the ''right'' answers. Unfortunately, a right answer may not exist for everyone or every situation; such is the nature of dilemmas. However, you can proceed from a basic framework that encourages you to look beyond your first thoughts or feelings to basic issues. A great deal has been written about the decision-making process in the last 2 decades—more in recent years than before. Along with this a number of models have been developed to assist us with ethical decision making (Curtin, 1978; Thompson & Thompson, 1981; Jameton, 1984; Milner, 1993). The steps identified below, gleaned from various approaches, offers a process you can use to help guide you in this task. In studying it, you will realize it is not much different than the nursing process with which you are already very familiar.

Identify and Clarify the Ethical Problem

To define the ethical problem with which you are struggling, you will need to review the situation and gain as clear a perception of the problem as possible. What is the decision to be made? You will need to clarify information about which you are not certain. Consider what ethical principles might be involved. Are those principles in conflict? Who are the relevant parties to this decision? What are their values? Ask yourself what your role and relationship to the problem is. Is this really someone else's decision, which you should not assume, or is it one in which a collaborative decision must be made? What are the time boundaries for making this decision? What other factors will influence the decision?

Gather Data

It is important to have as much information about the unique situation as possible. The facts of the situation will make a difference in what possible options exist. Remember that there is no magic pattern or formula to facts in most situations; they are screened through each person's background and experience. What clearly appears to be a ''true fact'' to one person may seem to be ''opinion'' to another. Therefore, seeking other viewpoints may help you to see the situation more clearly. You need to identify the relevant people in the situation and understand their concerns and perspectives as much as possible. Consider whether legal cases might affect decision making in this case.

Identify Options

Most ethical problems have more than one possible solution. If there were only one solution, there would be no ethical dilemma, because there would be no choice. In some cases more than one solution may be satisfactory; in others, none of the options will seem satisfactory. The more options you can identify, the more likely you are to find one you can support. What are the range of actions that could be taken? What would be the anticipated outcome of those actions? For each option consider its impact on each person involved. Also think about the impact on society as a whole if this option were to be chosen. Consider the ethical theories presented and ask yourself how each particular option compares with the basic principles of each theory. In this way you might determine that one option is basically a utilitarian approach (seeking the greatest good for the greatest number), whereas another is clearly supporting a deontological position of doing one's duty. Is there one approach that is more appropriate than another in this situation? Is this approach in keeping with your own moral and ethical position?

Make a Decision

At some point, you will have to make a decision. This is often difficult and in some instances painful. However, refusing to make a decision that is yours is not a responsible position and, in fact, doing nothing is indeed making a decision. There will never be enough time, enough data, or enough alternatives in some situations. No matter how thorough your analysis or how carefully you weigh all competing claims, you may still be left with uncomfortable feelings.

Act and Assess

Once you have chosen a course of action, you must carry out your decision. This may involve working with others or carrying out plans yourself. Assess the outcomes as you proceed. Unforeseen outcomes are common in ethical situations. Share your thoughts and concerns with others as you proceed, and continue to seek new insights into the situation. As you assess the outcome in this particular situation, consider its relevance for a wider range of situations and concerns. Use this situation as a foundation from which to grow and develop. Ask yourself, ''What have I learned from this experience that will be useful in the future?'' ''What would I do in another situation?'' ''What would I change?''

SPECIFIC ETHICAL ISSUES RELATED TO THE PROFESSION OF NURSING

Some of the ethical issues of concern to nurses relate specifically to the nursing profession; others relate to bioethical issues confronting all of society. In this section we discuss the issues facing nurses through commitment to the patient, commitment to personal excellence, and commitment to the nursing profession as a whole. Bioethical issues that relate to the whole society are discussed in Chapter 10. We present a definite viewpoint regarding ethics in the nursing profession. We feel strongly about the individual nurse's responsibility for nursing practice and place high value on personal integrity in professional relationships.

Commitment to the Patient

Nursing has a strong history of being committed to the well-being of patients who need care. Both the ANA Code for Nurses and the International Code for Nurses, presented earlier in this chapter, clearly point out the nurse's obligation to fulfill this commitment. This obligation has been used to try to persuade nurses that they must not be concerned for themselves, their working conditions, their salaries, or other aspects of their employment. This is not realistic, and may even be counterproductive to the development of effective, autonomous nurses. However, rejection of the handmaiden philosophy does not require rejection of a basic philosophy that nursing is focused on providing patients and their families with support for growth toward maximum health and well-being. Patients can never become objects for nursing, but must be approached as unique individuals who deserve concern, respect, and the best we have to offer.

Recommending a Care Provider

Patients and acquaintances may ask you to recommend a physician or other type of care provider because they believe that, as a nurse, you have special knowledge and insight in such matters. In the past, nurses were admonished not to express opinions about care providers and were encouraged to direct patients to the yellow pages, directories, or hospitals that referred patients to staff physicians on a rotating basis. If you have no personal knowledge about the requested information, then this would be a reasonable approach, or you might honestly tell an individual requesting information that you have no personal or professional knowledge regarding a particular care provider. But if you do have knowledge, it seems inappropriate to sidestep the issue. You could recommend several competent persons, pointing out characteristics of each that might be factors in personal choice. For example, if you were asked to recommend an obstetrician, you might recommend three. You could then further state that Drs. A., B., and C. are all board-certified specialists in obstetrics. You might add some information about their practices: Dr. A. is an older physician with a more traditional approach to childbirth; Dr. B. is a young and innovative physician who strongly advocates father participation and the Lamaze natural childbirth method; Dr. C. is new in the community but appears to allow patients a great deal of choice in their approach to childbirth. The patient can further research these physicians and make a personal choice.

If you are specifically asked about a physician whose care you believe to be less than satisfactory, you are faced with a different dilemma. Making severely critical statements might leave you open to a legal charge of slander by the physician (see Chapter 8). However, saying nothing is ethically a problem because you are not acting to protect the patient. A safe approach is to state, "I personally would not choose Dr. X. as my physician. Instead I would prefer to see Dr. N. or Dr. O." If pressed to give reasons, you are legally more secure if you say that you would prefer not to discuss specifics.

You do need to be careful that any recommendations are not based on hearsay or gossip. If you do not have solid information on which to base a referral, do not be drawn into making one. Being a nurse does not obligate you to be an expert on all health care questions.

Confronting Substandard Care

The day has passed when nurses could be expected to provide unwavering support of all members of the health care team, whatever their actions and whatever the outcome for the patient. Concern for the welfare of patients requires that nurses acknowledge the existence of substandard care and work toward change. We see the issue in terms of the form and extent the involvement should take, rather than whether the nurse should become involved.

A BASIC PATTERN FOR ACTION

The first step in any situation in which you believe substandard care exists is to collect adequate, valid information. Do not make decisions based on gossip, hearsay, or a single isolated instance. If you do, you may create problems for yourself rather than solving problems for the patient. Sometimes a single incident is serious enough that you want to act, but before taking action be sure of your facts.

Your second step is to be certain you understand both the official and the unofficial systems of authority and responsibility within your facility—the formal and the informal operations of the organization. You need to know which people have the authority to make decisions and changes, what the official prescribed route of change is, and what the hidden priorities of the institution might be. For example, the official lines of authority may provide the physician who has been elected chief of staff with authority within the medical group. Your knowledge of the informal system may reveal that a certain respected physician who does not have an official position actually is able to exert more influence for change. Within the nursing chain of responsibility, you may be aware that the head nurse of your unit, although officially having authority, in reality refers all decision making to the supervisor. The head nurse's role may actually be one of information gatherer and sharer.

It is most commonly recommended that you take concerns to your immediate supervisor first. Many people believe that reporting to a supervisor fulfills your ethical responsibility as well as your legal responsibility. If the system always worked effectively, your supervisor would forward the concern until it reached the individual or committee with the authority and duty to act. However, in some states, laws exist that require that poor practice be reported directly to the relevant licensing board. You need to know the hospital policies and the regulations of the state in which you are employed.

ALTERNATIVE APPROACHES FOR ACTION

There are times when the system does not always work as expected. Your concern regarding what you perceive as poor practice may be dropped or ignored at any one of many points. You may never learn what was done, even when positive action was taken, because of the constraints of confidentiality. Occasionally, results emerge only much later, when a change in procedure and policy occurs.

Often there are good reasons for this. Perhaps the persons in authority want to collect more specific data about a situation, with as little general discussion as possible. Sometimes there are aspects of a legal contract or a collective bargaining contract of which you are unaware that must be considered in the actions that are taken. Other times, professional confidentiality may make it seem that nothing is being done when, in fact, steps have been taken to correct a situation. It is easy as a newcomer to the health care scene to see only part of a picture.

However, there are times when an alternative initial approach is more appropriate to the situation. There are a number of ways you can bring about change. You may volunteer to serve on committees that deal with peer review. If there are no such committees, you may work to have them established, perhaps through a bargaining unit. This route of action will require a considerable investment of your own time and effort. The cry of ''Why doesn't somebody do something?'' may often be answered ''Because nobody takes the time.'' This is a real constraint on action.

Another initial approach is to use the informal system within the facility. You may discuss your concern with a trusted person (or mentor) who has influence within the system. You may learn that you are not alone in your concerns, that efforts toward change are being made, and that your input of data is welcomed. Another approach would be to seek the assistance of another individual with power within the organization. However, we must caution you about using informal systems; informal systems can backfire. If your immediate superior learns that you went over his or her head with your concerns, he or she may direct anger at you. Additionally, the person with whom you choose to share your concern may recognize that you have ''skipped a step'' in the reporting process and send you back to your supervisor.

If your initial approach is not effective, a formal route for seeking further change would lead you through the official lines of authority within your facility. After discussing your concern with your immediate supervisor and receiving no satisfactory response, you would tell the supervisor formally that you intend to carry your concern to the next higher authority. Technically you could proceed in this manner until you reached the administrator or even the board of directors.

Another formal route for seeking further change is through designated committees or procedures within your facility. As hospitals move into models of shared governance this may be your best alternative. Discussing or sharing a problem with a particular committee might require a carefully written documented report explaining your concern. You might then be called to answer questions that the committee believe it is important to ask.

A final alternative to a problem in your work setting is to offer your resignation if a change is not made. Continuing to work in an environment in which poor practice exists may place you in conflict with your ethical standards and values. If you find it necessary to do this, be careful that you do not jeopardize your own future with angry letters or intemperate remarks. The old saying, ''Don't burn your bridges behind you'' is relevant in such a situation. Render your resignation in a polite and professional manner even when expressing dissatisfaction with the system.

Reporting directly to a state licensing board or professional organization's disciplinary committee is an avenue of action outside of the employment setting. These organizations and agencies usually deal with serious problems that represent a breach of the public trust or serious harm. They may not have the capacity or desire to pursue minor (though still important) problems. The same constraints apply when reporting to these organizations. Remember that their investigation and decisions may be done in a judicial or legal manner. This may involve the requirement that you provide legal testimony in regard to your complaints.

PERSONAL RISKS IN REPORTING

If you decide to pursue any of these routes, you need to be fully aware of the possible consequences. You may be labeled a troublemaker, or worse. You may lose the opportunity to be promoted because you are seen as being antagonistic to the system. It is even possible that you could lose your job for creating too many waves. Officially this should not happen, but in reality it can and does. We do not mean to be unduly discouraging, but we want to warn you that the role of change agent is not easy, and you should be aware of and weigh the consequences before you decide to act. And above all, be certain that your perceptions are correct and that you are well-grounded in your concerns.

Commitment to Personal Excellence

To meet the commitment to a patient, each individual nurse must be committed to personal excellence. Basic to moving toward personal excellence is a willingness to engage in self-evaluation and assume responsibility in the work setting.

SELF-EVALUATION

Self-evaluation is discussed throughout this text in relationship to personal career goals, legal concerns, and continuing education. The health care professional also has a strong ethical responsibility to practice self-evaluation. You are the one who is best able to identify your weaknesses and practice deficits as well as your strengths. Your careful self-evaluation is the patient's best protection against poor or inadequate care.

Self-evaluation is not always an easy or pleasant task. If we are truly honest with ourselves, we will be likely to uncover areas we wish were not there. Remember, done informally, these do not have to be shared with anyone; that is one of the beauties of self-evaluation. On the other hand, do not hesitate to ask for assistance if you think you need it. One is seldom criticized for trying to do a better job. Many institutions are now including self-evaluation in the formal evaluation of employees. If this is the case, you may be asked to prepare a written self-evaluation that will be shared with at least your immediate supervisor.

One approach to self-evaluation is the use of the nursing process format. Begin with a thorough personal assessment. To do this you will have to gather data about your own performance. This requires a level of objectivity that is not easy. You might outline areas in which you want to gather data and actually keep notes on yourself.

After data have been collected, you will need to give yourself time to reflect on it and analyze it thoroughly. The self-assessment outline includes questions you should ask yourself; however, the criteria that you use to determine whether your answers reflect the quality of performance you want to attain are not included. Those specific criteria must be individualized to the setting in which you work and the nature of your role in that setting. The breadth of data that represent excellent practice for the nurse in the emergency department differs from what would represent excellence for the nurse working in a rehabilitation setting. The amount of decision making in which the patient participates differs between the post-anesthesia recovery room and the outpatient clinic.

Your analysis can reveal strengths, weaknesses, and areas for growth or improvement. Congratulate yourself on the strengths identified and then clearly delineate those areas in which you want to change. As in nursing care planning, clearly identifying and stating the problems or growth needed helps you to plan more effectively.

After you have identified your problems or areas for growth, it is appropriate to establish a plan of action. The plan is more helpful to you if it contains clearly defined goals. What is a realistic expectation for yourself? When is an appropriate time to reach that expectation? As part of realizing these goals, you might find it helpful to establish criteria you will use to identify your progress. Once the goals are set, you are better able to plan appropriate action to meet them. You might consider such things as requesting in-service education, taking continuing education courses, consulting with colleagues, and doing independent reading and study. Some plans need to include specific things to do in your daily nursing care for improvement. To do this you may want to request assignments that will provide opportunities for practice of skills.

All this planning should not go to waste. Implementing this plan will require you to remain focused on what you are trying to accomplish. Keeping records on yourself is often helpful. It also provides very positive reinforcement when you realize that some of your goals have been met.

DISPLAY 9-4
Self-Evaluation Plan

ASSESSMENT OF PATIENTS

- Do I gather enough breadth of data about patients and families, including both strengths and deficits?
- Do I gather data in great enough depth?
- Do I listen closely to the patient and attend to what is being said?
- Do I regularly use all available sources for information about my patients? (patient, family, other staff, chart, Kardex, and so forth.)
- Have I recognized problems quickly so that they did not become worse through inattention?
- Do I recognize physiological, social, and psychological problems?

PLANNING FOR PATIENT CARE

- Do I routinely seek more information on which to base decisions about patient care?
- Do I include the patient in decision making whenever possible?
- Do I consult with others on the health care team when planning?
- Are my written plans clear, concise, and reasonable to carry out?
- Do I take into account the realities of the situation when planning care?
- Are my plans for care sound and appropriate to the individual patient?
- Do I employ principles from the biological and social sciences in planning?

INTERVENTION

- Is my work organized and finished on time?
- Do I maintain optimum safe working habits?
- Do I perform technical skills in an efficient and safe manner?
- Do I communicate clearly and effectively with patients, family, and staff?
- Do I use therapeutic communication techniques appropriately and effectively?
- Do I use teaching approaches appropriate to the individual patient and family?
- Do I keep accurate and complete written records?
- Do I understand and perform any administrative tasks which are my responsibility? (ordering supplies, planning for laboratory tests, and so on.)
- Do I make the effort to learn about new techniques and procedures?

EVALUATION

- Do I routinely evaluate the effectiveness of the nursing care I give?
- Do I effectively assist in evaluation of the patient's response to medical care and to ordered therapies?
- Do I encourage the patient to participate in evaluating both the process and the outcomes of care?
- Is self-evaluation a planned part of my activities?
- Do I use data collected during evaluation for the improvement of my own functioning and patient care?

(continued)

DISPLAY 9-4
Self-Evaluation Plan (continued)

PERSONAL GROWTH AND RELATIONSHIPS

- Have I established a sound trust and working relationship with co-workers?
- Do I support and assist my co-workers when possible?
- Do I communicate effectively with others on the health care team?
- Have I sought opportunities for learning and personal growth?
- Is my attitude helpful and productive?
- Do I have sound working habits? (appearing on time, limiting coffee and lunch breaks to the correct time, and so forth)
- Is my appearance appropriate to the working environment?
- Do I use appropriate channels of communication within the institution correctly?
- Do I handle criticism constructively?
- Am I doing my share in overall professional activities such as serving on committees or assisting with development projects?
- Am I honest with myself, being neither too harsh nor too easy going?

Periodic evaluation of your progress is necessary so that you do not become discouraged. Any records you have kept will be valuable for this purpose. Sometimes it is hard to identify gradual change. You might even plan rewards for yourself for improvement that occurs. Try not to become discouraged if you do not see the improvement you desire. Remember that just as a reassessment and a new plan are often necessary in patient care planning, a revised plan may be needed in the self-evaluation process. Keep in mind that your overall goal is personal excellence in nursing practice. Display 9-4 suggests questions that can be asked in a self-evaluation plan.

RESPONSIBILITY FOR SUPPLIES

Pilfering includes stealing in small amounts or stealing objects of little value. Many people who are otherwise scrupulously honest do not recognize that taking small items from a place of employment is indeed theft. Employees often take home adhesive bandage strips, pens, and other such objects so routinely that they do not even consider whether this is right or wrong. With the large number of employees in modern agencies, this constant petty theft may total thousands of dollars. The cost of this must be passed on to those who pay the bills—the patients. As a leader in the care setting, the registered nurse is often in a position to clearly communicate to all employees that pilfering is unacceptable. The nurse can set an example of careful stewardship of the hospital supplies.

Sometimes removing supplies is an oversight rather than a planned action (Fig. 9-3). To make efficient use of time, nurses commonly place many small items such as alcohol wipes, extra needles, and pens in their pockets. One hospital unit found that their yearly

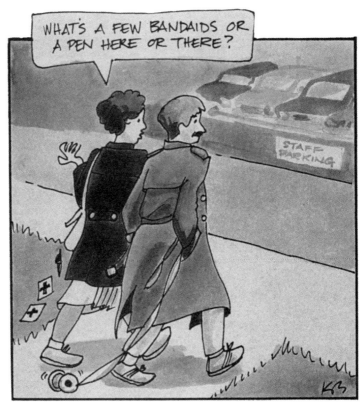

FIGURE 9-3
Many people who are otherwise scrupulously honest do not recognize that taking small items from a place of employment is theft.

supply budget for black pens was almost exhausted in the first 6 months of the year. The simple action of placing a basket in the lounge into which nurses dropped everything from their pockets before leaving cut the pen costs dramatically. Perhaps you can be equally creative in helping to solve such problems in your work setting.

Commitment to the Nursing Profession

Commitment to the nursing profession requires that each individual nurse be concerned not only about personal performance, but also about how nursing is practiced. This involves participation in formal and informal evaluation of nursing care, dealing with poor care, and identifying the impaired nurse. Nurses always have evaluated one another in both formal and informal ways. Some people think that evaluation implies noting error or deficiency. Good evaluation is much broader than this. The main purpose of peer evaluation is to maintain consistent high-quality nursing care. This is an ethical, professional obligation.

INFORMAL EVALUATION

Methods of evaluation vary. An important component of peer evaluation is actual obser-vation of the performance of others. Often coworkers are the ones who are best able to observe a nurse's performance. Watching other nurses will also help you to grow in your own practice. When you observe coworkers, you need to strive for objectivity. A common mistake is to let personal feelings, likes, and dislikes influence our observations so that we see only what we want to see. We may view a close friend only in a positive light, whereas we see only the negative aspects of a nurse with whom we have a poor personal relationship.

Another important aspect of evaluation is examining results or outcomes of care. Two nurses may use different approaches or techniques in similar situations, but both may achieve positive results.

Evaluation is not negative. As you observe behavior and outcomes in nursing practice, you will most often see good nursing care. Do not hesitate to commend others and share your positive feelings. Everyone benefits from positive reinforcement of skill; it helps nurses to create a good climate for personal growth and sharing.

DEALING WITH POOR CARE

An ethical dilemma arises when you observe a colleague practicing what you think is poor patient care, such as poor sterile technique. Various avenues of action are available to you. What you choose to do depends on the seriousness of the situation you have observed. We suggest the following pattern for action as one that may assist in correcting a problem and, at the same time, maintaining positive working relationships.

Usually the simplest and most effective solution to any problem is to go directly to the person involved and to state: "I observed this specific incident, and it seemed to me that it was not in the best interest of the patient because . . . . How do you feel about it?" This does not level accusations of bad nursing and it does allow the nurse to give rationale for the action taken; when you understand the situation more fully, you may have a different point of view. If you disagree with your colleague and the situation is not critical, you might want to simply state that you do disagree. Sometimes just calling an incident to the attention of the person will result in a change in behavior, even if there is no open agreement that a change is needed.

If you observe poor care a second time, you might again approach the person. State what you have seen, and note that it is the second time. If the person still disagrees that a problem exists, state that you feel obligated to discuss this with your immediate superior, because it is not in the best interest of the patient. You should then follow through on this.

When you approach a supervisor, you need to give specific information with dates, situations, and the action you took. You should not indulge in generalities or sweeping statements, but should stick to specific observed instances. Let the supervisor know that you have talked with the person under discussion and have informed the person that you would speak with the supervisor. It is important to specify the action you would like to see occur. You might ask the supervisor to discuss the matter with both of you to clarify the correct nursing procedure. Or you might ask that the supervisor talk about the matter with the other nurse or observe the nurse. A vague declaration of "You should do something about this!" is not helpful. It is also important to remember that once you have initiated this action, you may be involved in some follow-up.

If your focus has been on enhancing the welfare of patients, and you have been quick to praise the good care provided by others, your action in response to poor care will be more readily accepted. Remember that your attitude when approaching another nurse is crucial. Facial expressions and tone of voice, as well as words, need to be considered. If you are perceived as friendly and caring, your comments probably will be accepted in a far different manner than if you are seen as being negative and critical.

But you cannot always count on this. Many nurses feel threatened by the idea of evaluation, or have had bad experiences in which evaluation only involved pointing out deficiencies. These nurses may be angry and upset with any colleague who considers evaluation part of the colleague role. There is a great deal of pressure in these situations to close your eyes to what is happening around you and concentrate only on your own care.

If you observe an incident that has the potential to cause a patient danger (such as an unreported medication error) or one that has legal ramifications (such as the falsifying of narcotic records), you have a legal as well as an ethical responsibility to go immediately to a supervisor with your information. In a situation that has the potential for legal involvement, it is prudent to keep an exact personal record of your observations and actions. Your record should include times and dates of incidents and of your reporting efforts (see Chapter 8).

FORMAL EVALUATION

Formal evaluation of nursing is occurring in most settings under the title of quality assurance and quality improvement. Quality assurance is a planned program of evaluation that includes ongoing monitoring of the care given and of outcomes of care. It includes a mechanism for instituting change when problems or opportunities for improvement are identified. Quality assurance programs are required by the Joint Commission on the Accreditation of Healthcare Organizations and by Medicare.

All types of evaluation first call for establishing specific criteria to be used in the evaluation. These criteria may refer to process, to outcome, or to both. The creation of the criteria is a professional nursing responsibility.

The first aspect of nursing care that is usually evaluated is whether nursing actions taken are complete and appropriate. Criteria developed to evaluate this aspect are called process criteria. One basis for developing process criteria is the "Standards of Clinical Nursing Practice" developed by the ANA (American Nurses Association, 1991). General standards refer to all settings, and more specific ones exist for gerontologic, maternal–child, community health, psychiatric–mental health, and other specialty areas of nursing. Some specialty organizations such as the Intravenous Nurses' Society have also published standards that refer to their specific specialty.

Another basis for formal evaluation is the use of outcome criteria for patient care. Outcome criteria are specific, observable patient behaviors or clinical manifestations that are the desired results of care. They usually are established by nurses working in groups. Nursing literature is consulted so that appropriate criteria are established.

A number of methods have been used to evaluate both the process and the outcomes of nursing care. Conferences designed to discuss the matter to be evaluated are personal and flexible but may lack objectivity. Simple interviews with either patients or staff also lack objectivity, although valuable insight and direction may be gained from them. Direct observation of patients provides an excellent means of evaluation if specific criteria are set up before the observation, but it is time consuming. The method that is gaining wider acceptance in nursing is the audit based on review of the patient's record. If information does not appear in the record, (other than situations in which "charting by exception" are employed) then, for the purposes of the audit, the appropriate observations were not made or the actions were not taken. This may come as a shock to nurses who reply, "But we always do that!"

The chart review involves comparing the patient record with the criteria. Often medical records personnel are responsible for this evaluation. The accuracy of the review depends on the adequacy of the charting. This is just one of the reasons why you must recognize the importance of your charting and make sure that you maintain a high standard in written records. If audits are being done at your institution, you should become familiar with the criteria being used. These criteria can serve as guidelines for you in evaluating your own care and record-keeping.

The chart review has raised serious concerns that have resulted in greater attention to documentation, and even revision of record systems. Once the information has been gathered, nurses again take the initiative in determining the meaning of the data and what the next step should be. Because the goal is improvement of patient care, it is hoped that the audit will result in plans to enhance patient well-being. Changes in policies and procedures and in-service education classes are some of the approaches that have been used. Once remedial action has been taken, reevaluation is done to determine its effectiveness. Formal evaluation of nursing care is successful only if all nurses recognize their individual responsibility and accountability for practice and are willing to learn and grow to enhance patient care.

The Chemically Impaired Professional

The *chemically impaired professional* is a term used to describe that person whose practice has deteriorated because of chemical abuse, specifically the use of alcohol and drugs. There is a strong possibility that each of you, if you remain active in the profession, will at some time find yourself working with a chemically impaired colleague; perhaps you already have.

One would like to believe that nurses, who have studied the physiologic effects of alcohol and drugs on the system, would avoid the chances of such abuse. This is not the case. Statistics regarding chemical dependency in nurses are flawed, owing to the social stigma and the subsequent efforts to protect the individuals involved (Sullivan, Bissell, & Williams, 1988). From September 1980 to August 1981 the National Council of State Boards of Nursing collected data on disciplinary actions from its member state boards. Of the cases reported during that period, it was determined that 67% of the disciplinary proceedings involving nurses were related to some form of chemical abuse (Sullivan, Bissell, & Williams, 1988). The state boards have not published data since that time. Several studies of alcoholic physicians and nurses have revealed that only a small percentage were ever reported to their respective state boards (Bissell & Haberman, 1984; Bissell & Skorina, 1987). In their discussion of chemical dependency in nursing, Sullivan and colleagues (1988) estimated the number of chemically dependent nurses based on statistics for the general population and the number of nurses in treatment. Although both physicians and nurses are overrepresented among those in chemical dependency treatment programs, it may be that they are more predisposed to enter treatment than the population at large. Sullivan and colleagues conclude that the percentage of chemically dependent nurses is at least as great as the percentage of chemically dependent people in the general population, and it may be that there is a greater percentage in the nursing population based on accessibility of drugs.

Recently studies have been done to assess probable alcoholism among nursing students. Marion and colleagues (Marion, 1996) reported that the use of alcohol by nursing students paralleled the alcohol consumption of other college students, an age group recognized as demonstrating high usage. Their findings indicate that there are significant drinking problems among the students sampled. Campbell and Polk (1992) have also expressed concern about substance abuse among students, and have encouraged nurse educators to identify students suspected of abuse and to educate students about the problem. Sullivan, Bissell, and Leffler (1990) reported that the addiction process was starting earlier, sometimes even prior to nursing school, and that younger nurses were more likely to use narcotics, resulting in serious problems in job performance.

Why are nurses affected by this problem? Factors that lead to chemical dependency include the stress that one encounters in the nursing profession, particularly in intensive care units and emergency departments. Frequent shift changes and staffing shortages add to the situation. Unrealistic personal expectations, frustration, powerlessness, anxiety, and depression contribute to the problem. Once the problem exists, denial is a big part of the disease.

Jefferson and Ensor (1982) provide the following information about addiction:

Addiction is an insidious process that occurs as the result of a) prolonged intake of a chemical, b) processes going on within the individual (including genetic, psychological, and chemical), and c) processes external to the individual (that is, the actions and reactions of family, friends, co-workers, supervisors, and society) .... Addiction is present any time a chemical interferes with any aspect of a person's life and that person keeps using the chemical.

All areas of the profession are impacted by the problem of chemical dependency in nursing. A significant financial impact is realized by institutions that employ nurses with dependency problems in the forms of sickness, absenteeism, tardiness, accidents, errors, decreased productivity, and staff turnover. Early recognition and treatment have been recommended to help offset this problem (LaGodna & Hendrix, 1989). Nurse managers who are confronted with the problem of impaired practitioners may begin to question the efficacy of treatment (Hendrix, Sabritt, McDaniel, & Field, 1987).

In 1981, the ANA appointed a Nursing Task Force on Addiction and Psychological Disturbance to develop guidelines for the treatment and assistance of nurses whose practice was impaired by alcoholism, drug abuse, or psychological dysfunction. The guidelines were designed for use by state nurses' associations. These guidelines served as a basis for state associations to approach chemical dependency in nursing from a treatment and rehabilitation viewpoint rather than from a punishment viewpoint. In 1990, the ANA developed suggested state legislation to respond to the problems of chemical dependency and drug diversion in nurses (American Nurses Association, 1990). The emphasis in this recommendation was on a voluntary treatment and monitoring program for nurses with problems rather than traditional legal proceedings.

The concerns about the chemically impaired nurse are twofold. The first is a personal concern for the nurse who is afflicted: the illness may go undetected and untreated for years.

The second concern is for the patient, whose care is jeopardized by the nurse whose judgment and skills are weakened.

Because nurses, by virtue of their education, are socialized into caring roles, they have not always dealt with the problem in a straightforward fashion. The impaired nurse was often protected, transferred, ignored, and, in some instances, promoted. None of these actions helped solve the problem.

What are some of the behaviors you will notice in a chemically impaired colleague? The following characteristics are commonly seen in alcoholic nurses:

- More irritable with patients and colleagues; withdrawn; mood swings
- Illogical and sloppy charting
- Excessive errors
- Unkempt appearance
- Social isolation; wants to work nights, lunches alone, avoids informal staff gatherings
- Elaborate excuses for behavior such as being late for work
- Blackouts: complete memory loss for events, conversations, phone calls to colleagues; euphoric or "glossed over" recall of events on floor (ie, arguments or unpleasant events)
- Frequent use of breath purifiers, drinks high volume of "sodas"
- Flushed face, red or bleary eyes, unsteady gait, slurred speech
- Signs of withdrawal; tremors, restlessness, diaphoresis (Washington State Nurses Association, 1992, p. 10)

A drug-addicted nurse commonly exhibits the following behaviors:

- Extreme and rapid mood swings, irritable with patients, and then calm again (after taking drugs)
- Wears long sleeves all of the time
- Suspicious behavior concerning controlled drugs:
- Consistently signs out more controlled drugs than anyone else
- Frequently breaks and spills drugs
- Purposely waits until alone to open narcotics cabinet
- Constantly volunteers to be the medications nurse
- Disappears into bathroom directly after being in narcotics cabinet
- Vials/medications appear altered
- Incorrect narcotic count
- Discrepancies between his/her patient reports and others' patient reports on effect of medications
- Patient complaints that pain medications dispensed by this individual are ineffective
- Defensive when questioned about medication errors
- Abnormal number of syringes being used or missing
- Frequent use of restroom by the nurse; evidence of broken syringes, bloody pieces of cotton in bathroom (Washington Health Professional Services, 1992)

Problems related to drug abuse are complicated by the fact that the nurse usually is obtaining drugs from the supply available on the hospital unit and is therefore in violation of the Controlled Substances Act.

In addition to personal behavior changes, job performance changes also occur in those with drug and alcohol problems. These job performance changes include:

- Doing the minimum necessary
- Difficulty meeting schedules and deadlines
- Illogical and sloppy charting
- Excessive medication errors
- Excessive incidence of controlled drugs broken or spilled
- Increasing absences without adequate explanation (Washington State Nurses Association, 1992, p. 11)

As a registered nurse, what should you do if you suspect that a colleague has a chemical dependency problem? First of all, you need to know what the law in your state requires of you. In many states every professional is legally obligated to report a chemically dependent health care professional. This reporting most commonly is done through channels at the place of employment, but may also be done directly to the State Board of Nursing. If you do not know the requirements, you should immediately learn what they are. In some states failure to report can result in disciplinary action toward you.

When planning to report you do not have to be sure beyond any doubt that a problem exists. You need to have enough data to represent a reasonable concern. The investigation to clearly establish the problem is the responsibility of the employing agency or the state board.

To establish reasonable concern, collect data and document it, including objective facts, dates, and times that support your concern. Do not confront or accuse the person whom you suspect. For at least several good reasons you should not confront the person whom you suspect at this time.

First, the person may become more secretive about the behavior because of the danger of being caught. This will make collection of data more difficult, if not impossible. Personal defenses and denial may become stronger. The suspected person may ask for a transfer to another shift or to a different part of the facility, or, if truly threatened, may seek employment in another facility.

Second, the person may feel attacked and rejected. To ensure that it not end in a disaster, a confrontation needs the support of a knowledgeable professional. With the support of the appropriate health care person, the individual may be guided to appropriate choices for treatment and rehabilitation.

We have already alluded to another reason you should not confront the suspected person at this time. You are still collecting data and documenting it. You cannot be sure from a single observation that a problem exists. There are often reasons why things are not the way we initially perceived them to be. If the person is someone you know well, who confides in you regarding personal problems, you might use those occasions to refer the individual to appropriate resources for personal assistance and counseling.

Once you feel you have data to support a realistic concern, you should report it to a supervisor to validate your observations. Usually once you have notified your supervisor, he or she will assume responsibility for the problem, but may ask for your continued assistance with data collection or with confrontation.

Once adequate information has been gathered, agency administrative personnel will notify the State Board of Nursing. In addition, they usually must notify the State Board of

Pharmacy if drugs are involved. More investigation will be carried out; records will be examined. If a problem exists, actions appropriate to the situation will be taken. These usually include a carefully planned confrontation by an intervention team, a requirement that treatment be sought, and a presentation of the consequences of not seeking treatment.

The worst thing you can do if you suspect a problem is to ignore it or help a colleague "cover" for inadequacies. The problem will not get better if it is not recognized and treated. The longer the delay, the greater the chance that an innocent patient will be placed in jeopardy.

Fortunately, help and rehabilitation are being made available to those who need it. Many states now have programs to provide support for treatment of health care professionals with chemical dependency. These programs usually provide a specific contractual agreement in regard to professional practice during the treatment and monitoring period. This is often done without formal disciplinary proceedings. The goal of this process is restoration of the individual to effective functioning. At the present time, 16 states have special programs for chemically dependent nurses that serve as alternatives to standard disciplinary action (Smith & Hughes, 1996).

In some states the licensing boards may institute formal disciplinary proceedings to suspend a license or issue a license with limitations on practice, and to provide monitoring and supervision while the individual seeks treatment. When treatment is completed, the board may reinstate the license with temporary limitations and continued monitoring and support. The goal is the eventual full rehabilitation of the health care professional to the service of the community. Baldwin and Smith (1994) reported a much higher treatment success rate in nurses than in the general population. These researchers further identified that successful recovery was most likely in those nurses who retained their employment during treatment. Therefore, reporting a chemically dependent colleague may be the most caring action you can take.

If, as a nursing student, you suspect that a fellow classmate (or worse yet, an instructor) has a problem with chemical abuse, you would be wise to discuss your concerns with your instructor or with the director of the program. Because such problems typically get worse with time, the earlier they are addressed and corrected the better it is for everyone. Again, it is important that you have accurate information to report, along with times and dates and examples of the behavior that caused your concern.

KEY CONCEPTS

- Ethics is a branch of philosophy referred to as moral philosophy. It seeks to provide answers to some of the questions of human conduct that arise in our life, and attempts to determine what is "right" or "good."
- Inherent in the study of ethics is an appreciation of individual values that are derived from societal norms, religion, and family orientation. We can get in better touch with our own value system through the process of values clarification.
- The basic ethical concepts of beneficence, nonmaleficence, autonomy, justice, fidelity, veracity and the standard of best interest underlie ethical decision making and may be in conflict in an individual situation.

- The ethical theories of utilitarianism, deontology, natural law, and social equity and justice may be used to examine the implications of ethical decisions.
- Ethical decision making may be based on personal religious and philosophical view-points, but must always be grounded in professional standards seen in the Codes for Nurses and the statements of patient rights.
- A variety of social and cultural factors including attitudes, science and technology, legislation, judicial decisions, and funding all influence ethical decision making.
- The nurse's status as an employee, collective bargaining contracts, collegial relationships, the authoritarian and paternalistic backgrounds of health care, deliberations of ethics committees, and consumer involvement create pressures in regard to ethical decision making.
- A basic framework for ethical decision making emphasizes identifying and clarifying the problem, gathering data, identifying options, making a decision, acting, and assessing.
- Nurses have ethical obligations to the patient, and must maintain an objective stance in regard to other health care providers, and when confronting substandard care. Commitment to personal excellence and to the profession of nursing also characterize the excellent nurse.
- The chemically impaired nurse is a concern to the profession and a danger to patients. All nurses have an obligation to report those who demonstrate chemical impairment and to assist impaired colleagues in finding treatment and rehabilitation.

Critical Thinking Activities

1. Identify four situations you might confront in nursing in which your personal religious or philosophical values would be involved. If they are in conflict, how will you deal with the differences? Are there any other alternatives? What might they be?
2. Identify ways in which the concept of beneficence has shaped medical and nursing care provided to patients. Do you believe this is a concept that will have the same impact in years to come? Provide a rationale for your response.
3. Of the ethical theories provided in this chapter, select the one that most appeals to you and describe the aspects of the theory that make it most attractive.
4. Identify two sociocultural factors with which you have had personal experience that could impact ethical decision making. How is your view of this different than it might have been five years ago? In what ways have your views remained the same? Why do you think your views have changed or remained the same?
5. Assume that you have serious concerns that a colleague is delivering poor patient care because of problems with chemical dependency. Where would you begin? What is your personal responsibility? What is your responsibility to your colleague? What is your responsibility to the patients? What steps should you take? Do you have a personal liability in the situation?

REFERENCES

Aiken TD, Catalono JT. Legal, Ethical, and Political Issues in Nursing. Philadelphia: F.A.Davis Company, 1994

American Hospital Association. A Patient's Bill of Rights. Chicago, IL: AHA, 1992

American Nurses Association. Standards of Clinical Nursing Practice. Washington, DC: American Nurses Association, 1991

American Nurses Association. Suggested State Legislation: Nursing Practice Act, Nursing Disciplinary Diversion Act, Prescriptive Authority Act (Publ. No. NP-78). Washington, DC: American Nurses Association, 1990

Baldwin L, Smith V. Relapse in chemically dependent nurses: Relevance and contributing factors. Issues 15(1):1, 4–5, 1994

Bissell L, Haberman PW. Alcoholism in the professions. New York: Oxford University Press, 1984

Bissell L, Skorina J. 100 alcoholic women in medicine. JAMA 257:2939–2944, 1987

Bok S. Lying: Moral Choice in Public and Private Life. New York: Pantheon Books, 1978

Buchanan A. Judging the past: The care of the human radiation experiments. Hasting Center Report 2(13):25–30, 1996

Cohen MM, Cohen EN, Thomasma DC. Making treatment decisions for permanently unconscious patients. *In* Monagle JF, Thomasma DC: Medical Ethics: A Guide for Health Professionals. Rockville, MD: Aspen Publishers, 1988

Campbell AR, Polk E. Legal and ethical issues of alcohol and other substance abuse in nursing education. Atlanta, GA: Southern Council on Collegiate Education for Nursing, 1992

Curtin L. A proposed model for critical ethical analysis. Nursing Forum 17(1):12–17, 1978

Davis AJ, Aroskar MA. Ethical Dilemmas and Nursing Practice, 3rd ed. East Norwalk, Connecticut: Appleton & Lange, 1991

DeGeorge RT. Business Ethics. Englewood Cliffs, NJ: Prentice-Hall, 1993

Detmer DE, Steen EB. Shoring up protection of personal health data. Issues in Science and Technology XII(4):73–78, Summer 1996

Firth R. Ethical absolutism and the ideal observer. *In* Sellars W, Hospers J: Readings in Ethical Theory. Englewood Cliffs, NJ: Prentice-Hall, 1970

Fung L. Implementing the Patient Self-Determination Act (PSDA): How to effectively engage Chinese-American persons in the decision of advance directives. Journal of Gerontological Social Work, 22(1–2):161–174, 1994

Hall JK. Nursing Ethics and Law. Philadelphia: W.B. Saunders Company, 1996

Hendrix M, Sabritt D, McDaniel A, Field B. Perceptions and attitudes toward nursing impairment. Research in Nursing and Health 10:323–333, 1987.

Jameton A. Nursing Practice: The Ethical Issues. Englewood Cliffs, NJ: Prentice-Hall, 1984

Jefferson LV, Ensor BE. Confronting a chemically impaired colleague. Am J Nurs 82(4):574, 1982

LaGodna G, Hendrix M. Impaired nurses: A cost analysis. J Nurs Admin 19(9):13–18, 1989

Lane SD, Rubinstein RA. Judging the other: responding to traditional female genital surgeries. Hastings Center Report 26(3):31–40, 1996

Marion LN, Fuller SG, Johnson NP, Michels PJ, Diniz C. Drinking problems of nursing students. J Nurs Educ 35(5):196–203, 1996

Miller FG, Brody H. Professional integrity and physician-assisted death. Hastings Center Report 25(3):8–17, 1995

Milner S. An ethical nursing practice model. J Nurs Admin 23(3):22–25, 1993

Neufedt V, Guralnik DN. Webster's New World Collegiate Dictionary, 3rd ed. New York: Macmillan Company, 1996:581

New encyclopedia of bioethics includes A.N.A. code. Am J Nurs 77(8):872, 1977

Rawls J. A Theory of Justice. Cambridge MA: Harvard University Press, 1971

Salk J. Phenomena of Life. Chicago: University of Chicago Press, 1982 as cited in Hasting Center Report 25(7):inside back cover.

Smith LL, Hughes TL. Re-entry: When a chemically dependent colleague returns to work. Am J Nurs 96(2):32–37, 1996

Stahl DA. Ethics in Subacute Care–Part I. Nurs Management 27(9):29–30, 1996

Steele SM, Harmon VM. Values Clarification in Nursing. New York: Appleton-Century-Crofts, 1979

Sullivan E, Bissell L, Leffler D. Drug use and disciplinary actions among 300 nurses. International Journal of the Addictions 25(4):375–391, 1990

Sullivan E, Bissell L, Williams E. Chemical Dependency in Nursing: The Deadly Diversion. Menlo Park, CA: Addison-Wesley, 1988

Thompson J, Thompson H. Ethics in Nursing. New York: Macmillan Publishing Company, 1981

Washington Health Professional Services. A Guide for Assisting Colleagues Who Demonstrate Impairment in the Workplace. Olympia, WA: Washington State Department of Health, 1992

Washington State Nurses Association. Handbook for Working With the Chemically Dependent Nurse. Seattle: Washington State Nurses Association, 1992

FURTHER READING

Bagwood T. Substance abuse and obligations to colleagues. Nurs Management 21(8):40–41, 1990

Beckel J. Resolving ethical problems in long-term care. J Gerontol Nurs 22(1):20–26, 1996

Bosek MSD. Nursing ethics. Optimizing ethical decision making: The decision analysis model. Medsurg Nurs 4(6):486–488, 1995

Bowden PL. The ethics of nursing care and ''the ethic of care.'' Nursing Inquiry 2(1):10–21, 1995

Browne A. A conceptual clarification of respect. Journal of Advanced Nursing 18(2):211–217, 1993

Browne AJ. The meaning of respect: A First Nations perspective. Canadian Journal of Nursing Research 27(4):95–109, 1995

Buchanan A. Judging the past: The care of the human radiation experiments. Hasting Center Report 26(3):25–30, 1996

Capron AM. Constitutionalizing death. Hastings Center Report 25(6):23–24, 1995

Conlon C. Developing ethical competence. Am Nurs 26(3):1, 11, 1994

Cunningham ME. Afrocentrism and self-concept. Journal of National Black Nurses' Association 7(1):15–24, 1994

Czerwinski BS. An autopsy of an ethical dilemma. J Nurs Admin 20(6):25–29, 1990

Erlen JA. Managed care and the nurse's ethical obligations to patients. Orthopaedic Nursing 14(6):42–45, 1995

Esterhuizen P. Is the professional code still the cornerstone of clinical nursing practice? J Adv Nurs 23(1):25–31, 1996

Evans LK. Knowing the patient: The route to individualized care. J Gerontol Nurs 22(3):15–19, 47–53, 1996

Farquhar M. Definitions of quality of life: A taxonomy. J Adv Nurs 22(3):502–508, 1995

Fealy GM. Professional caring: The moral dimension. J Adv Nurs 22(6):1135–1140, 1995

Freedman B. Respectful service and reverent obedience: A Jewish view on making decisions for incompetent parents. Hasting Center Report 26(4):31–37, 1996

Gilfand G, Long P, McGill D, Sheerin C. Prevention of chemically impaired nursing practice. Nurs Management 21(7):76–78, 1990

Gobis IJ. Computerized patient records: Start preparing now. J Nurs Admin 24(9):15–16, 60, 1994

Greipp ME. Culture and ethics: A tool for analyzing the effects of biases on the nurse-patient relationship. Nursing Ethics: An International Journal for Health Care Professionals 2(3):211–221, 1995

Grossman D. Cultural dimensions in home health nursing. Am J Nurs 96(7):33–36, 1996

Hendin H. Selling death and dignity. Hasting Center Report 25(3):19–23, 1995

Hughes TL, Smith LL. Is your colleague chemically dependent? Am J Nurs 94(9):30–35, 1994

Kikuchi JF. Multicultural ethics in nursing education: A potential threat to responsible practice. J Prof Nurs 12(3):159–165, 1996

Kroeger-Mappes EJ. Ethical dilemmas for nurses: Physicians' orders versus patient's rights. *In* Mappes TA, Zembaty JS: Biomedical Ethics, 2nd ed. New York: McGraw-Hill, 1986:127

Laffey J. Bioethical principles and care-based ethics in medical futility. Cancer Practice 4(1):41–46, 1996

Laischenko J. Artificial personhood: Nursing ethics in a medical world. Nursing Ethics 2(3):185–196, 1996

Johnson E. Cultural diversity: Considerations for ethical and culturally sensitive practice. Md Nurs 14(1):6, 1995

Katims I. The contrary ideals of individualism and nursing value of care. Scholarly Inquiry for Nursing Practice 9(3):231–244, 1995

Lippman H. Addicted nurses: Tolerated, tormented, or treated? RN 55(4):36–41, 1992

McAlpine H. Critical reflections about professional ethical stances: Have we lost sight of the major objectives? J Nurs Educ 35(3):119–126, 1996

McGee P. The concept of respect in nursing. British Journal of Nursing 3(13):681, 683–684, 1994

McGrath P. It's ok to say no! A discussion of ethical issues arising from informed consent to chemotherapy. Cancer Nursing 18(2):97–103, 1995

Merrell J, Williams A. Beneficence, respect for autonomy, and justice: Principles in practice. Nurse Researcher 3(1):24–34, 1995

Milner S. An ethical practice model in the age of empowerment. Miss RN 57(5):16, 1995

Morrissey J. Data Security. Modern Healthcare 26(40):32–40, 1996

Morrissey J. Patient privacy requires cultural revolution. Modern Healthcare 26(40):36, 1996

Parmee R. Patient education: Compliance or emancipation? Nursing Praxis in New Zealand 10(2):13–23, 1995

Reckling JB. Conceptual analysis of rights using a philosophic inquiry approach. Image 26(4):309–14, 1994

Sherry D. Autonomy vs. beneficence. Home Healthcare Nurse 8(6):13–15, 1990

Smith G. Attitudes of nurse managers and assistant nurse managers toward chemically impaired colleagues. Image 24(4):295–300, 1992

Smith KV. Ethical decision-making in nursing: Implications for continuing education. Journal of Continuing Education in Nursing 27(1):42–45, 1996

Schneiderman LJ, Jecker NS. Wrong Medicine. Baltimore, MD: Johns Hopkins University Press, 1995

Spindel PG, Suarez SH. Informed consent and home birth. Journal of Nurse-Midwifery 40(6):541–554, 1995

Sugirtharjah S. The notion of respect in Asian traditions. British Journal of Nursing 3(14):739–741, 1994

Tallon RW. Computer-based patient records: Hype versus reality. Nurs Management 27(3):53–56, 1996

Taylor C. Medical futility and nursing. Image: Journal of Nursing Scholarship 27(4):301–306, 1995

Taylor SL. Quandary at the crossroads: Paternalism versus advocacy surrounding end-of-treatment decisions. Am J Hosp Palliat Care 12(4):43–46, 1995

Wennerstrom PA, Rooda LA. Attitudes and perceptions of nursing students toward chemically impaired nurses: Implications for nursing education. J Nurs Educ 35(5):237–239, 1996

Whitbeck C. Ethics as design: Doing justice to moral problems. Hastings Center Report. 26(3):9–16, 1996

10

Bioethical Issues in Health Care

Ironically, while the desire for progress leads to greater knowledge and innovation, it also raises the general level of discontent with the status quo, which tends to be seen as inadequate in light of the future possibilities.
(Callahan, 1997)

Objectives

After completing this chapter, you should be able to:

1. Discuss major bioethical issues and give examples of nursing involvement.

2. Outline the history of family planning in the United States and discuss how various value systems and beliefs have affected it.

3. Analyze the controversy surrounding the Human Genome Project and its relationship to genetic screening.

4. List some of the possible ethical and legal problems associated with artificial insemination, surrogate motherhood, and in vitro fertilization.

5. Discuss the problems associated with determining when death has occurred.

6. Review and examine multiple factors in right-to-die issues, including the difference between active euthanasia and passive euthanasia.

7. Discuss the major issues related to withholding or withdrawing treatment, and patients' rights with regard to informed consent and treatment.

8. Identify the major concerns associated with organ transplantation.

9. Discuss the factors that make it difficult to establish firm rules regarding the treatment of the mentally ill.

10. Outline concerns related to the rationing of health care.

KEY TERMS

Abortion (spontaneous, therapeutic, elective)
Advance directives
Age of consent

Amniocentesis
Artificial insemination
Assisted death
Behavior control

Bioethics
Death
Durable power of attorney for health care
Emancipation of a minor
Eugenics
Euthanasia
Genetics
Genetic mother
Gene therapy
Genetic screening
Gestational mother
Family planning
Futile treatment
Informed consent
In vitro fertilization

Living will
Mature minor
Negative euthanasia
Negative right simpliciter
Organ procurement
Organ transplantation
Patient self-determination (PSD)
Property rights
Right to die
Positive euthanasia
Scarce medical resources
Spare-the-mother syndrome
Surrogate mother
Withdrawing/withholding treatment
Wrongful birth
Xenografts/xenotransplantation

*B*ioethics is the study of ethical issues that result from technological and scientific advances, especially as they are used in biology and medicine. This area of study may also be called biomedical ethics because of its association with medical practices. It is a subdiscipline within the larger discipline of ethics, which (as discussed in Chapter 9) is the philosophical study of morality—or what is right and what is wrong. Today more than ever, nurses and their patients need to keep pace with the technologic changes occurring in health care. There are choices that must be made that patients and caregivers did not have to face years ago.

This chapter discusses some of those choices and should be read, studied, and discussed within the framework of the information concerning ethical decision making that was provided earlier. It should provide a basis on which you can look at judicial rulings, legal mandates, and social standards, and how they can be used to assist in resolving some of the concerns with which we are faced in health care delivery. You have had some experience in looking at what is right or wrong with regard to your personal professional practice. This chapter examines more specifically those issues that apply to the bioethics of patient care.

MAJOR AREAS WHERE BIOETHICS ARE APPLIED

The bioethical issues surrounding the delivery of health care are numerous and multifaceted. They also are always in the process of changing and taking on new dimensions. At an earlier point in time most of the truly serious debates related to birth, death, or the processes that bring a person to either point. Today, issues related to birth and death represent just the ''tip of the iceberg'' as we explore such concerns as universal access to health care, rationing of health care, cost containment, where and how federal dollars should be spent with regard to the nation's health, and the obligation of others to assist the homeless.

There are a number of reasons why we are confronted with these concerns. As a nation, our population is getting older and living longer. Because of life style changes and medical breakthroughs, today many persons live to reach old age. Life expectancy has increased a year or two in each recent decade; today the average life span is 75.5 years, compared with 47 at the beginning of the 20th century. Diseases such as Alzheimer's and acquired immunodeficiency syndrome (AIDS), for which no cures exist at this time, have increased in prevalence. New technologies have resulted in treatments that were not available 15 years ago. Many of the treatments require use of technologies so expensive that they are priced beyond what an individual or family can afford without help from third-party payers. Finding new and better ways to treat life-threatening conditions challenges medical researchers, and the treatments that become available often invite debate among bioethicists. For example, the use of *xenografts* (animal-organ transplants) has been suggested as a way to meet the increasing demand for healthy organs, but many question this practice.

Some would indicate that the "birth of bioethics" occurred with the publication of an article in Life Magazine titled "They Decide Who Lives, Who Dies" (November 9, 1962). This article told the story of a group of individuals in Seattle whose duty it was to select patients for a recently opened hemodialysis program in the city. Many more patients needed treatment than could be accommodated; those not selected would likely die. This event was followed several years later by an article regarding the ethics of medical research that provided impetus for examining these issues. When Christiaan Barnard performed his first heart transplant in 1967, the world again responded with awe and concern. Who was the donor? Where did he come from? Was he truly dead? (Jonsen, 1993).

Centers for research in bioethics emerged, most notably the Institute of Society, Ethics, and the Life Sciences, located in Hastings-on-Hudson, New York (often called The Hastings Center), and the Kennedy Institute Center for Bioethics, located at Georgetown University in Washington, DC. Journals such as the *Hastings Center Report* and the *Journal of Medicine and Philosophy* have come into being and an encyclopedia, *The Encyclopedia of Bioethics*, has been published. Today bioethicists are included in many important task forces and special committees.

Entire textbooks have been devoted to bioethical considerations. Initially most of these were written for medical students, but now just as many are written for nursing students. Some nursing programs include a course in ethics and bioethics as a part of the curriculum. This chapter will only introduce the topic and, we hope, broaden your perspective and deepen your interest. You are encouraged to read about and study these issues further as they affect your practice as a nurse.

As we mentioned earlier, most of the bioethical issues with which we wrestle were not a concern 20 or even 10 years ago. They are a product of the technological advances that have occurred in medical practice and research. Table 10-1 lists some of the significant medical milestones that have occurred since 1920, some of which we have come to take for granted (eg, antibiotics and DNA).You readily can see that in 1960 there was no quest for human organs or critical decisions with regard to the life status of a possible donor. We were not able to fertilize ova outside the human body and reimplant fertilized eggs in a woman's uterus until 1978. Certain lifesaving machines (such as ventilators) and miracle drugs (such as some of the chemotherapeutic agents used today) were not available to offer extension of life. Technologies such as magnetic resonance imaging (MRI), which gives us information about the structure of tissues and allows for early diagnosis and treatment, were not available. Concerns related to the quality of life were often more clear-cut. As advances occur in medical practice, we must challenge ourselves to think through our own beliefs and feelings with regard to these practices.

It is our intent in this short section to share with you some of the major bioethical issues confronting the new graduate today. You will have an opportunity to gain informa-

TABLE 10-1. Some Medical Milestones of the 1900s

When	Who	What
1928	Alexander Fleming	This British bacteriologist noticed that one of his culture plates had grown a fungus and the colonies of staphylococci around the edge of the mold had been destroyed. Because this fungus was a member of the *Penicillium* group he named it penicillin.
1938	Howard Florey & Ernst Chain	These two pathologists took up the work of Fleming and demonstrated the efficacy of penicillin in treating infection. In 1945 the three were jointly awarded the Nobel Prize for Physiology of Medicine.
1951	Forrest Bird	The first Bird breathing device was developed (Bird Mark 7) and breathing treatment machines were introduced. Inhalation (respiratory) therapy rapidly developed as a health profession (Pilbeam, 1992).
1953	James Watson & Francis Crick	These two geneticists deciphered DNA's double-helix structure. Researchers began to focus on the internal functioning of the cell and molecular biology developed as a specialty.
1954	Physicians in Boston	Transplanted the kidney from one twin to the other, thus moving kidney transplantation from the experimental stage it had occupied since 1902. Kidney transplantations have been the most successful of transplantations (Miller-Keane, 1992).
1955	Jonas Salk	Public health officials began immunizing children against polio with Dr. Salk's vaccine, which contained dead virus.
1957	Albert Sabin	A polio vaccine was developed, which was based on weakened live virus, that could be administered orally.
1967	Christiaan Barnard	This South African surgeon performed the first human-heart transplant.
1972	British engineers	The computer tomography (CAT) scanner was developed in England, which assembles thousands of x-ray images into a highly detailed picture of the brain. It was later expanded to provide scans of the entire body.
1978	English physicians	The process of in vitro fertilization was developed and Louise Brown became the first person to be conceived in a test tube, then implanted into the mother's uterus.
1979	World Health Organization	This group declared that smallpox had been eradicated 2 years after the last known case was identified. This occurred because of world-wide immunization against the disease.
1981	Physicians in San Francisco and New York	Doctors from these two cities reported the first cases of what would later become known as acquired immunodeficiency syndrome (AIDS). To date, there exists no cure.
1982	The U.S. Food and Drug Administration	The first drug developed with recombinant-DNA was approved by this group. It was a form of human insulin; it's availability saves thousands of lives.
1995	Duke University surgeons	Hearts from genetically altered pigs were transplanted into baboons, proving that cross-species transplantations can be done. Within two years they plan to give pig hearts to humans.

Much of the material for this table was gathered from an article by Sherwin B. Nuland, *Time Special Issue,* Fall 1996.

tion, explore philosophical and religious issues, and integrate your own beliefs into your role as a nurse (see Table 10-1).

BIOETHICAL ISSUES CONCERNING THE BEGINNING OF LIFE

A number of bioethical issues with which we wrestle are focused on the process by which conception occurs, the products of conception, and the beginning of life, including whether it should occur. Much of the early debate related to family planning and conception.

Family Planning

The modern population control movement probably can trace its beginnings to the writings of a minister in the Church of England. In 1798, Thomas Malthus, in an essay titled ''On Population,'' expressed deep concern about a population that was growing faster than were the resources to support it. To offset this problem he advocated late marriage, no marriage, or sexual abstinence in marriage. No forms of contraception as we know them today were available, although women sometimes developed homemade devices in an effort to prevent pregnancy. Most commonly these devices were sponges dipped in various herbs and other substances that, when inserted in the vagina, soaked up or inactivated semen.

In the United States another approach was taken that undoubtedly led to some of the controversy related to the issue of birth control. In 1873, Congress passed the Comstock Act, prohibiting the sale, mailing, or importing of any drug or article that prevented conception. This resulted in the illegal importation and distribution of contraceptive devices. You may have read about Margaret Sanger (1883–1966), a nurse who championed for contraceptive practices at a time when such activities and viewpoints were extremely unpopular and illegal. Although charged and sentenced for disseminating information on birth control, she went on to establish the National Committee on Federal Legislation for Birth Control, the forerunner of the Planned Parenthood Federation.

It was not until 1965 that a clear, legal concept of planned parenthood was developed, when the Supreme Court of the United States established the right of the individual to obtain medical contraceptive advice and counseling in the case of *Griswold and Buxton v. the State of Connecticut* (Hayt, 1977).

Additional controversy over birth control is related to the theological teachings of some religious groups, who believe interference with procreative powers is wrong. Encyclicals from popes of the Roman Catholic Church from early times to the present have forbidden the use of artificial birth control. The Catholic Church strongly advocates the natural use of reproductive powers to ensure the propagation of the human race; anything that impedes attainment of the purpose for which these organs were created (ie, reproduction) is considered immoral. We see high birth rates in countries that are predominantly Catholic. Orthodox Judaism has specific rules about when sexual intercourse may or may not occur; these rules are geared toward increasing the Jewish population. The Orthodox Jewish population is so small, in proportion to other groups, that the impact is not significant. The members of the Church of Jesus Christ of Latter Day Saints (Mormons), although less adamant in their teachings, also discourage the use of artificial birth control under normal circumstances.

Some conservative Protestant Christians and conservative Muslims also advocate allowing God to plan families and do not use birth control methods.

When caring for patients whose personal beliefs prohibit the use of artificial birth control, you must be knowledgeable about natural methods of family spacing, such as fertility awareness methods, that will meet the patient's needs. If your personal views regarding contraception differ, your views must be set aside as you focus on assisting the patient in selecting a method that is compatible with the patient's personal values and beliefs.

Among the methods of birth control available to those who have no religious sanction against their use, not all methods are acceptable to all people. For example, some find the intrauterine device unacceptable because they believe that interfering with a fertilized egg should be viewed as abortion (researchers are not entirely sure how the intrauterine device works, but some suggest that it prevents the fertilized egg from implanting in the wall of the uterus). The other extreme is represented by those who find abortion an acceptable method of coping with an unwanted pregnancy. During your career as a nurse you will care for patients who represent many differing viewpoints.

Central to all discussions of contraception is the issue of freedom to control one's body. This immediately raises a second question: who has that right? Is it the woman's right because it is her body? Avid feminists would answer with a resounding ''yes.'' What if the partners disagree about family planning practices? Does one have more say than the other? What if one partner wants to have a family and the other does not? It is not within the scope of this chapter to explore the ramifications of all these concerns, but nurses working in this area need to be aware of the many issues that are present.

Largely because of personal values, there is disagreement over how contraception should be practiced, by whom, and at what age. In general, it is assumed that adults are capable of giving free and informed consent. The ability to procreate precedes what is generally considered legal age, however, and we find ourselves grappling with problems related to age of consent, its definition, and the role of the parents and the family.

Problems of Consent and Family Planning

In legal terms, the *age of consent* is ''the age at which one is capable of giving deliberate and voluntary agreement, especially to marriage or to unlawful sexual intercourse'' (Thomas, 1993). This implies physical and mental ability and the freedom to act and make decisions. Until they reach the age of consent, parents are required to give consent for the care of their children. Implicit in this is the assumption that the parents have the best interests of the child at heart and that they are better qualified than the child to make decisions in the child's best interest. (Do you see how this generates the concept of ''paternalism'' that has been discussed in other parts of the book?) The authority to give consent goes along with the understanding that the parents are responsible for the care (including medical costs) and education of the minor. However, trends today cloud the issue, and legislators and concerned citizens continue to struggle with legislating ''rights'' through arbitrary criteria such as age. In former times, the age of 7 was considered an appropriate age at which to give consent, because by age 7 children were expected to know right from wrong and to have reached the age of reason. Although few of us would think that this is an age at which a child should be responsible for consenting to medical treatment, guidelines of the Department of Health and Human Services have allowed that this age is sufficient for refusing consent, despite parental opinion (Hellegers, 1975).

The trend recently has been toward the concept of the ''emancipated minor.'' An *emancipated minor* is a child legally under the age of majority who is recognized as having the legal capacity of an adult under circumstances prescribed by state law. Emancipated minors may give consent for medical treatment regardless of their parent's or legal guardian's knowledge or agreement (Kelley, 1994). Most states recognize some form of emancipation of minors.

Another term we often hear is *mature minor*, a relatively new concept. This term is applied to ''youths who are sufficiently mature and intelligent to understand the nature and consequences of a treatment that is for their benefit'' (Mancini, 1978, p 126). Under this definition, a minor who wants birth control devices because he or she is sexually active demonstrates the ability to make a mature decision, although the parents may not agree with the decision. The mature minor also may consent to therapy for sexually transmitted disease, drug abuse, and pregnancy care. Health care workers have no legal obligation to inform parents of any such treatment. The most liberal legislation applies to the treatment of sexually transmitted disease and is endorsed by most states. Minors of any age can consent to diagnosis and care for sexually transmitted disease. The following illustrates this situation.

> An 11-year-old girl sought treatment for gonorrhea. At her insistence the physician promised to honor her legal right to confidential health care and not to inform her parents. Later, a public health nurse who was working with the girl learned that the child was being repeatedly sexually assaulted after school by a 16-year-old neighbor while her parents were still at work. The nurse also felt bound to a pledge of confidentiality but was able, with encouragement, to get the child to discuss this with her parents and enlist their support. In this instance the statute that protected the ''rights'' of the child may have led health care professionals to become involved in activities that did not serve the best interests of the child.

In 1973, the American Academy of Pediatrics developed the Model Act, which addresses the issue of consent of minors for health care. This act recommends that minors be allowed to give consent for health services when they are pregnant or afflicted with reportable communicable disease (including venereal diseases) or drug or substance abuse (including alcohol and nicotine). It is generally accepted that the age of the patient is not to be considered for some treatments, but that parental consent is automatically required for other treatments (when the patient is younger than 18). Certainly there will be times when physicians' ethical and moral convictions will prevent them from complying with adolescents' requests for care. This occurs most commonly in response to requests for contraceptive pills and abortions. In such cases, physicians often discuss their beliefs with the adolescent, and frequently refer the patient to a medical colleague for assistance.

A major controversy exists around the role of the school in the sex education of high school students and the dispensing of contraceptives. Those who are concerned about the rising incidence of teenage pregnancies and sexually transmitted diseases argue that the information must be disseminated, regardless of who does it. Conservatives think that this is an erosion of the role of the family, and worry that the indiscriminate dispensing of contraceptives encourages promiscuity among teenagers. Concern about the spread of AIDS has done much to liberalize thinking, particularly in regard to the dispensing of condoms.

Abortion

What has been said about contraception becomes an even greater issue when related to abortion. In medical terms, abortion is the termination of pregnancy before the viability of the fetus—that is, any time before the end of the sixth month of gestation. An abortion may occur spontaneously as a result of natural causes (*spontaneous abortion*). A pregnancy may be interrupted deliberately for medical reasons (*therapeutic abortion*), or for personal reasons (*elective abortion*). It is these last two classifications (especially the latter) that induce bioethical debate. Ethically, the entire debate revolves around the definition of human life and when the fetus should be considered a human being. There exist two schools of thought about the nature of the fetus: one supports the belief that new life occurs at the moment of conception; the other contends that human life does not exist until the fetus is sufficiently developed biologically to sustain itself outside the uterus.

The legal aspects of abortion were clarified on January 22, 1973, when the U.S. Supreme Court ruled that any state laws that prohibited or restricted a woman's right to obtain an abortion during the first 3 months of pregnancy were unconstitutional. The following excerpt details the case of *Roe v. Wade*, in which the Supreme Court recognized that, during the first trimester of pregnancy, a privacy right exists that allows an individual woman to make the final decision with regard to what happens to her own body (*Roe v. Wade*, 1973).

> "Jane Roe" was the fictitious name Norma McCorvey used when two young attorneys, both women, filed her lawsuit. A pregnant, divorced waitress, and a victim of a gang rape and beating, Jane Roe sued the State of Texas because she could not obtain a legal abortion in that state and was too poor to travel to New York or California, where abortion was legal. Without access to abortion, she had the baby, whom she placed for adoption. Four years later, the Supreme Court struck down the laws that prevented her seeking abortion. Certain time limitations as to when an abortion can be performed were determined to be necessary, because of the state's interest in protecting potential life; at the period of viability, the state's interest took precedence over the mother's desire for an abortion. Supreme Court Justice Blackmun, in writing an opinion that met with agreement from six other justices, decided that a woman's decision to terminate a pregnancy was encompassed by the right to privacy, up to a certain point in the development of the fetus (Blackmun, 1981); it was established that this lasted until the end of the first trimester. Thus, the courts ruled that the state could not prevent abortions during the first trimester, but could regulate abortions in the second and third trimesters of pregnancy, at which point the interests of the fetus took precedence over those of the mother.

Despite these rulings, the issue of abortion versus right to life continues to surface, with new legislation and rulings being considered each year. The legal positions also do little to help us deal with bioethical concerns. Many people view termination of life at any point after conception as murder. The Roman Catholic Church firmly upholds its traditional position on abortion. Many conservative Protestant Christian groups are also active in opposing abortion.

Some believe that although abortion is not desirable, under certain circumstances it would be justifiable—for example, in cases of rape or incest, or in instances where amniocentesis indicates that a fetus would be born retarded or genetically defective. Others think that early termination of a pregnancy might be acceptable, but that termination after the fourth month would not be appropriate.

Those who support abortion without restriction usually do so because they believe that women should have control over their own bodies. They further argue that the quality of life of an "unwanted" child, or a child born with a deformity or genetic defect, may be minimal. Interesting and challenging cases have emerged with respect to this concept. These are generally known as *wrongful birth* cases, and are based on the principle that it is wrong to give birth to children (such as those with birth defects or limitations that can be diagnosed or anticipated before birth) who will not have the same quality of life as other children.

As a nurse, these issues may present some difficult questions you will need to answer. To what extent do you believe you can personally participate in the abortion procedure? You may find it easier to assist with an abortion performed as a dilation and curettage at 10 weeks' gestation, in a doctor's office or clinic, than to assist with a saline abortion carried out at $5\frac{1}{2}$ months' gestation in a hospital labor room. The products of conception aborted at 10 weeks have little that is lifelike in their appearance. The fetus aborted at $5\frac{1}{2}$ months appears much like a premature infant. Certainly, as a nurse, you have the right to refuse to be involved in abortion procedures or the care of patients seeking abortion. However, employment in certain areas (for example, labor and delivery rooms) may rest on the nurse's willingness and ability to assist with abortions and to give conscientious care to the patient who has had an abortion. Some religiously affiliated hospitals have elected to close their labor and delivery suites rather than perform abortions.

Attention has been focused on incidents in which an abortion was attempted toward the end of the fifth or sixth month of gestation, and the fetus was born showing signs of life. Is the doctor or nurse obligated to try to keep the infant alive? Is the doctor or nurse guilty of malpractice, or even murder, if he or she does anything to hasten the infant's death? Should this infant be considered a human being? Does the infant have "rights"? Does the mother have legal possession of and responsibility for the child if, in fact, she attempted to abort the fetus? This issue, like so many others, probably will be settled in a court of law while we continue to debate it ethically.

The abortion issue is also complicated by consent problems. Many states have recognized the special problems related to parental consent for teenagers and to health care involving pregnancy and have legislated special exceptions.

In the last few years, the abortion issue has been made more complex by research that would use the fetal tissue resulting from an abortion for therapeutic purposes. Research has suggested that implantation of fetal brain tissue (recovered at the time of abortion) may be helpful in the treatment of Parkinson's disease, if implanted in the brain of the Parkinson's patient. The ramifications of this type of research and treatment are so great that a special committee has been appointed to develop guidelines to govern future research and treatment activities requiring the use of fetal tissue.

As a society, it seems likely that we will continue to debate the issue of abortion. Ultimately, the decision rests with the individual who must make the choice. Certainly the legal entanglements become more complex with each court ruling, and will be limited only by our willingness to challenge other aspects of the question.

Amniocentesis, Prenatal Diagnosis, and Genetic Screening

A major breakthrough in our ability to detect genetic abnormalities before birth occurred in the 1970s with the development of techniques to carry out *amniocentesis*. An amniocentesis is performed between 14 and 20 weeks after the last menstrual period. This test is performed after identifying the placental site and locating a pocket of amniotic fluid via an ultrasound scan; a 22-gauge needle is then inserted through the pregnant woman's abdomen and uterus, and 15–20 mL of fluid is removed and analyzed. From these cells a number of genetic problems can be diagnosed prenatally, among them such conditions as Down syndrome (which accounts for about one third of the cases of mental retardation in western countries), hemophilia, Duchenne's muscular dystrophy, Tay-Sachs disease, and problems related to the brain and spinal column (eg, anencephaly and spina bifida).

Down syndrome, a condition occurring with higher frequency in mothers in their early 40s and older, is the most common reason for seeking amniocentesis. When genetic screening reveals a genetic disease, a woman will often choose to have an abortion. Rothstein (1990, p. 39) reports that ''termination rates for muscular dystrophy, cystic fibrosis, and alpha and beta thalassemia are nearly 100%; they are 60% for hemophilia; and 50% for sickle cell anemia.'' Some couples request amniocentesis if they are in an ''at-risk'' group, but state that they would not abort the fetus under any circumstances; instead they believe that an additional 5 months will give them time to adjust to the presence of a disease before the baby is born. Usually doctors are reluctant to do an amniocentesis under these circumstances, because the risk of performing the procedure, although small, does not seem justified.

Some people are concerned about this procedure because of where it might lead. Is mass genetic screening a possibility? Ethicists have expressed concern about the possibility of the government making diagnostic amniocentesis and abortion of all defective fetuses mandatory. Others argue against genetic counseling and amniocentesis because of the stress it places on a marriage, and because of the guilt placed on the partner carrying the defective gene (in cases in which that can be determined). Their argument is that there are some things we are better off not knowing. Genetic screening also may result in at least one of the partners (often the carrier) seeking voluntary sterilization to prevent pregnancies with less than favorable outcomes.

Amniocentesis does have some positive aspects. Prenatal diagnosis, for example, may save more fetal lives than it terminates. Many women carrying fetuses at high genetic risk might resort to abortion if diagnostic techniques were not available. Such women, unwilling to take a chance, would rather abort a healthy fetus than risk bearing a defective one.

The advent of amniocentesis has heralded the development of yet another medical specialty: that of prenatal surgery. Although the specialty is still new, some corrective surgery is being performed on infants while they are in their intrauterine environment.

As a nurse, you may care for clients with varying viewpoints regarding amniocentesis and abortion, and you will also have your own values to consider. Will your values conflict with those of your clients? Are you obligated to advocate for a client when the client's request is squarely in opposition to what you believe to be right? Should you try to sway a woman who is indecisive toward either decision?

Sterilization

For years, surgical operations resulting in permanent sterilization have been performed for therapeutic purposes. Examples of this include the removal of reproductive organs to halt the spread of cancer or other pathologic processes. Although problems may arise for the patient and family as a result of such surgeries, usually they are resolved without serious ethical debate (depending on the family's religious values, the patient's body concept, family plans, and personal values).

With increasing frequency, voluntary sterilizations have been requested by couples to terminate reproductive ability. These surgical procedures, performed on either men or women, should, for all intents and purposes, be considered permanent and irreversible. For those who are satisfied with the size of their family, sterilization may pose few problems. In most cases, full and informed consent is obtained from both partners before the surgery is performed. Some people question whether a man or woman is free to make an independent decision regarding sterilization without consulting the partner. Although many people see this as the prerogative of a couple, others find any type of sterilization in conflict with their religious and moral beliefs. A few states still have laws forbidding voluntary sterilization for contraceptive purposes, but these laws may not be enforced.

Eugenics

Most controversial is any type of sterilization performed for eugenic purposes, especially if there is any question about the procedure being voluntary. *Eugenics* is the movement devoted to improving the human species through genetic control. The practice of eugenics is not new. The idea of improving the quality of the human race is at least as old as Plato, who wrote on the topic in his *Republic*. The modern eugenic movement is thought to have started in the 19th century. Charles Darwin's theory of evolution was advanced by his cousin Francis Galton, who created the term *eugenics*. Key to this were philosophical beliefs of certain 18th century thinkers about the notion of human perfectibility. When Mendel's law provided a framework for explaining the transmission and distribution of traits from one generation to another, the eugenics movement took hold. Organizations focusing on eugenics were created around the world.

The center of the eugenics movement in the United States was the Eugenics Record Office in Cold Spring Harbor, New York, and its leader was geneticist Charles Davenport. Until the early 1930s, the eugenics movement grew. Eugenicists presented a two-part policy. Negative eugenics advocated the elimination of unwanted characteristics from the nation by discouraging ''unworthy'' parents. This included a variety of approaches such as marriage restriction, sterilization, and permanent custody of ''defectives.'' Many eugenicists were actively involved in other issues of the day, including prohibition, birth control, and legislation that would outlaw miscegenation (marriage between two persons of different races, especially between white and black people in the United States). During this time, states passed compulsory sterilization bills affecting certain developmentally disabled groups. By 1929, California, for example, had sterilized approximately 6,250 people, almost twice as many as all other states combined (Kevles, 1993).

Also passed at this time was the Immigration Restriction Act of 1924, which dramatically limited the immigration of people from southern and eastern Europe on the grounds that they were "biologically inferior."

Positive eugenics encouraged increasing the desirable traits in the population by urging "worthy" parents. "Superior" couples were encouraged to have more children.

The eugenics movement grew in Germany as well as in the United States. In 1933, Hitler sanctioned the Hereditary Health Law, or the Eugenic Sterilization Law, which ensured that the "less worthy" members of the Third Reich did not pass on their genes. It resulted in the sterilization of several hundred thousand people and helped lead to the death camps.

By the late 1930s, eugenics in the United States began a tremendous decline. Americans became concerned about the concept of a "master race." At the same time, psychologists and anthropologists were conducting research that indicated that culture and environment also had great influence over human development.

When the eugenic movement was rekindled in the 1960s, it had a different focus—one related to genetic counseling and genetic research. Today, a couple who gives birth to a child with a congenital anomaly (or who realizes that one of them is carrying a genetic trait that could cause a child to have a congenital anomaly) might voluntarily seek genetic counseling, and possibly opt for the sterilization of one of the partners. Again, this approach offends the religious and moral values of some, but generally it is viewed as the couple's prerogative.

Problems are created when the concept of eugenics is applied to minors or to institutionalized people. Problems also arise in the language of laws in certain states that would include "epileptics, habitual criminals, and moral degenerates" among those eligible for compulsory sterilization. Some states extended compulsory sterilization to include those who might become wards of the state (Hayt, 1977). In the case of epilepsy, modern medical advances have changed our understanding of the role of heredity in the disease and our attitudes toward people who are affected. The trend in recent years has been for states to modify, repeal, or ignore their eugenic sterilization laws.

In states that still permit compulsory eugenic sterilization, questions can be raised as to who may request sterilization, who may sign the consent, and who must fund the procedure. As the result of a court decision, federal monies may not be used for this purpose (Hellegers, 1975). However, the taxpayer contributes to the cost of institutionalizing people who are not capable of living independently in today's society, and caring for those with severe illnesses and disabilities. The question must also be raised regarding the ability of two individuals who are mentally retarded to care for children they may parent. Therefore, it is not only a personal concern but also society's concern.

The sterilization of sex offenders has also been discussed recently. In some instances, sterilization has been recommended for individuals convicted of repeated sexual offenses, particularly those against children. Because sex crimes are related to power and aggression, and not just to sex drive, this remains a controversial issue.

The Human Genome Project

A *genome* may be defined as all the genetic material in the chromosomes of a particular organism. You will remember from your biology classes that the human genome consists of 46 chromosomes: 22 pairs of autosomes and a pair of sex chromosomes. Genomes have been studied for many reasons, including disease prevention, determination of the effects of radiation and chemicals on living species, and more recently, genetic therapy.

The Human Genome Project was first proposed by Nobel prize-winning virologist Renato Dulbecco in 1986. The actual project officially started in 1990. Its cost is estimated at $3 billion and it is expected to last for 15 years. The project has two goals: to develop detailed maps of the human genome (genetic makeup) and the genomes of other well-studied organisms, and to determine the order (sequence) of the individual nucleotides in the DNA of these genomes (Rossiter & Caskey, 1993).

This research is inspired by the discovery that an estimated 4,000 disease genes reside within the human genome. Identification and isolation of defective genes, and their replacement with functional genes (*gene therapy*), could result in the elimination of diseases that have plagued society for years. Several significant conditions currently under study are cystic fibrosis, Huntington's disease, myotonic dystrophy, gout, and adult polycystic kidney disease.

Gene therapy can be divided into two categories. The first kind is an alteration in germ cells (sperm or ova) that results in a permanent genetic change in a whole organism and subsequent generations. For ethical reasons this is not currently being considered for human beings. The second is called "somatic cell gene therapy," and is similar to an organ transplant. Several cases of somatic cell gene therapy have been initiated, most relating to treatment of cancers and blood disorders (Rossiter & Caskey, 1993).

The Human Genome Project brings the promise of improved diagnosis and of possible treatment measures for many inherited diseases (Fig. 10-1). Most people are initially excited at the possibility of preventing such diseases as diabetes or cystic fibrosis. Then they begin to think about other ramifications. What would be the effects of manipulating stature, intelligence, or sex? Do we run the risk of creating "super-babies?" What might be the advantages and disadvantages of knowing the diseases to which you are susceptible? With whom should that information be shared? Employers? Insurance companies? The government? Does this project represent eugenics revisited? Thus, this project carries with it vast and controversial bioethical challenges. How can its misuse be prevented? Should couples with family histories of certain disease conditions be required to participate in genetic screening? If the screening is done and the results indicate a one-in-four chance of bearing a child who will have the disease, what next? These and many other questions are yet to be answered. Students interested in having more extensive knowledge of this project are encouraged to do research in their school or local library.

In Vitro Fertilization

In 1978 in England, much attention was focused on the birth of the first child who was conceived in a test tube, a process we refer to as *in vitro fertilization (IVF)*. Owing to a blockage in the mother's fallopian tubes, conception in her tubes was impossible. The ovum was removed from the mother, united with the father's sperm in a laboratory test tube, and then implanted in the mother's uterus, where it grew to term and was delivered by cesarean section. Today IVF and similar procedures (Table 10-2) help many infertile couples (approximately 26,000 so far) to become parents. An additional 40,000 have found the procedure to be unsuccessful (Grady, 1996).

Many herald this as one of medical science's great advances. For others it raises many concerns. If more than one fertilized ovum is returned to the uterus, it is possible for the

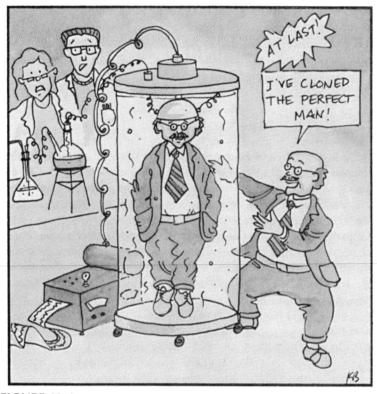

FIGURE 10-1
Another interesting issue involves the creation of life or, more correctly, the circumstances under which it may occur

mother to have multiple births. Multiple births seldom go full term, resulting in financial and emotional costs. When the number of implanted embryos is too great, consideration is given to aborting several of them; this creates additional ethical dilemmas for the family. What should be done with fertilized ovum that are not returned to the uterus? Should they be thrown away? Given to a donor? Used for research? Should tax dollars be used to fund this type of research? If frozen, how long should they remain frozen? What should be done with them at the end of this time? In England in 1996, 3,300 embryos were allowed to defrost and die because of a 1990 law that limits storage time to five years unless donor couples seek an extension (English cardinal . . . , 1996).

Despite the objections raised against IVF, it is now recognized as a viable alternative for many couples who would otherwise be childless (at least as far as natural parenting is concerned). Reproductive problems often stem from blocked fallopian tubes. By harvesting the eggs, fertilizing them in a laboratory, and implanting them in the woman's uterus, this problem can be bypassed.

Other offshoots of in vitro fertilization allow people who are carrying a severe genetic disease to be assured that their children will not be affected by the condition or carry the defective gene.

TABLE 10-2. Types of Assisted Reproductive Techniques

Name	Initials	Description	First Used With Humans
Artificial Insemination: Homologous	AIH	Husband's semen is collected and then deposited at the cervical os or in the wife's uterus by mechanical means.	1884 United States
Artificial Insemination: Donor	AID	Donor's semen is collected and deposited at the cervical os or in the woman's uterus by mechanical means.	1884 United States
In Vitro Fertilization	IVF	After heavily medicating the woman with hormones to trigger ovulation, eggs are harvested and fertilized with father's sperm in a laboratory. Several of the resulting embryos are implanted in the mother's uterus.	England, 1978
Gamete Intrafallopian Transfer	GIFT	Eggs and sperm are inserted directly into the woman's fallopian tubes using a laparoscope. Embryos travel to the uterus for implantation.	United States, 1984
Zygote Intrafallopian Transfer	ZIFT	Eggs and sperm are combined in the laboratory. The resulting zygotes are then inserted into the woman's fallopian tubes and travel to the uterus for implantation.	Belgium, 1989
Preimplantation Genetic Diagnosis	PGD	Egg and sperm are united in the laboratory and the embryo is allowed to develop to 4–8 cells. One or two cells are removed and examined for harmful genes. Defective embryos are discarded; healthy ones are implanted in the woman's uterus.	United States, 1991
Immature Egg Harvest	IEH	Similar to IVF, the eggs are harvested from the ovaries while still immature, are cultured in the laboratory, fertilized, and transferred into the woman's uterus.	South Korea, 1991
Intracytoplasmic Sperm Injection	ICSI	In a laboratory setting, a single sperm cell is injected into an egg and then both are implanted in the woman's uterus.	Belgium, 1992

A Louisiana couple decided, after the death of their 3-year-old daughter from Tay-Sachs disease, not to risk having more children. They learned that they both carried one copy of the Tay-Sachs gene, which would result in a 1-in-4 chance of their conceiving a child with the disease. Shortly thereafter, the couple were notified that a procedure had been developed through IVF and high-tech genetic testing (known as preimplantation genetic diagnosis [PGD]) whereby technicians can remove one or two embryonic cells from those fertilized in vitro and test for the harmful gene. This allows only healthy embryos to be transferred back to the woman's uterus. This procedure resulted in the birth of a healthy child for this couple, and one who is not a carrier of Tay-Sachs disease.

As wonderful as this may seem, concerns exist regarding what some would call the misuse of IVF. In Italy, a 62-year-old woman became pregnant using donated eggs and IVF before implantation in her uterus. She gave birth by cesarean section in 1994. A 59-year-old woman in England delivered twins by this method. More recently, a new record was set for what is thought to be the oldest woman in the world to give birth to a healthy infant. In April 1997, it was announced that a 63-year-old woman had given birth via cesarean section on November 7, 1996. The woman, married and previously childless, is said to have told doctors she was 50 and had medical records attesting to that age. (The medical center where the IVF occurred sets an age limit of 55 on accepting patients.) A donor egg and the husband's sperm were used for the IVF (Roan, 1997).

In some countries legislation is being passed that will prevent such situations. In January 1994, the French Senate opted to prohibit the use of reproductive options in certain cases (Capron, 1994). One can readily identify some of the difficulties in starting the mothering process at age 62 or 63, not the least of which would be living long enough to see the child reach adulthood. Quality-of-life issues may also be involved. If the mother is 62 when the child is born, she will be 67 or 68 when the child starts school and 78 when the child becomes a teenager.

Other concerns focus on the fear that PGD will be used to make "perfect babies," or for sex selection, even when there is not a medical reason (such as hemophilia) for such action.

Artificial Insemination

Other discussions revolve around the topic of *artificial insemination*, which is the planting of sperm in the woman's body to facilitate conception. Although we tend to think of this as a fairly new procedure, the first time artificial insemination is said to have been used was in Philadelphia in 1884 (Fromer, 1981). There are two different kinds of artificial insemination: homologous (AIH), in which the husband's sperm is used, and heterologous (AID), in which a donor's sperm is used. Using the husband's sperm is by far the most common and creates the fewest problems legally, ethically, and morally. In some instances, the sperm from the husband and the sperm from a donor with similar physical characteristics are mixed together. As a result, if conception occurs, the couple could easily believe it was the husband's sperm that was accepted by the ovum.

Although some religious groups may have objections, few concerns arise when the husband's sperm is used. That is not true with donor sperm. If the woman is artificially inseminated with donor sperm without the knowledge and consent of her partner, the problems are multiplied. One of the major questions raised is that of adultery, which is considered a criminal act in most states. If conception occurs and the child is not biologically that of the husband, can one say that adultery has occurred? In at least one instance, the wife was found guilty of adultery after being artificially inseminated with donor sperm (Hayt, 1977). Others question whether the child should be legally adopted by the husband, an act that, to some extent, helps to clarify issues of inheritance, child support (if the couple should later divorce), and the legal status of the child.

Single Parents

Another ethical issue has emerged as our society has granted greater acceptance to single-parent families. More single women are trying to adopt children, and some see artificial insemination as a logical solution. In some instances, these women are also lesbians. One of the couple will seek artificial insemination with a donor sperm; the child is then raised as family in the lesbian relationship. Providing a parenting option to lesbians is totally unacceptable to many people. Aside from the emotion that the issue of a lesbian relationship may introduce, there is the argument against the artificial insemination of any single woman—on the basis that the traditional two-parent family composed of a man and woman is in the best interest of all children.

Surrogate Mothers

Unique problems arise with surrogate mothering, a practice by which a woman agrees to bear a child conceived through artificial insemination and to relinquish the baby at birth to others for rearing. This practice has occurred with increasing frequency and in a variety of relationships. The following represents one such situation.

> A 47-year-old woman agreed to serve as gestational surrogate for her own daughter, whose uterus had been removed because of disease. The daughter's eggs were inseminated with her husband's sperm and the embryos were then implanted in the mother, who gave birth to triplets when she was 48. Thus, this woman became the gestational mother and the genetic grandmother to triplets.

As you see, these artificial means of reproduction have complicated even the language that we are accustomed to using. The term *biological* is no longer adequate for making some critical conceptual distinctions. Macklin (1991, p. 6) states, ''The techniques of egg retrieval, in vitro fertilization (IVF), and gamete intrafallopian transfer (GIFT), now make it possible for two different women to make a biological contribution to the creation of a new life.'' Macklin further believes that the woman who contributes her womb during gestation is also a biological mother. We find terms such as *genetic mother* used to refer to the individual contributing the ovum, and *gestational mother* used to refer to the individual who provides the uterus in which the child develops. In some instances the surrogate mother is both.

Surrogate mothering within a family has caused fewer problems than have been seen when a stranger serves as the surrogate mother. The majority of serious conflicts have occurred in situations in which a woman has been paid to serve as a surrogate mother. A formal, contractual relationship is usually established. The couple who wish to have the child agree to pay all expenses associated with the pregnancy, and to pay the surrogate mother an agreed sum for her time and involvement. The contract must be carefully drawn up because it is illegal in all states to sell a child.

What happens if the child is born with an anomaly, as occurred with a New York couple in 1982? How are these dilemmas to be solved? What is to happen to the child? Who bears the responsibility?

> A gentleman paid a woman to be artificially inseminated with his sperm and to carry his child. When the child was born with microcephaly, the man rejected the infant, stating that he could not be the father. The surrogate mother and her husband also did not want to accept the responsibility for parenting the child.

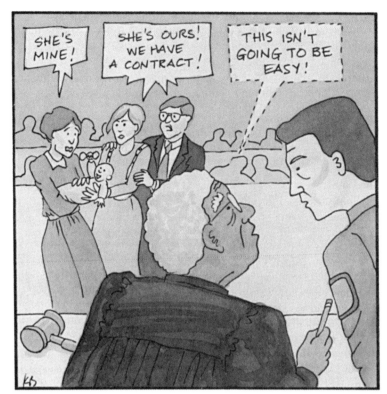

FIGURE 10-2
Complexities arise when surrogate mothers are unwilling to relinquish the infant after birth.

Recently, problems associated with surrogate mothering have centered around the surrogate mother's unwillingness to give up the child after birth (Fig. 10-2).

//B aby M,'' as the court calls her, was born to a surrogate mother after she was impregnated with the sperm of a man for whom she agreed to bear the child. This man's wife, a pediatrician, chose not to bear a child because she had multiple sclerosis. Although signed agreements existed, the surrogate mother broke the contract within days of the baby's birth and asked for custody of the child.

Such instances create great controversy, and pain for those involved. There are no easy answers.

Sperm Banks

Another aspect of the artificial insemination issue is that of sperm banks. Sperm banks have been established in different parts of the United States for various reasons. Men who want to have a vasectomy may contribute to a sperm bank ''just in case'' they change their minds at some future time. Men who will be exposed to high levels of radiation in their work, or during treatment of disease, may wish to have sperm stored because radiation may cause mutation of the genes or result in sterility. In most cases, sperm banks are established by the medical community so that sperm is available for artificial inseminations. In California, a sperm bank was started that contains sperm of only outstanding and brilliant men. The idea was to create children with this sperm who will be genetically endowed with greater intelligence and creativity. Many find this unacceptable because it brings up the issue of creating a super race. Concerns have also been raised regarding the possible number of offspring in a single community who might be genetically related without knowing it. Some ask how a man can ethically father offspring and have no responsibility for their well-being.

The Right to Genetic Information

All the issues of artificial insemination with donor sperm, surrogate mothering, single parenting, and sperm banks are further complicated by a recent trend toward providing individuals with information regarding their genetic background, makeup, and history. You can readily anticipate the problems that would be created if donor sperm were used for insemination. In some instances no record has been maintained with regard to who donated the sperm.

How many individuals would be willing to donate sperm if it were to include a detailed genetic background? What might be the ultimate legal involvement? On the other hand, what are the rights of the child with regard to knowing what genetic factors he or she carries? Whose rights should take precedence?

BIOETHICAL ISSUES CONCERNING DEATH

One of the most important areas of ethical debate involves the topic of death and dying. As mentioned earlier, the advent of lifesaving procedures and mechanical devices has required redefinition of the term *death*, caused us to examine the meaning of ''quality of life,'' and created debates about ''death with dignity.''

Also associated with the issue of death are a number of companion concerns that did not exist before we had some of the technological advances that have occurred within the past 10 years. Some of these concerns relate to euthanasia, the right to refuse treatment, and the right to die. Other concerns relate to organs retrieved from the dying, because of the scarcity of these medical resources. Generally, the demand for donated organs far exceeds the number of organs available to meet the needs. Superimposed on all these issues is that of informed consent.

Death Defined

Until recently the most widely accepted definition of death was from *Black's Law Dictionary*, which defines death as the irreversible cessation of the vital functions of respiration, circulation, and pulsation (Rothman & Rothman, 1977). This traditional view of death served us well until the development of ventilators, pacemakers, and other advances in medical science made it possible to sustain these functions indefinitely. We also have learned that various parts of the body die at different times. The central nervous system is one of the most vulnerable areas, and brain cells can be irreversibly damaged if deprived of oxygen while other parts of the body will continue to function.

Newer definitions of death have been built around the concept of human potential— meaning the potential of the human body to interact with the environment and with other people, to respond to stimuli, and to communicate. When these abilities are lacking, there is said to be no potential. Because this potential is directly related to brain function, the method most often used to assess capability is electroencephalography. Brain activity, with few exceptions, is said to be nonexistent when flat electroencephalographic tracings are obtained over a given period of time, often 48 hours (Rothman & Rothman, 1977). At this point the person may be considered dead, although machines may be supporting the vital functions of respiration and circulation. Many institutions now accept this definition of cerebral death and use it as a basis for turning off respirators and stopping other treatments. It is also used as a basis for determining death when there is a desire to recover organs from the patient.

Planning for End-of-Life Issues

Increasing emphasis is being placed on prior planning for end-of-life issues. One aspect of this is identifying futile treatments. Another important consideration relates to patient self-determination in regard to these issues. Many hope that the use of such planning will decrease the ethical dilemmas present in end-of-life situations.

FUTILE TREATMENTS

Futile treatments are those that ''cannot, within a reasonable possibility, cure, ameliorate, improve or restore a quality of life that would be satisfactory to the patient'' (Hudson, 1994b). For example, when an individual is dying of terminal cancer, treatment for a respiratory infection may be deemed futile because it will not alter the fact that the person is dying and will not restore a satisfactory quality of life. Identifying whether further treatment is futile may be extremely difficult. However, Schneiderman and Jecker (1993) suggest that if, in the last 100 cases of the same nature, there was no change in the outcome based on the treatment, it can be considered futile. Others take a position that treatment never can be declared futile. In their thinking the future cannot be predicted accurately, and if there cannot be absolute certainty about the outcome, then futility cannot be clearly identified.

Other problems may arise when futility is declared. Does a patient have a right to treatment even if it has been identified as futile? What about cost considerations? Should insurance companies be required to pay for treatment that has been classified as futile? What about Medicare or Medicaid? Should there be differences in decisions based on age or quality of life?

PATIENT SELF-DETERMINATION

When end-of-life concerns do arise, the patient is often unconscious or not able to participate in decision making. This raises the question of obtaining consent. Does the responsibility for action, or the lack of action, then fall to the family, the physician, or the nurse? The law in each state specifies who may give consent when an individual is incapacitated and there is no directive as to the patient's choice for a surrogate decision maker. Would the ethical answer to this question be the same as the legal answer? Who is to decide?

In an attempt to gain greater control over the area of dying, many people are now completing a variety of documents that have been titled *advance directives.* An advance directive is a legal document that indicates the wishes of an individual in regard to end-of-life issues.

In the fall of 1990, Congress took a major step regarding this issue by passing legislation that requires all Medicare and Medicaid providers to inform patients, on admission, of their right to refuse treatment. In December 1991, this federal Patient Self-Determination Act (PSDA) went into effect. The intent of this legislation was to enhance an individual's control over medical treatment decisions by promoting the use of advance directives. The PSDA requires individual institutions to inform patients of state law regarding directives, to document the existence of directives in their medical records, and to educate the community. An "interim final rule" gave considerable latitude to institutions regarding the ways that requirements could be met. Many institutions have used this as an opportunity to promote patient decision making. The entire process has not been without its problems. The time of admission to a health care facility is often filled with anxiety, making it almost impossible to consider such matters. Most patients indicate that they prefer to discuss these matters with a doctor or nurse who is involved in their care, but in some settings this task is delegated to an admissions clerk (Hudson, 1994a).

A *living will* is a document that has been widely used as an advance directive (Fig. 10-3). In a living will, a person requests that no extraordinary measures be implemented to sustain life if he or she becomes terminally ill. Although the living will is not necessarily considered legal consent, it does reveal the desires of the person receiving care. It may help families to more confidently make decisions. Another approach that is being used with increasing frequency is the signing of a *durable power of attorney for health care.* In this type of an agreement, an individual (referred to as the "principal") may designate another person to have the power and authority to make health care decisions for the principal, should the principal be unable to make those decisions for himself or herself. The durable power of attorney does not go into effect until after the principal is no longer capable of making decisions. These forms can be purchased in most office supply stores and become valid if signed before a notary public. However, it is best to consult an attorney before entering into such an arrangement (Figure 10-4).

Since 1985, New York has had a Task Force on Life and the Law, which has dealt with issues related to organ procurement and distribution, the determination of death, and surrogate motherhood. The group has also worked on the issue of appointing a surrogate to make health care decisions for an incapacitated adult patient who lacks a precise advance directive or a previously appointed health care agent.

In 1991, the American Nurses Association developed *A Position Statement on Nursing and the Patient Self-Determination Act*, which was revised in 1995. They believe that nurses should play a primary role in implementation of the Act, should facilitate informed decision making for patients, and should occupy a critical role in education, research, patient care, and advocacy (ANA, 1995b).

Euthanasia

Euthanasia, meaning "good death," may be classified as either negative or positive. The word, as it is generally applied, refers to the act or method of causing death painlessly so as to end suffering.

**TO MY FAMILY, MY PHYSICIAN, MY LAWYER, MY CLERGYMAN
TO ANY MEDICAL FACILITY IN WHOSE CARE I HAPPEN TO BE
TO ANY INDIVIDUAL WHO MAY BECOME RESPONSIBLE FOR MY
HEALTH, WELFARE OR AFFAIRS**

Death is as much a reality as birth, growth, maturity and old age—it is the one certainty of life. If the time comes when I, _____
can no longer take part in decisions for my own future, let this statement stand as an expression of my wishes, while I am still of sound mind.

If the situation should arise in which there is no reasonable expectation of my recovery from physical or mental disability, I request that I be allowed to die and not be kept alive by artificial means or "heroic measures". I do not fear death itself as much as the indignities of deterioration, dependence and hopeless pain. I therefore, ask that medication be mercifully administered to me to alleviate suffering even though this may hasten the moment of death.

This request is made after careful consideration. I hope you who care for me will feel morally bound to follow its mandate. I recognize that this appears to place a heavy responsibility upon you, but it is with the intention of relieving you of such responsibility and of placing it upon myself in accordance with my strong convictions, that this statement is made.

Signed _____

Date _____

Witness _____

Witness _____

Copies of this request have been given to _____

_____

_____

_____

FIGURE 10-3
The living will.

NEGATIVE EUTHANASIA

Negative, or passive, *euthanasia* refers to a situation in which no extraordinary or heroic measures are undertaken to sustain life. The concept of negative euthanasia has resulted in what are called "no codes" (also designated as DNR—do not resuscitate) in hospital environments, situations in which hospital personnel do not attempt to revive or bring back to life persons whose vital processes have ceased to function on their own.

It is difficult to describe what constitutes extraordinary measures, and to determine on whom they should or should not be used. Is it one thing to defibrillate a 39-year-old man who is admitted to an emergency department suffering from an acute heart attack, and quite another to defibrillate a 90-year-old man whose body is riddled with terminal cancer and whose heart has stopped? Often people who are involved in giving medical and emergency

[PLEASE NOTE: This is a standardized legal document that may not be appropriate for a person in your particular situation. You should consult your attorney before signing this or any legal document.]

DURABLE POWER OF ATTORNEY FOR HEALTH CARE DECISIONS

I, _____ as principal, domiciled and residing in the State of Washington, hereby enter into a Durable Power of Attorney to provide informed consent for health care decisions pursuant to the laws of the State of Washington.

1. **Designation.** I designate _____ , if living, able and willing to serve, as my attorney-in-fact. If he or she is not living, able and willing to so serve, then I designate _____ , if living, able and willing to serve, as my attorney-in-fact.

2. **Powers.** The attorney-in-fact, as fiduciary, shall have all powers to provide informed consent for health care decisions on principal's behalf.

3. **Effectiveness.** This power of attorney shall become effective upon the disability or incompetence of the principal. Disability shall include the inability to make health care decisions effectively for reasons such as mental illness, mental deficiency, physical illness or disability, advanced age, chronic use of drugs, chronic intoxication, confinement, detention by a foreign power or disappearance. Disability may be evidenced by a written statement of a qualified physician regularly attending me. Incompetence may be established by a finding of a Court having jurisdiction over me.

4. **Duration.** This power of attorney shall remain in effect to the extent permitted by RCW 11.94 notwithstanding any uncertainty as to whether the principal is dead or alive.

5. **Revocation.** This power of attorney may be revoked in writing by notice mailed or delivered to my attorney-in-fact, and by recording the written instrument of revocation in the office of recorder or auditor of the county of my residence.

FIGURE 10-4
Durable power of attorney for healthcare.

care develop an almost automatic response to lifesaving procedures and have difficulty accepting dying as an inevitable part of the life process. It is difficult to know when it is permissible to omit certain life-supporting efforts, or which efforts should be omitted. If the 90-year-old man who is dying of terminal cancer were also to develop pneumonia, should his physician prescribe antibiotics? This brings us to the distinction between stopping a particular life-supporting treatment or machine, or withdrawing treatment, and not starting a procedure in the first place—that is, withholding treatment.

POSITIVE EUTHANASIA

Positive, or active, *euthanasia* occurs in a situation in which the physician prescribes, supplies, or administers an agent that results in death. In the case (cited later in this chapter) in which parents choose to let a newborn with Down syndrome and an intestinal blockage

6. **Termination.**

    a. By Appointment of Guardian The appointment of a guardian of the person of the principal terminates this power of attorney. The appointment of a guardian of the property only does not terminate this power of attorney.

    b. By Death of Principal. The death of the principal shall be deemed to revoke this power of attorney upon proof of death being received by the attorney-in-fact.

7. **Reliance.** The designated and acting attorney-in-fact and all persons dealing with the attorney-in-fact shall be entitled to rely upon this power of attorney so long as neither the attorney-in-fact nor person with whom they were dealing at the time of any act taken pursuant to this power of attorney had received actual knowledge or actual notice of the revocation or termination of the power of attorney by death or otherwise, and any action so taken, unless otherwise invalid or unenforceable, shall be binding on the heirs, devisees, legatees, or personal representatives of the principal.

8. **Indemnity.** The estate of the principal shall hold harmless and indemnify the attorney-in-fact from all liability for acts done in good faith and not in fraud on behalf of the principal.

9. **Applicable Law.** The laws of the State of Washington shall govern this power of attorney.

10. **Execution.** This power of attorney is signed on this _____ day of _____, 199 _____ , to become effective as provided in Paragraph 3.

                          Signature: _____

                          Print name: _____

STATE OF WASHINGTON)

) ss.

COUNTY OF KING   )

I certify that I know or have satisfactory evidence that _____ is the person who appeared before me, and said person acknowledged that _____he signed this instrument and acknowledged it to be h_____ free and voluntary act for the uses and purposes mentioned in the instrument.

FIGURE 10-4
(continued)

die, positive euthanasia would have occurred if the doctors had hastened the infant's death with medication. There may well be more instances of positive euthanasia than we know about publicly.

The issue of positive euthanasia is cloudy. On some occasions, a physician will prescribe strong narcotics for a terminally ill patient and will request that the medication be given frequently enough to "keep the patient comfortable." Nurses often are reluctant to administer a medication that they realize has a potentially fatal effect when given in that dosage. In such cases, the ethical intent of the action is often considered. Medications given for the comfort of the dying patient may be ethically justifiable even if they hasten death to some extent. When nursing staff have difficulty with this issue, a patient conference with an oncology specialist or with a nurse skilled in the area of death and dying will help the staff to clarify values and deal with individual feelings.

Right-to-Die Issues

Right-to-die issues are gaining much more attention than in previous years. Kass (1993, p 37) identifies four reasons for such a right to be asserted:

- fear of prolongation of dying due to medical interventions; hence, a right to refuse treatment or hospitalization, even if death occurs as a result;
- fear of living too long, without fatal illness to carry one off; hence, a right to assisted suicide;
- fear of the degradations of senility and dependence; hence, a right to death with dignity;
- fear of loss of control; hence, a right to choose the time and manner of one's death.

Much debate currently rages around the issue of maintaining the lives of persons considered to be in a persistent vegetative state (PVS). Some of the issues that arise are the patient's rights, the family's wishes, and the cost to society. In most cases, the problems emerge when the life of a family member is being maintained through support measures that might be considered extraordinary.

In 1991, St. Francis-St. George Hospital in Cincinnati was sued in one of the first cases of its kind. The suit charged that the nurses should not have resuscitated an 82-year-old man when he suffered a heart attack. In so doing they disregarded a "no code" status of the patient (Hospital sued . . . , 1991).

WITHHOLDING TREATMENT

Withholding treatment could be considered negative euthanasia. A historic case occurred in 1963.

A couple on the East Coast gave birth to a premature infant who was diagnosed as having Down syndrome, with the added complication of an intestinal blockage. The intestinal blockage could have been corrected by surgery with minimal risk; without surgery the child could not be fed and would die. The Down syndrome, however, would have resulted in some degree of permanent mental retardation. The severity of the retardation could not be determined at birth, but would range from very low mentality to borderline subnormal intelligence.

The parents, who had two normal children at home, believed that it would be unfair to those children to raise a child with Down syndrome, and refused permission for the corrective operation on the intestinal blockage. Although it was an option, the hospital staff did not seek a court order to override the decision. The staff believed it was unlikely that a court would sustain an order to operate on the child against the parents' wishes, because the child had a known mental handicap and would be a burden to the parents financially and emotionally, and perhaps a burden to society. The child was put in a side room (an interesting action) and was allowed to die, a process that took 11 days. When confronted with the possibility of giving medication to hasten the infant's death, both doctors and nurses were convinced that it was clearly illegal (Gustafson, 1973).

The situation above stimulates both ethical and legal questions. Would the approach have been the same if the infant had not been mentally retarded? Would the staff have been guilty of murder if the infant had been given medication to hasten death? If a court decision to proceed with the surgery had been requested and granted, who would have been responsible for the costs incurred? What are the rights of the child? Who advocates for those rights if the child is unable to do so?

WITHDRAWING TREATMENT

In some instances, a family has sought court orders to have extraordinary life-support measures discontinued. A landmark case is that of Karen Quinlan.

> Karen Quinlan was a young woman left in a vegetative state after suffering severe brain damage from chemical abuse that involved both drugs and alcohol. She was placed on a respirator, and her physicians believed that she would live only a short time if it were to be removed. Her parents requested that the respirator be discontinued, but because she continued to manifest a minor amount of brain activity, their request was refused. After previous petitions to the Supreme Court of New Jersey had been rejected, the courts ruled on March 31, 1976, that her parents could exercise her privacy right on her behalf, and the respirator was discontinued. Much to everyone's surprise, Karen continued to live after the respirator was stopped, although she never emerged from her comatose condition; she died in 1986.

This case represents a situation in which treatment was withdrawn even though the treatment was not futile and the individual was not considered immediately terminal. Such cases represent hard decisions for all involved and evoke legal, moral, and ethical questions in almost all instances. A similar case that attracted much attention was that of Nancy Cruzan.

> In March 1988, Joe and Joyce Cruzan requested through the Jasper County Missouri Probate Court that they be allowed to remove the gastrostomy tube that kept their daughter Nancy alive. Nancy had been in a persistent vegetative state since an automobile accident in 1983. Although the request was granted, Missouri's attorney general appealed the decision, asking for a clear precedent from a higher court. In June 1990, the U.S. Supreme Court effectively denied the request in asking for "clear and convincing" evidence of the patient's view. In reaching this point, a fine line was drawn between initially withholding medical treatment and later withdrawing it. In Missouri, once the family gives initial consent for treatment, they forfeit all power to undo that consent or to stop treatment. No other state has such a law (Colby, 1990). Treatment can be stopped only two ways: if it can be demonstrated that it causes pain, or if the patient left behind clear and convincing evidence of his or her wishes prior to incompetency. The first was not an option because of Nancy Cruzan's persistent vegetative state. Therefore, her parents presented a state court with testimony from her physician and three friends that Nancy would not have wished to continue existing with irreversible brain damage. The Circuit Court judge ruled that this met the test and Nancy's feeding tube was removed on December 14, 1990. She died on December 26th.

Other cases have reached the headlines as individuals and families have striven to have more voice in determining issues related to the right to die. In all cases, much conflict exists in the arguments put forth by those supporting the right-to-die and right-to-life movements. In the fall of 1990, Congress took a major step regarding this issue by passing legislation that requires all Medicare and Medicaid providers to inform patients, on admission, of their right to refuse treatment. The matter is far from settled and is discussed in greater detail later in this chapter.

Of particular concern to nurses are their own feelings when a decision is reached to remove life-supporting measures, whether they are tube feedings or ventilators. Strong emotional attachments often form between the nurse and patient, even when the patient is in a vegetative state. Nurses who have worked to preserve the patient's dignity have great difficulty ''letting go.'' In some instances, patients are transferred to other facilities to die in an environment where the nurses are not so emotionally involved with the patient.

POSITIONS ON WITHHOLDING AND WITHDRAWING TREATMENT

Several organizations and groups have issued guidelines for their members, and others who would find them useful, with regard to the issue of withholding or withdrawing treatment. Key to all of these guidelines is whether the patient is legally *competent* (able to make decisions for herself or himself), or *incompetent* (in need of someone else to make those decisions). Table 10-3 outlines the date, organization and major tenets of some of those positions.

ASSISTED DEATH

The activities of a retired Michigan pathologist, Jack Kevorkian, who is alleged to have assisted patients in their suicide, have received much media attention in the past few years. Although charged on several cases, to date he has not been found guilty. The first case involved an Oregon woman, who was said to be suffering from Alzheimer's disease.

> A woman in Oregon sought the assistance of the physician, who assembled intravenous equipment and prepared medication in the back of his Volkswagen van. She initiated the administration of the solution that would allow her to end her own life. The courts decided the woman's death was a suicide. Michigan has since passed legislation outlawing assisted suicide.

In 1991, the Washington legislature wrestled with a referendum initiative sponsored by the Washington Citizens for Death with Dignity that would allow patients who are in a medically terminal condition to request and receive ''physician aid-in-dying.'' The initiative permitted a medical procedure to be performed by a physician that would end the life of a ''qualified'' patient, and changed Washington State's Natural Death Act to the Death with Dignity Act. Both this bill and a similar one in California were narrowly defeated, in part because they were badly drafted laws.

The American Nurses Association has developed a position statement on assisted suicide in which they state that the nurse should not participate in assisted suicide. Such an act is viewed as a violation of the *Code for Nurses*. The role of the nurse in providing comprehensive and compassionate end-of-life care is emphasized, stressing the promotion of comfort and relief of pain, and at times, the foregoing of life-sustaining treatment (ANA, 1994).

TABLE 10-3. Positions on Withholding And Withdrawing Treatment

Date	Organization	Position
1983	President's Commission Report—*"Deciding to Forego Life-sustaining Treatment"*	Focused on the ethical, medical, and legal issues in treatment decisions. Distinguished between withholding (not starting) and withdrawing (stopping after it started) treatment without making a moral distinction between the two. Suggested that withholding may require more justification because the positive effects would not be known.
1986	American Medical Association—*"Statement on Withholding or Withdrawing Life-prolonging Medical Treatment"*	Stated that life-prolonging medical treatment and artificially or technologically maintained respiration, nutrition, and hydration, could be withheld from a patient in an irreversible coma even if death was not imminent (Fry, 1990).
1986	Office of Technology Assessment of the U.S. Congress—*"Life-sustaining Technologies and the Elderly"*	Issued the results of its study on the use of life-sustaining technologies on the elderly. Report noted that the most controversial of the technologies was that of nutritional support. Identified that the most troublesome aspect of nutritional support is whether it is intravenous feeding and hydration or a tube feeding (Fry, 1990).
1987	Hasting's Center—*"Guidelines on the Termination of Life-sustaining Treatment"*	Provided clear definitions of key terms and a general guideline for making decisions regarding treatment. Viewed nutrition and hydration as medical interventions, much as other life-sustaining measures. Placed emphasis on the patient's ability to make decisions and required case-by-case assessment (Fry, 1990).
1988	American Nurses Association—*"Guidelines on Withdrawing or Withholding Food and Fluid"*	Indicated that there were few instances under which it would be permissible for nurses to withdraw food or fluid from their patients. No distinction was made between withdrawing and withholding (ANA, 1988).
1995	American Nurses Association—*"Position Statement on Foregoing Medically Provided Nutrition and Hydration"*	Stated that the decision to withhold medically provided nutrition and hydration should be made by the patient or surrogate with the health care team. The nurse continues to provide expert and compassionate care to patients who are no longer receiving medically provided nutrition and hydration. Distinguished between medically provided nutrition and hydration and the provision of food and water (ANA, 1995a).

THE RIGHT TO REFUSE TREATMENT

The right to refuse treatment is an issue closely aligned with the right to die. However, it carries some special implications that require separate consideration. Although we discussed some of the parameters of this issue in the previous section on the right to die, other aspects can create even bigger problems for the nurse. The moral, if not legal, precedent for refusing treatment occurred in 1971.

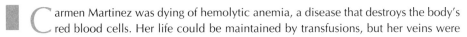

C armen Martinez was dying of hemolytic anemia, a disease that destroys the body's red blood cells. Her life could be maintained by transfusions, but her veins were such that a "cut-down" (a surgical opening made into the vein) was necessary to accomplish the transfusions. Finally Martinez pleaded to have the cut-downs stopped and to be "tortured" no more. The physician, fearful of being charged with aiding in her suicide, asked for a court decision. The court ruled that Martinez was not competent to make such a decision and appointed her daughter as her guardian. When the daughter also asked that no more cut-downs be performed, the compassionate judge honored the daughter's request. He decided that although Martinez did not have the right to commit suicide, she did have the "right not to be tortured." She died the next day (Veatch, 1976).

People working in the health care professions are frequently confronted with such dilemmas. Cases in which a patient refuses to have a leg amputated, even though not having the surgery will undoubtedly result in death, frequently make the news. The right to refuse treatment can take on additional implications when the patient, by refusing one type of treatment, is essentially demanding alternative medical management. Our support of the right to refuse treatment is based on a basic belief in and respect for the autonomy of the patient. When the refusal of medical intervention means that the individual is no longer a patient, it is known as a *negative right simpliciter* by bioethicists. In these cases the patient's physician need only do nothing, as in cases in which the patient discharges himself or herself from the hospital. When the patient refuses treatment, but does not withdraw from the role of being the patient, the matter becomes more complex. An example would be the patient who refuses to have a gangrenous toe surgically removed and demands to have it treated otherwise. These are referred to as positive rights. In the case of a gangrenous toe, one form of treatment may be more accepted than the other, but both may be successful. A case illustrating this right occurred in late 1993 in Chicago, and attracted national attention.

A Pentecostal Christian mother refused to have a cesarean section when physicians recommended the procedure because her fetus was being deprived of oxygen and would die if delivered vaginally. The courts upheld the patient's right to refuse the surgery. She later gave birth to an apparently healthy boy.

When children are involved, it is even more newsworthy, and again points out that there is as yet no consensus about when minors should be allowed to refuse treatment.

In November 1994, 16-year-old Billy Best made national news when he ran away from home to avoid another five months of chemotherapy and radiation. Suffering from Hodgkin's disease, the high school junior was experiencing nausea, aching and fatigue, as well as hair loss, from the treatment. He stated, ". . . I could not stand going to the hospital every week. I feel like the medicine is killing me instead of helping me." (Dorning, 1994).

Often in such cases the parents refuse to have the treatment started, many times because of religious beliefs. The courts usually become involved in reaching a decision. A case in Illinois in 1952 is typical.

Eight-day-old Cheryl suffered from erythroblastosis fetalis (Rh incompatibility). Her parents, who were Jehovah's Witnesses, refused to authorize the administration of blood necessary to save her life. The judge in the case ruled that Cheryl was a ne-

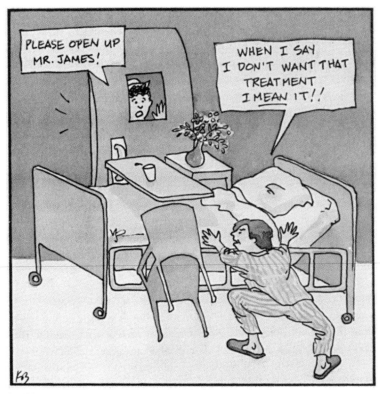

FIGURE 10-5
People working the health care field are frequently confronted with the dilemma of patients who may wish to refuse treatment.

glected dependent and overrode the parent's refusal. In such instances, the child is usually made a temporary ward of the court and legal documents are attached to the record authorizing the needed treatment. Such court decisions usually have been based on the premise that the right to freedom of religion does not give parents the right to risk the lives of their children or to make martyrs of them (Veatch, 1976).

Sometimes, when time is not a factor, the court will recommend that treatment be delayed until the child is aged 15 or 16 and can make a decision as an older minor. Other judges will rule just the opposite, deciding that it is cruel to place the burden of the decision on this older minor.

Situations like those that have been cited are always difficult for the people involved. Because nurses have the most contact with patients, they must examine their own feelings and attitudes. Nurses must recognize that patients also have the right to attitudes and beliefs. If a nurse decides that his or her own feelings are so strong that they might interfere with the ability to give compassionate care, it would be wise to ask to be assigned to other patients (Fig. 10-5).

ADDITIONAL BIOETHICAL CONCERNS

Most of you will probably find the area of bioethics interesting. Although many topics are central to the area of bioethics, such as the right to die, the right to refuse treatment, and all the issues related to conception, a number of less well-defined concerns are encountered in our health care delivery system. We cannot discuss all of these without creating a separate bioethics textbook; however, several deserve some review.

Organ Transplantation

Developments in the area of *organ transplantation* have created a number of issues deserving consideration. As discussed earlier in this chapter, it has in many ways necessitated a clearer definition of death. The supply of organs that can be used for transplantation has not been able to keep up with the demand. This is a result of the larger variety of organs that can be transplanted today. It is also a result of the decreased availability of organs as modern technology is increasingly being used to save more lives.

CONCERNS ABOUT PROCUREMENT

It has been estimated that between 1990 and 1995, an annual average of 4,835 people donated organs for use after their deaths. But many more, about 48,000 individuals, remain on organ waiting lists (Cimons & Maugh, 1996). Conflicts of interest between the potential donor and the person receiving the donor organ are easy to anticipate. Certainly no one would want to remove an organ from a donor as long as that person had any potential for recovery; on the other hand, it is imperative that donor organs be removed immediately after the death of the donor, before the organ to be removed becomes unusable.

Although there is lack of uniformity in the definition of death throughout the 50 states, it is generally accepted that organs can be removed from donors who have a flat electroencephalogram. This action is based on the 1975 definition of death, which states: ''For all legal purposes, a human body with irreversible cessation of total brain function, according to usual and customary standards of medical practice, shall be considered dead'' (Capron, 1978, p. 300).

The idea of consent again becomes important when we talk about organ transplantation. It is preferable to have the consent obtained from the donor. This has been facilitated in many states by the Uniform Anatomical Gift Act, which was drafted by a committee of the National Conference of the Commissions of Uniform State Laws in July 1968, and adopted in all American jurisdictions in 1971 (Hayt, 1977). People who are willing to donate parts of their bodies after death may indicate the desire to do so in a will or other written documents, or by carrying a donor's card. Many states now provide a space on driver's licenses where individuals can authorize permission for organ donations.

The spouse or the next-of-kin can also grant permission for the removal of organs after death. However, the time factor is crucial; the deaths are often accidental, and the relatives are often so emotionally distressed at the time that the process of obtaining permission may be difficult. Most medical personnel have at least some initial hesitancy in requesting permission for donor organs at this critical time. As we have gained more experience in this

Consent for Removal of Organs from the Deceased

I, _____ , next of kin (_____)
    Name   *Relationship*

of _____
                    Name of Donor

for humanitarian reasons hereby give consent for removal of _____

_____ from
            Names of Organs and Tissues

_____
                    Name of Donor

after his or her death for the purpose of transplantation, or for the retention of such organs and tissues for any other scientific or therapeutic purposes.

I understand that some of the procedures necessary for determination of suitability for transplantation will include testing for HBsAg (hepatitis B virus) and human immunodeficiency virus (AIDS virus antibody). I further authorize the release of medical information gathered in this process to the physicians involved in transplanting the above stated organs and tissues.

_____
                    Signature

_____
                    Date

_____
    Witness

_____
    Witness

FIGURE 10-6
Organ donation, consent form. (English version)

process, we also have developed better ways to deal with delicate issues. It is generally recommended that two groups of personnel be involved in requesting organs. The first group (usually nurses or medical personnel) helps the family realize that death has occurred or is imminent. This allows the family to grasp the reality of the situation. The second group, often referred to as the procurement team, requests the organ donation; these are persons skilled in recognizing the stress being felt by the family and experienced in providing information that will be important to them. The accompanying figures show both English and Spanish versions of the typical form that the family would be requested to complete (Figs. 10-6 and 10-7).

Some states have regulations that will allow donation of organs from an unidentified donor. Once a diligent search has been completed for next-of-kin, organs can be recovered. A coroner's consent is required in cases of accidental death, homicide, suicide, or any questionable cause of death.

Consentimiento para Remover los Órganos de la Personal Fallecida

Yo, _____ , familiar (_____)
               Nombre   *Relación*

de _____
                                Nombre del donador

consiento por razones humanitarias, la extracción de_____

_____ de
                          Nombrar órganos y tejidos

_____
                          Nombre del donador

posterior a su muerte para el propósito de trasplantes, o para la retención de dichos órganos y tejidos para cualquier otro propósito científico o terapéutico.

Entiendo que se requieren ciertos procedimientos para determinar si el trasplante es adecuado, estos incluyen las pruebas de HBsAg (virus de la hepatitis B) y del virus de immunodeficiencia humana (anticuerpo del virus del SIDA). También autorizo que los médicos que van a trasplantar los órganos y tejidos antes mencionados, tengan toda la información médica obtenida en este proceso.

_____
Firma

_____
Fecha

_____
Testigo/a

_____
Testigo/a

Source: Certified as a correct Spanish translation of all relevant information from the English original by Sarina Cats Frank, Notary Public.

FIGURE 10-7
Organ donation consent form (Spanish version).

In response to the inadequate supply of organs to meet societal needs—a situation referred to as *scarce medical resources*—some states have passed legislation requiring that donor organs be requested of the family when it is apparent that the patient has no chance for survival. This brings forth other problems. Who is to be responsible for approaching the family and requesting the organs? Must it be the family's physician? Would critical time be saved if it were the emergency department nurse or hospital social worker? A growing number of hospitals are designating a nurse as transplantation coordinator to facilitate this process. An interesting and controversial case occurred in California in 1990.

An 18-year-old woman, an only child, was diagnosed as having chronic myelogenous leukemia. Although this form of leukemia responds favorably to bone marrow transplants, no compatible donor could be found after testing the girl's family and contacting the National Marrow Donor Program. In desperation, the parents decided to have another child with the hope that the new baby would have genetically matching tissue type. This required that the father have a vasectomy reversed and that the mother, age 43, go through another pregnancy that terminated in a cesarean section. The baby provided a good match and was able to provide donor tissue for her sister. The case drew considerable attention as medical ethicists voiced concern about creating one child to save another. Citing Immanuel Kant, they argued that the baby was conceived, not as an end in itself, but for utilitarian purposes. Some medical ethicists argue in favor of the rights of the individuals involved, saying that it is not the concern of biomedical ethicists to intrude into matters affecting private citizens, especially when that intrusion approaches "intruding into a couple's bedroom." Still others say that striking cases must be brought before the public because an obligation to inform society exists.

The critical need for human organs also causes us to challenge previous decisions. A good example is that raised when considering organs removed from an anencephalic infant. An anencephalic infant is one born with only enough brain to support such vital functions as heartbeat and respiration. It has been estimated that about 60% of these infants are stillborn, and of those born alive only about 5% will live more than 3 days. Because anencephaly affects only the brain, other organs can be used for transplantation if the infant is kept alive on a respirator until a donor is located. This challenges our definitions of death. How can current definitions of ''brain'' death be applied to a condition in which there is no brain as we normally recognize it?

Other problems also arise with regard to organ transplantations, especially because there are more people who need organs than there are organs available. The skill of modern technology has resulted in the development and implantation of artificial organs such as the heart. Such technological advances were once viewed as science fiction. As a result, historic cases such as the implantation of an artificial heart in Barney Clark received a great deal of publicity. Over the years the use of artificial organs has not proven effective, and the practice of implanting artificial organs is not common today. This is not true of artificial parts. The use of artificial joints, heart values, and other prostheses continues to grow.

MINORITY ATTITUDES TOWARD ORGAN DONATION

Another issue that has emerged is that of minority differences in regard to organ donation. A growing number of minorities are now on waiting lists for transplantation. The risk of end-stage renal disease for African Americans and Native Americans is three to four times higher than for the white population (Kasiske, Neylan, Riggio et al., 1991). Minority organ donations lag behind those from the white population with 78.5% cadaver donations coming from caucasians, 11.4% from the black population, 8.2% from hispanics, and 1.0% from Asians (Wheeler & Cheung, 1996). Some of this difference is attributed to the fact that minority groups have been found to lack education and information regarding organ donation.

Minority groups have also identified religious beliefs and cultural customs as forbidding organ donation, although no major Western religion prohibits organ donation. African Americans listed distrust of the medical community, fear of premature death, and racism as major barriers. Hispanics experienced language barriers and identified the importance of having the entire extended family involved in all decision making regarding donations. Puerto Ricans verbalized denial of death and fear of mutilation of the body as critical factors. Barriers to organ donation in the Asian American cultures included the belief that the body should remain intact to the grave and lack of respect during the handling of the body after death. Although Native Americans are supportive of organ donations, their rate of donation is low, probably due to lack of knowledge (Wheeler and Cheung, 1996). While no single approach to organ donation will fit all groups, efforts to decrease barriers to donation are being instituted.

CONCERNS ABOUT XENOTRANSPLANTATION

Xenotransplantation refers to the practice of using animal organs, cells, and tissues for transplantation into human beings. The most recent case receiving national publicity was that of an AIDS patient in San Francisco who received the transplant of baboon bone marrow to bolster his weakening immune system. Of particular concern was the possibility of transmitting serious animal viruses and other microbes to people.

In September, 1996, the federal government proposed strict safeguards to provide protection. The guidelines were developed by representatives from the Food and Drug Administration (FDA), the Centers for Disease Control and Prevention, and the National Institutes of Health. The guidelines urged that patients and their families be fully informed of potential risks and further required that any planned procedure be thoroughly screened and approved by a series of local institutional review boards, and by the FDA. The recommendations also require that transplants take place at a clinical center associated with an accredited biology and microbiology laboratory.

Animal-rights activists also have expressed concern about the process. For them, the transplantation experiments are viewed as costly, cruel, and hopeless.

CONCERNS ABOUT ALLOCATION

How will we determine who will receive donated organs? Is there any "elitism" in their distribution—that is, does a white-collar worker have a better chance to receive an organ than a blue-collar worker? Medicaid and most insurance policies refuse to pay for the cost of many organ transplants, although the costs of corneal transplants and kidney transplants are usually covered by Medicare. Transplants are expensive procedures, often running into several hundreds of thousands of dollars. If money is required "up front," as it sometimes is, where can the needy person procure such funds? Other questions involve both donor and recipient. Should the donor or the donor's family be able to say who will receive the organ? How can one "get in line" for an organ, and how can that need be made known? What about selling a healthy organ, such as a kidney?

Much has been written about the problem of selecting recipients for organ transplantation when the number of applicants exceeds the number of available organs. Many criteria have been suggested, and as one might anticipate, these criteria have received arguments both pro and con; the criterion requiring medical acceptability is probably the only exception. Many transplants require that compatibility exist in the tissue and blood type of donor and recipient. It would not be logical to give a much needed organ to a person whose body would automatically reject it.

The criterion of the recipient's social worth is probably one of the hardest to defend, although it was used in the Pacific Northwest in the early 1960s to decide who should be allowed to live by kidney dialysis. Social worth, including past and future potential, was considered, and even such factors as church membership and participation in community endeavors were considered.

Some suggest a form of random selection, once the criterion of medical acceptability has been met. This could be either a natural random selection of the first come, first served variety, or an artificial selection process such as a lottery. A criticism of this method is that it removes rational decision making from the process.

We offer no suggestions to solve this problem, but merely demonstrate the difficulty it presents. Even the issue of who should serve on the decision-making committee can be touchy. The problem of personal biases is a big concern.

In an effort to gather donations and disseminate information about people who need various organs, an Organ Procurement Program was started in Pittsburgh, Pennsylvania. This program was established to facilitate the matching of donor with recipient and to provide a central listing agency for those in need of transplants. Today organ procurement agencies are located in all regions of the country. These groups carry out many activities related to organ procurement, including establishing groups for individuals who have received donated organs and their families, publishing newsletters and developing educational materials, increasing public awareness of the need for organs, and serving as a clearinghouse for organ procurement and matching. They are connected through the federally funded United Network for Organ Sharing.

CONCERNS ABOUT INDIVIDUAL PROPERTY RIGHTS

Concern for an individual's property rights in regard to human tissues has also attracted attention. Biotechnological developments allow profit-oriented companies to use human tissue to generate lucrative products such as drugs, diagnostic tests, and other medically related materials. The modern legal system has consistently held that no property rights are attached to the human body (Swain & Marusyk, 1990). In 1990, a Seattle man sued the University of California, two researchers, and two biotechnology and drug companies, because in 1976 he had sought treatment for hairy cell leukemia and subsequently had his spleen removed (which is the standard treatment). It was later discovered that the removed spleen contained unique blood cells that produced a rare blood protein used experimentally in the treatment of certain cancers and possibly AIDS. The patient was never told that his cells had great potential value, although he was brought from Seattle to Los Angeles frequently for blood and other tests. His cells were then developed into a self-perpetuating cell line to mass produce the rare blood protein. The patient's suit claimed that the defendants wrongfully converted to their own use his personal property (ie, the blood cells) and that this was done without his consent.

Truth-Telling and Health Care Providers

The issue of ''to tell'' or ''not to tell'' may not carry the emotional and bioethical impact that one experiences with concerns such as euthanasia, but it is one that is frequently encountered in the health care environment. Although informed consent has forced a more straightforward approach between physician and client, the problem of having the patient fully understand the outcome of care still exists. Sometimes the question about telling the client the expected outcome of care results from a request made by a close relative, but most of the time it results from the persistence of past medical practices.

In such instances the physician operates in a paternalistic role in relation to the client. Under this model of care, the locus of decision making is moved away from the client and resides with the physician. ''Benefit and do no harm to the patient'' is the dictum often cited as the ethical basis for this approach. It rationalizes that complete knowledge of his or her condition would place greater stress on the client. More recent discussions of medical ethics explore the rights of clients, particularly their right to make their own medical decisions. These discussions emphasize that in our pluralistic society, which has also fostered medical specialization to keep up with advances in knowledge and technology, physicians may be unable to perceive the ''best interests'' of their clients and to act accordingly.

Physicians do not agree on how much patients should know about their conditions. We usually experience a major controversy relating to this issue when a client has a terminal diagnosis such as cancer. Because, ideally at least, physicians are committed to protecting their clients from potential harm, both physical and mental, many have difficulty sharing bad news that will result in unhappiness, anxiety, depression, and fear. These physicians are concerned that if a client knows he or she is suffering from a terminal illness, the client will give up. After all, medical science might be wrong, or research may develop new cures that would change the course of the disease.

Physicians who argue the other side of the issue state that there exists a common moral obligation to tell the truth. They believe that the anxiety of not knowing the accurate diagnosis is at least as great as knowing the truth, especially if the truth is shared in a humane manner. These physicians also argue that one needs to have control over one's life and, if the news is bad, to have time to get personal affairs in order.

Although to tell or not to tell is a problem that exists between client and physician, nurses often become involved in it. First of all, the nurse may have definite personal feelings one way or the other. For example, if the physician has decided not to tell the client, or to delay sharing this information until later, and the nurse believes that the client has the right to be informed, the nurse may be in a frustrating situation and may even be angry with the physician. Because the nurse is in contact with the client for a more extended period of time, he or she may be put on the spot by the client's questions. The nurse may feel that hedging on a response is a compromise of the ethics of nursing practice. In such instances a conference, whether formal or impromptu, that would involve the physician, nurses, and other appropriate members of the health team, may help everyone deal with the situation. The nurse who is a novice in the health care system should realize that anyone can initiate a client care conference, although appropriate channels of communication should be followed in organizing it.

Thus far we have discussed situations in which information regarding a terminal illness may be shared with the client and family. At least one other circumstance that involves telling the truth is worth mentioning, although many examples could be included. One that we often see in the obstetric area of the hospital deals with sharing information with the parents of a newborn who is critically ill or who has a malformation. Sometimes physicians may want to spare the mother unpleasant news until she is stronger. This occurs frequently enough for obstetric nurses to have labeled it the *spare-the-mother syndrome*. In some instances, the physician may want to delay giving information until suspicions can be validated. If the doctor is waiting for the return of laboratory tests to confirm suspicions of genetic abnormalities, several days may be required. If good communication exists between nurse and physician, so that the nurse is well-informed, the nurse can provide emotional support and meet the client's need for information. Once again, a team approach usually is most effective.

The question of whether "to tell" or "not to tell" has been applied to another issue in the health care delivery system in recent years. That controversy pits the rights to privacy of the individual who is HIV positive against society's right to be protected. Dr. Cary Savitch, who has treated AIDS patients since 1981, advocates universal testing. Dr. Savich (1996, p. 140) states, "Controlling the epidemic is the only means to limit needless suffering and death. Controlling the epidemic will not come at the hands of a vaccine or miracle drug. Controlling the epidemic requires prevention. Prevention requires knowing who is communicable. Knowing who is communicable requires universal testing."

Many express concerns about privacy and confidentiality. If universal testing for AIDS is mandated, what would be next? Others argue that if health care providers exercise proper precautions, little danger exists. Still others would find the cost of universal testing be too great to make it realistic. There is no agreement among health care providers, activists, civil libertarians, and all concerned citizens regarding this issue, but it is certain to continue.

Ethical Concerns and Behavior Control

Before leaving this discussion of bioethical issues, we should say a few words in relation to behavior control. Many people experience extreme discomfort when contemplating research into human behavior. Although it may be one thing to work with atoms, molecules, and genes, it seems quite another to look at the science of human behavior.

Some of the problem seems to center around the fact that people define "acceptable behavior" in different and sometimes conflicting ways. When is behavior deviant? When is the client mentally ill? An excellent example is that of homosexuality, which at one time was listed by the American Psychiatric Association as a mental illness. Although many people may not approve of homosexuality, they would not classify all homosexuals as being mentally ill. Increasingly, society looks on sexual orientation as a personal matter.

The world has benefited from the work of many people whose behavior might not be looked upon as normal. Van Gogh cut off his ear; Tchaikovsky had terrible periods of depression; Beethoven was known for his uncontrollable rages. Some have suggested that Florence Nightingale's flights into fantasy could better be described as neurosis. Should this behavior have been changed and by what methods?

We can now change behavior by a variety of methods. Certainly one of the most common methods in which nurses will be involved is the administration of pharmacologic agents. Tranquilizers are now one of the largest classifications of drugs in the United States. Other chemicals, such as alcohol, marijuana, cocaine, and lysergic acid diethylamide (LSD), also change behavior. Some of these are considered socially acceptable, whereas others are not. Some are socially acceptable to some people or to some whole cultures, yet unacceptable to others cultures.

Electroconvulsive therapy (ECT), known earlier as electric shock therapy (EST), has been used for years to treat severe depression. Although antidepressant drugs are more commonly used today, ECT is still used in many areas of the country for depression that does not respond to drugs. Opponents of this form of therapy, who see it as inhumane, are becoming an organized political force. Proponents point out that with the current safeguards, it can be an effective therapy.

Psychosurgery—for example, frontal lobotomy (portrayed in *One Flew Over the Cuckoo's Nest*)—was used in the 1930s. This is undoubtedly one of the most criticized of treatment modalities because of its effect on the person. It is rarely used today, although another type of brain surgery is now being suggested for obsessive–compulsive disorder.

Psychotherapy can change other behavior. Techniques include verbal and nonverbal communication between the client and the therapist. Although psychotherapy requires considerable time, it is widely used.

When are any of these methods justified? Who makes the decision? What behavior is beyond the realm of acceptability? Who determines this? How does behavior control mesh with our beliefs about the autonomy of the individual or with concepts of self-respect and dignity? The issues of power and coercion pose a concern at this point. Problems related to involuntary commitment have moved this from the arena of ethics to that of legal determinants.

Halleck (1981, p. 268) has defined behavior control as treatment ''imposed on or offered to the patient that, to a large extent, is designed to satisfy the wishes of others. Such treatment may lead to the patient's behaving in a manner which satisfies his community or his society.'' Halleck goes on to point out that the question of behavior control has become more critical because newer drugs and new behavior therapy (such as aversive therapy and desensitization) make it possible to change specific behavior more rapidly and effectively. Traditional psychotherapy, which works slowly, offers the patient time in which to contemplate the change and reject it if it is unacceptable.

Dworkin (1981, p. 278) has proposed a set of guidelines that preserve autonomy in behavior control, as briefly stated here.

> We should favor those methods of influencing behavior that support the self-respect and dignity of those who are being influenced.
>
> Methods of influence that destroy or decrease a person's ability to think rationally and in his or her own interest should not be used.
>
> Methods of influence that fundamentally affect the personal identity of the person should not be used.
>
> Methods of influence that deceive or keep relevant facts from the person should not be used.
>
> Modes of influence that are not physically intrusive are preferable to those that are (such as drugs, psychosurgery, and electricity).
>
> A person should be able to resist the method of influence if he or she so desires, and changes of behavior that are reversible are preferable to those that are not.
>
> Methods that work through the cognitive and affective structure of a person are pref-

erable to those that "short-circuit" his beliefs and desires and cause him to be passively receptive to the will of others.

Rationing of Health Care

As we move into the 21st century, perhaps no issue in health care will receive more attention than the rationing of health care. Technology has allowed people to live longer. New treatment modalities have become more expensive. Dollars do not exist within our current social system to make all forms of health care available to all who wish to receive it. What should be treated and what should not? Who should receive the treatment and who should not? Should age be a factor? Mental status? Ability to contribute to society?

A number of states have begun to address these issues. In 1989, the Oregon legislature passed several statues that, among other things, created a process by which health care priorities would be established so that Medicaid and state-encouraged private coverage could provide the most cost-effective and beneficial forms of care for the largest number of persons. Implicit in this legislation was the involvement of the public in the process of building consensus on the values to be used to guide health resource allocation decisions. Oregon has continued to lead the nation in health care reform, especially at the consumer involvement level.

In Vermont, a statewide public education and discussion project was initiated that was designed to explore public attitudes and values that underlie health care and the public's priorities in the allocation of health resources. The project focused on the need for individuals to make known their preferences with regard to personal treatment.

In New Jersey, a Citizens' Committee on Biomedical Ethics has taken the position that citizens have the right and responsibility to insist that their preferences and values influence the development of health care policies and the allocation of medical resources. They have launched a community health program to clarify the ethical and social issues surrounding the provision of health care in that state.

Other states are following the examples set. Citizens are being asked to make informed decisions regarding health care. As a nurse, you have a vital role to play in the sharing of information regarding the delivery of health services. It is critical for you to anticipate some of the questions you may be asked and to analyze your own values.

KEY CONCEPTS

- Bioethics is the study of ethical issues that result from technologic and scientific advances, especially in biology and medicine. The number of bioethical issues surrounding the delivery of health care is growing.
- The leading bioethical issues can be divided into two major categories: those related to the beginning of life and those related to the end of life.
- Family planning (and the associated concern regarding age of consent) is one issue related to the beginning of life. Personal preferences and religious beliefs are critical determinants and nurses should be prepared to meet the needs of all clients without imposing their personal values on clients.

- Abortion, amniocentesis, prenatal diagnosis, genetic screening, sterilization, the concept of eugenics, the Human Genome Project, in vitro fertilization, artificial insemination, surrogate mothers, single parents, sperm banks, and the right to genetic information are additional topics presenting concerns.
- Fundamental bioethical issues concerning death are the changing definition of death and the decision about when it occurs.
- End-of-life issues include identifying futile treatment and establishing patient self-determination.
- Although negative euthanasia has been accepted by many courts based on individual circumstances, positive euthanasia remains very controversial.
- Surrounding the discussion of right-to-die are many issues, including those related to withholding treatment, withdrawing treatment, assisted death, and the right to refuse treatment.
- Bioethical concerns associated with the process of organ transplantation include procurement of organs, minority attitudes, allocation of organs, individual property rights, and the appropriateness of xenotransplantations.
- Debate and controversy have long surrounded determining what degree of information should be shared with clients and their families.
- The area of behavior control is subject to bioethical review, and guidelines have been established to preserve autonomy in behavior control.
- Rationing of health care commands major attention at the present time. Many states have begun to establish citizen committees to respond to this concern.

Critical Thinking Activities

1. Select one of the positions taken regarding abortion. Defend your position, providing a strong rationale for your thinking. Discuss this with a classmate who holds a different position, remembering that all persons are entitled to their own viewpoints.
2. hat do you see as the major issues associated with the Human Genome Project? What do you see as the major benefits to come from it? Weigh the problems against the benefits and take a position with regard to how far it should be developed.
3. What safeguards would you recommend with regard to in vitro fertilization, artificial insemination and surrogate mothers to ensure sanctity of human life? Be specific about how you believe these safeguards would be effective.
4. Have you signed an organ donation card? If not, discuss the reasons why you have chosen not to. If you have, discuss the reasons why you have. Is there a possibility you will change your mind? Why or why not?
5. What do you see as the major issues regarding the rationing of health care? Develop a list of the major health conditions for which you believe care should be funded. Identify those that should receive partial funding. List those that you believe should not be funded. Give a rationale for placing the various conditions on one of the three lists.

REFERENCES

American Nurses Association. Position Statement on Foregoing Medically Provided Nutrition and Hydration. Washington, DC: American Nurses Association, 1995a

American Nurses Association. Position Statement on Nursing and the Patient Self-Determination Act. Washington, DC: American Nurses Association, 1995b

American Nurses Association. Position Statement on Assisted Suicide. Washington, DC: American Nurses Association, 1994

American Nurses Association. Guidelines on Withdrawing or Withholding Food and Fluid. Washington, DC: American Nurses Association, 1988

Blackmun H. Majority opinion in Roe vs Wade. *In* Mappes TA, Zembaty JS: Biomedical Ethics, 2nd ed. New York: McGraw-Hill, 1981:478–482

Callahan D. The goals of medicine: Setting new priorities. Special Supplement, Hasting Cent Rep 26(6):51–528, 1997

Capron AM. Grandma? No, I'm the Mother! Hastings Cent Rep 24(2):24–25, 1994

Capron AM. Death, definition and determination of: Legal aspects. *In* Reich WT: Encyclopedia of Bioethics, vol 1. New York: Free Press, 1978

Cimons M, Maugh II,TH. Rules outlined for transplants from animals. Transplant: Safeguards drafted on animal-to-human treatments. *Los Angeles Times*, September 21, 1996: A1, A15

Colby WH. Missouri stands alone. Hastings Cent Rep 20(5):5–6, 1990

Dorning M. Teen-agers refusal of treatment stirs debate. *San Diego Union Tribune*, November 13, 1994:A8

Dworkin G. Autonomy and behavior control. *In* Mappes TA, Zembaty JS: Biomedical Ethics, 2nd ed. New York: McGraw-Hill, 1981:273–280

English cardinal bucks Vatican on destroying embryos. *The Herald,* August 1, 1996:7A

Fromer MJ. Ethical Issues in Health Care. St. Louis: CV Mosby, 1981

Fry ST. New ANA guidelines on withdrawing or withholding food and fluid from patients. *In* Lindeman CA, McAthie M: Readings: Nursing Trends and Issues. Springhouse, PA: Springhouse, 1990:499–507

Grady D. How to coax new life. *Time Special Issue,* Fall 1996:37–39

Gustafson JJ. Mongolism, parental desires, and the right to life. Perspect Biomed, Summer 1973:529

Halleck SL. Legal and ethical aspects of behavior control. *In* Mappes TA, Zembaty JS: Biomedical Ethics, 2nd ed. New York: McGraw-Hill, 1981:267–273

Hayt LR. Medicolegal Aspects of Hospital Records, 2nd ed. Berwyn, IL: Physicians' Record Company, 1977:397

Hellegers AE. Bioethical debates in gynecology and obstetrics. *In* Romney SL, et al: Gynecology and Obstetrics: The Health Care of Women. New York: McGraw-Hill, 1975:36

Hospital sued for ''wrongful life.'' Am J Nurs 91(5):111, 1991

Hudson T. Advance directives: Still problematic for providers. Hospitals and Health Networks 68(6):46, 48, 50, 1994a

Hudson T. Are futile-care policies the answer? Hospitals and Health Networks 68(4):26–32, 1994b

Jonsen AR. The Birth of Bioethics. Special Supplement to Hastings Cent Rep 23(6):S1–S4, 1993

Kasiske BL, Neylan JF, Riggio RR, et al. The effect of race on access and outcome in transplantation. N Engl J Med 324:302–307, 1991

Kass LR. Is there a right to die? Hastings Cent Rep 23(1):34–43, 1993

Kelly SJ. Pediatric Emergency Nursing (2nd ed.). Norwalk: Appleton & Lange, 1994

Kevles DJ. Social and ethical issues in the Human Genome Project. National Forum LXXIII(2): 18–21, Spring, 1993

Macklin R. Artificial means of reproduction and our understanding of the family. Hastings Cent Rep 21(1):5–11, 1991

Mancini M. Nursing, minors, and the law. Am J Nurs 78(1):124–127, 1978

Miller-Keane Encyclopedia & Dictionary of Medicine, Nursing, & Allied Health, 5th ed. Philadelphia: WB Saunders Company, 1992

Nuland SB. An epidemic of discovery. *Time Special Issue:* 8–13, Fall 1996

Pilbeam SP. Mechanical Ventilation: Physiological and Clinical Applications, 2nd ed. St. Louis: Mosby Year Book, 1992:17

Roan S. Woman gives birth at 63: Ethical questions raised. *Los Angeles Times*, April 24: A1, A31, 1997

Roe v. Wade, 410 U.S. 113 (1973)

Rossiter BJF, Caskey CT. Medical consequences of the Human Genome Project. National Forum LXXIII(2):12–14, Spring, 1993

Rothman DA, Rothman NL. The Professional Nurse and the Law. Boston: Little, Brown, 1977

Rothstein MA. The challenge of the new genetics. National Forum 69(4):39–40, 1990

Savitch C. The Nutcracker is Already Dancing: The HIVs and the HIV-Nots. Ventura, California: The Teague House Press, 1996

Schneiderman LF, Jecker N. Futility in practice. Arch Intern Med 153:437–440, 1993

Swain MS, Marusyk RW. An alternative to property rights in human tissue. Hastings Cent Rep 20(5): 12–15, 1990

Thomas CL. Taber's Cyclopedic Medical Dictionary, 17th ed. Philadelphia: FA Davis, 1993

Veatch RM. Death, Dying and the Biological Revolution. New Haven, CT: Yale University Press, 1976

Wheeler MS, Cheung A. Minority attitudes toward organ donation. Critical Care Nurse 16(1): 30–34, 1996

FURTHER READING

American Nurses Association. Position Statement on Promotion of Comfort and Relief of Pain in Dying Patients. Washington DC: American Nurses Association, 1994

American Nurses Association. Position Statement on Nursing Care and Do-Not-Resuscitate Decisions. Washington DC: American Nurses Association, 1995

Arras GJ. Crazy making: Embryos and gestational mothers. Hastings Cent Rep 21(1):35–38, 1991

Arras JD. Anencephalic newborns as organ donors: A critique. JAMA 259:2284–2286, 1988

Bailey LL. Organ transplantation: A paradigm of medical progress. Hastings Cent Rep 20(1):24–28, 1990

Berrio MW, Levesque ME. Advance directives; most patients don't have one. Do yours? Am J Nurs 96(8):24–29, 1996

Callahan D. Medical futility, medical necessity: The problem without a name. Hastings Cent Rep 21(4):30–35, 1991

Chafey K. ''Caring'' is not enough: Ethical paradigms for community-based care. N & HC Perspective on Community 17(1):10–15, 1996

Chervenak FA, McCollough LB. Justified limits on refusing intervention. Hastings Cent Rep 21(2): 12–18, 1991

Colbert T. Public input into health care policy: Controversy and contribution in California. Hastings Cent Rep 20(5):21, 1990

Cranford RE. A hostage to technology. Hastings Cent Rep 20(5):9–10, 1990

Crawford KF. How ethical dilemmas are resolved. Journal of Long-Term Care 22(3):4–9, 1994

Crawshaw R. A vision of the health decisions movement. Hastings Cent Rep 20(5):21–22, 1990

Daniels N. Duty to treat or right to refuse? Hastings Cent Rep 21(2):36–46, 1991

Downes J. Ethical issues. The ethical dilemmas of mandatory prenatal and newborn HIV testing. Nursing Connections 8(4):43–50, 1995

Dunn DG. Bioethics and Nursing. Nursing Connections 7(3):43–51, Fall 1994

Ellman IM. Can others exercise an incapacitated patient's right to die? Hastings Cent Rep 20(1): 47–50, 1990

Freda MC. Childbearing, reproductive control, aging women, and health care: The projected ethical debates. JOGNN 23(2):144–152

Garland MJ, Hasnain R. Health care in common: Setting priorities in Oregon. Hastings Cent Rep 20(5):16–18, 1990

Gaylin W. Fooling with mother nature. Hastings Cent Rep 20(1):17–21, 1990

Greer MB. Factors affecting opinions on life support issues in the elderly. Issues on Aging 18(2): 19–23, 1995

Guido GW. Legal Issues in Nursing: A Source Book for Practice. Norwalk, CT: Appleton & Lange, 1992

Hill TP. Giving voice to the pragmatic majority in New Jersey. Hastings Cent Rep 20(5):20, 1990

How far should we push Mother Nature? *Newsweek* 17:54–57, January 1994

Jecker NS, ed. Aging and Ethics: Philosophical Problems in Gerontology. Clifton, NJ: Humana Press, 1991

Kowalski S. Withdrawal of nutritional support: A family's choice. Gastroenerology Nursing: 19(1) 25–28, 1996

Lauritzen P. What price parenthood? Hastings Cent Rep 20(2):38–46, 1990

Lippman H. After Cruzan: The right to die. RN 54(1):65–68, 73, 1991

Lynn J, Glover J. Cruzan and caring for others. Hastings Cent Rep 20(5):10–11, 1990

Markowitz MS. Human fetal tissue: Ethical implications for use in research and treatment. AWHONNS Clinical Issues in Perinatal and Women's Health Nursing 4(4):578–588

Moody HR. Ethics in an Aging Society. Baltimore/London: Johns Hopkins University Press, 1992

Moss RJ, La Puma J. The ethics of mechanical restraints. Hastings Cent Rep 21(1):22–25, 1991

Nurses seek a voice in right-to-die cases. Am J Nurs 91(3):26, 1991

Oregon Nurses Association. Death with Dignity Act Position Statement. Oregon: Oregon Nurses Association, 1995

Overall C. Selective termination of pregnancy and women's reproductive autonomy. Hastings Cent Rep 20(3):6–11, 1990

Pence T. Ethics in Nursing: An Annotated Bibliography, pt 2. Publication No. 20-1989. New York: National League for Nursing, 1986

Pinch WJ, Dougherty CJ, McCarthy V. Ethics in nursing practice: Confidentiality for women and their children with HIV/AIDS. Medsurg Nurs 4(6):452–457, 1995

Powledge TM. Capital report—springtime for fetal tissue research? Hastings Cent Rep 21(2):5–6, 1991

Reich WT. Encyclopedia of Bioethics. New York: Macmillan, 1982

Robertson JA. Cruzan: No rights violated. Hastings Cent Rep 20(5):8–9, 1990

Rothman, DJ. Strangers at the Bedside: A History of How Law and Bioethics Transformed Medical Decision Making. New York: Basic, 1991

Rousseau PC. How fluid deprivation affects the terminally ill. RN 54(1):73–74, 1991

Taylor SL. Quandry at the crossroads: Paternalism versus advocay surrounding end-of-treatment decisions. American Journal of Hospice and Palliative Care 12(4):43–46, 1995

Vernale C, Packard SA. Organ donation as gift exchange. Image 22(4):239–242, 1990

Weber LJ, Campbell ML. Ethics and the law. Medical futility and life-sustaining treatment decisions. Journal of Neuroscience Nursing 28(1):56–60, 1996

Wendling EM. Anencephalics as organ donors. Imprint April/May 1990:47–48

Wurzbach ME. The dilemma of withholding or withdrawing nutrition. Image 22(4):226–230, 1990

Zerwekh Z. Do dying patients really need IV fluids? Am J Nurs 97(3):26–31, 1997

Career Opportunities and Professional Growth

In this unit we present basic information about the employment world you will find in nursing. This will help you as you move from the student role to the role of the registered nurse employed within the health care delivery system. Chapter 11 looks at your personal relationship with this new role; in Chapter 12, we present ways that you can affect the nursing environment in which you practice through collective bargaining, shared governance activities, and participating in committees to develop policies and procedures.

Unit IV

Beginning Your Career as a Nurse

The knowledge, skills, competencies, values, flexibility, commitment, and morale of the health professional workforce serving the systems of care will become the most important factors contributing to the success or failure of the system.
(Pew Health Professions Commission, 1995)

Objectives

After completing this chapter, you should be able to:

1. Describe a variety of employment opportunities available to nurses today.

2. Explain the common competencies needed by the new graduate as outlined by the job analysis study.

3. Analyze the eight common expectations employers have of new graduates and relate them to your own background and education.

4. Develop a list of your personal short- and long-term career goals.

5. Describe how you plan to maintain your competence in nursing.

6. Create a personal resumé; sample letters of application, follow-up, and resignation; and a plan for your personal responses in an employment interview that can be used when you seek employment.

7. Explore strategies that you might personally use to prevent or alleviate reality shock.

8. Analyze your own values and life situation in relationship to your personal potential for burnout.

9. Discuss three areas of concern relative to sex discrimination in nursing.

10. Identify hazards to the health of both yourself and others in the nursing workplace and ways that you can act to protect yourself.

KEY TERMS

Burnout
Comparable worth

Competency
Cover letter

Discrimination	**Proficiency**
Expert	**Reality shock**
Long-term goals	**Resumé**
Novice	**Short-term goals**
Occupational hazard	**Stereotype**

A fter completing an educational program, you, as a new graduate, will want to get out into the real world and practice your nursing skills. In the past such a goal was rather simple and straightforward, but a nursing career is now much more complex.

HISTORICAL EMPLOYMENT OPPORTUNITIES IN NURSING

Early in the 20th century, almost all graduate nurses performed private-duty nursing. The nurse was hired by a client or family to provide care during a particular episode of illness or disability. Some nurses specialized in maternity cases, in which they cared for new mothers and infants; others specialized in caring for persons with long-term illnesses, such as strokes. The nurse was expected to live at the client's residence and assume 24-hour responsibility for the client's care. This might even include preparing special foods for the convalescing client and the family. Nurses hired as graduate nurses in hospitals usually were head nurses, supervisors, or directors. Client care was usually provided by students (see Chapter 4).

By the 1930s, the employment situation began to change. More graduate nurses were hired to provide client care. Employment practices became modernized, and nurses were no longer expected to be on duty 24 hours a day when engaged in private-duty nursing. Most nurses were employed in a hospital or an institution. Regular work schedules were established in hospitals. Nurses still worked split shifts—morning and evening of the same day with several hours ''off duty'' in the afternoon. There were few employee benefits (paid holidays, vacations, insurance, and retirement plans), but the beginnings of change were there.

World War II had a major impact on nursing. Because women were essential to the war effort, it became acceptable for married women to continue working. Women nurses were valued members of the armed forces and attained elevated status by becoming officers in the military. These nurses had to learn to be assertive in managing their responsibilities, and many brought this quality back to the hospital. Wanting to be of service to a country at war, women who might never have considered nursing because of its previous status now entered the profession.

The expansion of the hospital or institutional job market for nurses was also influenced by population growth. Advances in medicine, which included more surgery being performed, resulted in special care that was available only in a hospital. The number of hospitals increased dramatically.

The noninstitutional job market also grew. Since the early 1900s, when Lillian Wald established a visiting nurse service, community health nursing has continued to develop. Nurses were pioneers in bringing health care to people's homes and in focusing on prevention of illness through consumer education.

Other areas of nursing in the community began to widen as well. More nurses were working in industry. Conditions for workers improved, and action regarding their health became part of law, custom, or contract. Nurses also worked in school districts, and the school nursing specialty started to expand.

Nurses began to provide primary health care. Primary care is that segment of health care that furnishes both the initial contact with the health care system and the longitudinal supervision of health care needs. Perhaps the first primary health care by nurses was provided by the midwives of the Frontier Nursing Service in Kentucky in the 1920s. These midwives assumed overall responsibility for the care of child-bearing women during pregnancy, delivery, and the postpartum period.

Another early group that expanded practice were the nurse anesthetists, who organized the Association of Registered Nurse Anesthetists in 1931 and assumed responsibility for accrediting programs to prepare nurses in this specialty field. At this time nurses employed outside of institutions were a minority.

After World War II, nursing grew geometrically, extending to many areas at once, and the nation experienced a shortage of nurses. Because of this shortage, many other categories of health care workers were created, but roles and relationships were not carefully planned. The majority of nurses continued to be employed in hospitals. As the supply of nurses grew, new patterns of care delivery that capitalized on the skills of the registered nurse developed and primary nursing became widespread.

EMPLOYMENT OPPORTUNITIES TODAY

The health care environment today is affected by all that has gone before. In some settings, there are remnants of the paternalistic attitudes that were prevalent in the years when women were expected to accept the hospital as the family surrogate during training and employment. This attitude may coexist with one that expects today's nurse to be an independent decision-maker. Emphasis is placed on the nurse's need for breadth and depth of theory to cope with the complexities of caring for the acutely ill. At the same time, pangs of nostalgia may be expressed for the days when nurses "really knew how to work" and did not worry much about "book learning."

Unlike graduates of the hospital programs of the past, you will have had fewer hours working in an employment-type situation. Your contact with employment settings may have been brief and you may not have experienced all of the many settings in which registered nurses are employed. You may have questions regarding employer expectations and your own role as a registered nurse employee.

As more care is delivered outside of acute care hospitals, the percentage of nurses working outside the hospital has increased. Home health care, hospice care, community mental health centers, women's health care delivery systems, maternal–infant care programs, outpatient and primary care, and long-term care facilities are hiring growing numbers of registered nurses as they care for patients with more complex needs. In Chapter 1 we discussed the many settings in which health care is delivered, and we also pointed out the nursing roles seen in those settings.

The growth of autonomy for the registered nurse has been even more marked outside the hospital setting than in it. Community health nurses have always operated much more independently than hospital nurses. The focus on health care is shifting from illness to health. Because many positions in the community require a baccalaureate degree, experience, or specialized educational programs, the new graduate is most often employed in the hospital or long-term care institution.

The number of positions for registered nurses in many settings other than those that provide client care has also grown. Health care-oriented businesses such as insurance companies and medical equipment supply companies have found that it is easier to teach nurses about business than to teach business people about health care. As a result, nurses are being employed in what some individuals see as non-nursing positions. Others argue that these, too, should be considered nursing positions, because the expertise that makes the individual successful is nursing expertise.

The number of men in nursing, which remained relatively small for many years, is beginning to grow as society reassesses its attitude toward labeling jobs as woman's or man's work. Men have been attracted by the opportunities and improving economic picture of nursing and in turn have not been reluctant to advance it still further.

The economic position of the nurse has improved for a variety of reasons. One reason is the extension of laws governing fair labor practices to nonprofit institutions and the advent of collective bargaining. Another major factor affecting the economic position of nurses was the nursing shortage of the 1980s. The demand for nurses rose faster than the supply; employers began increasing salaries and benefits to attract nurses. This was especially notable in urban communities.

Then in the 1990s, the pressures of a changing health care system and cost containment created still more changes for nursing. Hospital stays shortened so dramatically that hospital censuses decreased across the country. The nursing shortage appeared to end abruptly as hospitals began reassessing their needs. Some hospitals have closed; many have downsized. In addition, many hospitals have restructured to employ more unlicensed assistive personnel. These factors have contributed to layoffs of nurses from hospitals. Long-term care and home care have increased, although funding of home care remains a problem.

All of these factors bring you, as a new graduate, into a world of uncertainty, but one also filled with opportunity and promise. Now you must determine your place in this world.

COMPETENCIES OF THE NEW GRADUATE

Recently you have heard the term *competency* used a great deal, especially as it applies to the new graduate. Competency, as used here, refers to the ability of the graduate to effectively and safely perform specified nursing skills, including the application of critical thinking skills. Some have differentiated "competency," which is an entry-level expectation, and "proficiency" which is expected of the expert and requires experience (Fig 11-1).

Competencies Identified By Nursing Organizations

The most definitive statement on the competencies needed by the newly registered nurse has been developed by the National Council of State Boards of Nursing (NCSBN), based on its job analysis study that serves as the basis for the NCLEX-RN licensing examination (Chornick, Yocom, & Jacobson, 1993).

This study was based on responses by a stratified random sample of newly licensed, entry-level registered nurses, most of whom were employed in acute care hospitals. Both the frequency of 270 nursing activities and their *criticality* were studied. Criticality refers to activities that cannot be delayed or omitted without a "substantial risk of unnecessary

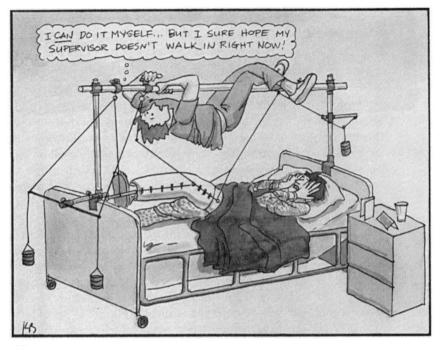

FIGURE 11-1
New graduates are expected to know both their own abilities and when to seek appropriate help.

complications, impairment of function, or serious distress to clients'' (Chornick, Yocum, & Jacobson, 1993, p 11).

Activities expected of newly licensed nurses that led the list for criticality were:

- Use universal precautions
- Report significant changes in the client's condition
- Perform cardiopulmonary resuscitation
- Perform Heimlich maneuver/abdominal thrust
- Provide emergency care for a wound disruption
- Recognize the occurrence of hemorrhage
- Manage a medical emergency until a physician arrives
- Implement measures to prevent circulatory complications (such as embolus, shock, hemorrhage, etc.)
- Respond to symptoms of fetal distress

Activities were further studied in terms of the frequency with which they were expected of newly licensed registered nurses. In all settings nurses were expected to:

- Coordinate care through working with others on the health care team and supervising delivery of care by assistive personnel
- Preserve the quality of care through such activities as acting as an advocate for needed changes in care, documenting errors or problems, and intervening in situations involving unsafe or inadequate care

- Maintain the safety of the client as exemplified by verifying, identifying, and reporting unsafe equipment, and following infection control guidelines
- Prepare clients and families for care that is to be done, including procedures and treatments; and help them to understand expected outcomes
- Carry out procedures in a safe, effective manner

Physiologic integrity and psychosocial integrity were supported by a wide variety of individual nursing actions. Some, such as assessing vital signs, seemed almost universal. Others, such as monitoring for side effects of radiation therapy, were needed in a small minority of settings. Allowing clients to talk about their concerns and assisting them to communicate effectively were again almost universal activities.

Activities that represent carrying out the nursing process in terms of assessment, analysis, planning, implementation, and evaluation applied to almost all settings.

In addition to this study, statements regarding competencies of new graduates have been developed by the various educational councils of the National League for Nursing (1991). Additionally, some states have developed statements of competencies for graduates of the nursing programs in those states. Similarities and patterns have emerged from all of these statements. The outline of theoretical knowledge and functioning in regard to the nursing process seems to be the most consistent. The most divergent opinions seem to be in the area of specific skill or task competency (Fig. 11-2).

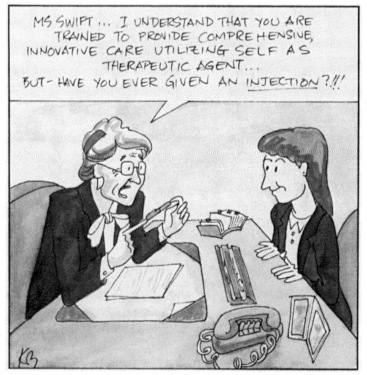

FIGURE 11-2
Employers are often concerned about an applicant's specific technical skills.

Employers' Expectations Regarding Competencies

Employers often ask for further clarification of competence. Have these graduates only the necessary theoretical knowledge regarding the skill? Have they actually performed the skill? If so, was it in a practice laboratory only, or was it in a client care situation? Does competence mean that the new graduate can function independently, or will some supervision still be needed?

Further complicating the picture is the confusion surrounding competencies of the graduates of the three types of nursing education programs preparing individuals for registered nurse licensure: the hospital-based diploma program, the associate degree program, and the baccalaureate degree program. Although statements by a variety of organizations have distinguished among levels of functioning, many employers do not differentiate expectations. Some employers state that new graduates from different types of programs have not clearly demonstrated differences in competencies. This has created confusion in the minds of nurses, employers, and the public over the role of the registered nurse prepared in each type of educational program.

What is expected of the new graduate varies in different health care agencies and in different geographical areas. Expectations are affected by various factors in the community, such as whether there are nursing programs in that community and whether new graduates come from one or from many different schools. The acuity of the client care load and the types of services offered by an agency may also affect expectations. The Joint Commission on the Accreditation of Healthcare Organizations (JCAHO) has a criterion requiring that accredited institutions monitor and assure the competence of their staff. This requires that an institution identify expected competencies for staff and then design an assessment method. As institutions move to comply with this standard, most are directing their initial efforts toward technical skills, because these are more easily identified and assessed. Other competencies will be more difficult to assess.

Based on the NCSBN job analysis study (Chornick and others, 1993), agencies that employ newly graduated registered nurses expect them to demonstrate the following competencies:

1. *Possess the necessary theoretical background for safe client care and for decision making.* Many employers believe that new graduates today are very competent in this area. For instance, the new graduate should understand the signs and symptoms of an insulin reaction, recognize it when it occurs, and know what nursing actions should be taken. The new graduate must know when an emergency or complication is occurring and secure medical help for the client when that is needed.

2. *Use the nursing process in a systematic way.* This includes assessment, analysis, planning, intervention, and evaluation. New graduates should be able to develop plans of care as well as follow plans such as care pathways that have been developed by the agency.

3. *Recognize own abilities and limitations.* To provide safe care, the nurse must identify when a situation requires greater expertise or knowledge and when assistance is needed. Employers may be able to assist if nurses ask for help and

direction, but cannot accept the risk to clients created by nurses who do not know their own limitations.

4. *Use communication skills effectively with clients and coworkers.* In every setting there are clients and families who are anxious, depressed, suffering loss, or experiencing other types of emotional distress. The nurse is expected to respond appropriately to these individuals and to facilitate their coping and adaptation. Effective communication skills are essential to the functioning of the entire health care team. Often the nurse is expected to help coordinate the work of others, and this cannot be done without effective communication skills.

5. *Understand the importance of accurate and complete documentation.* Employers generally recognize that the new graduate must be given time to learn the documentation system used in the facility. However, the new graduate is expected to recognize the need for recording data. It is anticipated that the nurse will keep accurate, grammatically correct, and legible records that provide the necessary legal documentation of care.

6. *Understand and have a commitment to a work ethic.* This means that the employee will take the responsibility of the job seriously and will be on time, take only the allowed coffee and lunch breaks, and will not take "sick days" unless truly ill. It also means that the new graduate recognizes that nurses may be needed 24 hours a day, 365 days a year, and that this may require sacrifices of personal convenience, such as working evening shifts or on holidays.

7. *Possess proficiency in the basic technical nursing skills.* This is an area in which a wide variety of expectations may be present. In most settings, proficiency in the basic skills required to support activities of daily living is expected. These skills include transferring, giving baths, and performing general hygienic measures. In some settings, nurses will be carrying out these tasks, whereas in others they will be directing or teaching others who do them, such as nursing assistants or family members. In either case, proficiency is essential to evaluating the care provided.

   The technical skills or tasks that are reserved for the registered nurse represent the area of widest diversity in the identification of essential skills. The settings in which nurses practice are diverse, and therefore technical skills may be needed in one setting but not in another. Some facilities provide extensive orientation programs in which every skill is checked before the new graduate is allowed to proceed independently. Other employers expect the new graduate to perform the skill if able, and be checked off as required, or to ask for help if unable to be independent. Often employers are flexible in their expectations, so that it may be acceptable if an individual seems to have competency in a reasonable percentage of the skills required by that agency; further development of skill competency will be supported by the institution. Other employers have a list of skills in which competency is mandatory at the time of hire, although speed may not be expected. Also, there may be a difference between what the employer would wish and what the employer will accept.

8. *Function with acceptable speed.* This is another area in which expectations differ greatly. Most employers state that they expect the new graduate will be slower;

however, they may vary in how much slowness is acceptable and how soon they feel that nursing actions should become more time efficient. Generally, an orientation period is planned—although, with the pressures on health care agencies, this often has been shortened considerably. An acceptable speed of function is reflected by the ability to carry out a usual registered nurse assignment within a shift. Thus, if the usual client assignment for a registered nurse is the care of six to eight moderately ill clients, the new graduate is expected to accomplish this by the end of the orientation period.

PERSONAL CAREER GOALS

In caring for clients, you are involved in the process of goal setting. Many nurses recognize the value of this in client care but never transfer the concept to their personal lives. Nursing as a profession offers many career options. Without carefully setting goals, you might drift for years.

Focusing Your Goals

You may want to focus on a broad area of clinical competency, such as pediatric nursing, or on a more restricted area, such as neonatal care. Clinical areas available for concentrated effort become more varied as health care becomes more complex. Emergency care, coronary care, neurologic and neurosurgical nursing, and specialties in the care of persons with ear, nose, and throat disorders are just a few of the clinical possibilities. Nurses specialize in aerospace nursing, enterostomal therapy, and respiratory care as well as operating room nursing and postanesthesia care. Opportunities for additional education and for practice in most clinical specialties are now available for any experienced registered nurse, regardless of the person's initial educational background.

Some specialty positions are in the primary care field, such as the woman's health care specialist, the family nurse practitioner, and the pediatric nurse practitioner. Increasing numbers of these programs require a baccalaureate degree for entry, but some admit registered nurses with experience in that specialty area.

Another approach may be to focus your goals on the setting in which care is delivered, such as acute care, long-term care, or community care. As health care needs expand, these separate realms of care delivery are all demanding more specialized knowledge. Even within the individual area of focus differences are present. For example, within the community are ambulatory care settings, public health nursing agencies, occupational health nursing departments, and day care facilities.

Yet another way of focusing your goals is according to functional categories. Although nurses are initially thought of as direct care providers, they are needed in many other positions. For example, there is need for those who would move into supervisory and administrative capacities, those who teach, and those who conduct nursing research. Nursing also lends itself to writing, to community service, and even to political involvement.

You may decide to set your goals in relation to all three types of foci. That is, you might identify a clinical area, a care setting, and a functional category.

Setting Your Goals

The first step in setting personal career goals is a thorough self-assessment. Determine how your abilities and competencies correspond to your own expectations, as well as to those of employers. Other factors to explore are your likes and dislikes and the situations or types of work you particularly enjoyed as a student. Also, it is important to recognize the area in which you were most comfortable. Were there areas in which you or your instructor felt that you were an above-average student? Consider your health and personal characteristics in relationship to types of work. Do you have physical restrictions? Do you prefer working independently or with others? How do you respond to close supervision or to relative freedom in the job setting? Do you prefer a work environment that is relatively predictable or do you thrive in a situation that changes frequently? Do you work well with long-term goals and a few immediate reinforcements, or do you need to see results quickly? Another factor to consider is your own geographic mobility: would you be willing to move or travel as part of a job? Both your personal responsibilities and preferences operate in this arena.

As you plan ahead, you need to examine many of the options offered by nursing. What types of jobs and opportunities are open to you? What education and personal abilities are needed in these areas? Are you interested? Does the education you have meet the educational requirements? Are avenues for additional education available to you? All of these considerations are important as you plan for the future.

Career goals need to be both short- and long-term. They will help you to plan your future constructively. This does not mean that goals are static. Just as client goals must be realistic, personal, and flexible, so must your own goals.

Short-term goals will encompass what you want to accomplish this month and this year. What do you want to do and what do you want to be in the immediate future? For example, one recent graduate stated that her short-term goal was to have 2 years of solid experience in a busy metropolitan hospital.

Long-term goals represent where you want to be in your profession 5 to 10 years from now. The long-term goal of the graduate referred to above was to work in a small, remote community in which she would have the opportunity to function autonomously.

Although both long- and short-term goals will be revised as your life evolves, they will guide you in making day-to-day decisions more effectively. In today's world of rapid health care change, you may need to keep your goals somewhat broad and flexible. Be ready to consider alternative goals and a variety of pathways to one goal. These approaches will be of value as you enter a system in transition.

Maintaining and Enhancing Your Competence

Every nurse has an obligation to society to maintain competence and continue practicing high-quality, safe care. Continuing education may occur through learning on the job, through reading of professional publications, or through attending classes. There are television courses, programmed instruction programs, and examinations related to journal articles. Any of these avenues may be appropriate, depending on the circumstances. Some nurses may want to advance through specialty or higher education. Included in your goal setting should be an approach to maintaining and enhancing your competence.

MAKING GOALS REALITY

Philosophical questions regarding goals must be resolved by practical approaches. As a new graduate, your first goal simply may be to get a job in nursing (especially if you live in one of the areas of the country that has more limited opportunities for registered nurses).

Whatever the situation, you are more likely to realize your goals if you are prepared to present yourself in the best possible way to a prospective employer. Many of you have held different jobs in the community as students and as adults. You may be familiar with and competent in the job search process. Others of you have never applied for the kind of job that truly could be considered the beginning of a career. Different expectations are held by employers and prospective employees in such a situation.

Identifying Potential Employers

In order to effectively begin your job search, you will need to identify potential employers. You might begin your review with those more familiar to you and gradually move outward in an ever widening circle to identify others.

The clinical sites where you had experiences as a student or where you worked when a student are good places to begin. You may know these agencies, be familiar with the type of care provided, and already be oriented to many of their policies and procedures. Your prior association with these agencies may provide you with ready access to their hiring procedures. If you worked as an employee in a health care setting before graduation, you may be given preference in hiring. This is one reason for seeking health care employment during your nursing education process.

Another source of potential jobs is the classified section of the local newspaper. There you are more likely to find single jobs in small facilities as well as general recruitment announcements from larger facilities. However, just because an agency does not advertise does not mean they will not be hiring any employees. Advertising is expensive and may result in an excess of applicants to screen. Therefore, some health care agencies do not advertise and rely on those who independently seek them out as potential employers.

The ''Yellow Pages'' of the telephone book may help you to locate smaller employers in your community. You could look under ''nursing homes,'' ''home care,'' ''nursing care'' and other such headings. This may help you to identify health care providers you were not aware of. Do not hesitate to call or even personally visit these settings in order to obtain information for a job application.

If you have the flexibility to move from your local area, you may expand your search for possible positions. The major nursing journals have sections in the back pages devoted to advertisements. Some of these advertise nursing positions. If you have a specific area in mind, you might visit your local library and consult the newspaper and the telephone directory for that area. Your nursing program may receive advertising magazines that are designed to present job opportunities for new graduates. These magazines provide a few articles about relevant job search topics, such as interviewing, as well as advertisements from health care agencies. These advertisements present information on the agency itself and how to contact them for possible application.

For those with electronic access to the World Wide Web, additional sources of potential jobs are available. Many governmental job openings also are posted online. Using your search engine, look for "employment opportunities," "jobs," or "careers." Some online service providers have additional support services for a job search that might include career guidance (for a fee), or sample documents such as resumés and cover letters.

Letter of Inquiry or Application

Writing a letter of inquiry is an excellent way to approach many prospective employers. (Display 11-1). This letter is often termed a "cover letter" because it is sent with your resumé (see below). You can present yourself positively through a well written letter. In addition, a letter may be dealt with at the recipient's convenience, whereas a telephone call may interrupt a busy schedule. There are fewer chances for misunderstanding if your request is in writing and if you receive a written reply.

Before you write your letter, you should make sure you have information about the prospective employer. What kind of facility is this? What types of clients do they serve, and what special services do they offer? It makes a poor impression to write to a prospective employer stating that your goal is to work in pediatrics when that facility does not provide any pediatric services. You might obtain this information by calling the human resources department of the facility or by contacting a public information office. In a small agency, you may simply speak with a receptionist or secretary. Be honest and straight forward in explaining that you are considering applying for employment and would like information about the agency before making that decision.

Another part of your advance planning is identifying how you will focus your letter on your special qualifications and what you want to highlight. You will want to focus on the skills or accomplishments related to the position you want. Your letter should be no more than one page in length, but be planned to present all essential information. Introduce yourself and your purpose for writing in the first paragraph so that the reader immediately has an understanding of why you are writing. You may want to briefly state your reasons for applying for a position with this particular employer. The more specific the reasons, the better the impression you are likely to make.

Briefly highlight your qualifications for the position. This should not be a simple recitation of what is in your resumé, but should either present the information in a slightly different light or add pertinent detail that is not in the resumé. If you are responding to an advertisement, you should respond to each of the qualifications listed in the advertisement. You might include personal qualities that would make you an effective employee in the position. You should relate your skills and abilities to the needs of this particular agency. If your health care experience is limited, you should point out skills you have gained from other jobs that would be useful in nursing. These might be interpersonal skills, management skills, adaptability or other such skills.

In the final paragraph, make a summary statement indicating why you want to work for this employer and ask for an appointment for an interview. Be sure to indicate the times you can be available and how and where you can be contacted if the employer so wishes. It is also wise to indicate that you will contact the person to whom the letter is addressed to request an appointment. This allows you to maintain some initiative in the process. Thank the person for considering your application, and close.

Another point to remember is that the letter's appearance as well as its content rep-

DISPLAY 11-1
Sample Letter of Application

Margery Hoskins
1625 13th Ave. N.E.
Seattle, WA 98105

June 8, 1998

[Individual's Name]
[Health Care Agency Name]
[Street Address]
[City, State/Province Zip/Postal]

Dear [Individual's Name]:

    I am interested in working as a *Registered Nurse* in your perioperative department. I am a *skilled operating room technician* with over *10* years of experience to offer you. I have now completed my associate degree in nursing. I will take my NCLEX examination on June 10 and expect to have my license by July 1. I enclose my resume as a first step in exploring the possibilities of employment with [name of agency].

    My most recent experience was working for an orthopedic surgeon. I was responsible for *assuring that the operating room was set up to facilitate his effective function, acting as scrub technician, and providing some surgical assistance.* In addition, *I worked collaboratively with the operating room staff and perioperative nurses.*

    As a *Registered Nurse* with your organization, I would bring a *focus on quality and effective problem solving.* Furthermore, I work well with others and recognize the value of team work.

    I will call you in a few days to arrange an interview at a convenient time for you. If you wish to contact me, I can be reached at the telephone number listed on my resume. Thank you for your consideration.

Sincerely,

Margery Hoskins

Margery Hoskins

---

resents you. You will be judged on spelling, grammar, clarity, and neatness as well as on the letter's content. Your letter of application should be written in standard business form on plain white or off-white business paper. Make it brief and clear. Ask a friend or family member to check your first draft if you have any questions about its correctness.

The Resumé

A resumé is a brief overview of your qualifications for a position (Display 11-2). Its purpose is to provide the employer with a way to quickly identify whether you have the basic

---

DISPLAY 11-2
Questions to Help You Plan a Resumé

1. What educational institutions have you attended? Dates? Degrees or certificates?
2. What credentials do you have that might be useful in a nursing employment setting?
3. What jobs have you held that you want to highlight? Were any of them health care related?
4. What specific skills did you apply in your workplace that would be transferable to nursing?
5. What skills, abilities, or personal characteristics do you want to draw the employer's attention to?
6. Have you had volunteer or community experiences that demonstrate positive personal attributes?
7. Have you had any awards or recognition that identify your positive abilities or attributes?

---

qualifications for a position, and to present you in the most positive light to be considered for the position in which you are interested. In most instances you will want to include your resumé with your initial letter. In addition, you may leave your resumé with the employer at the end of your interview.

APPEARANCE

The appearance of your resumé is important because it presents your initial image to the prospective employer. You will want its appearance to reflect a competent, professional image. It is not necessary to have a professionally produced resumé. Nursing employers, when asked, have indicated that it neither adds to nor detracts from their impression to read a resumé that has been produced by some professional printing method. The important point is that it be a somewhat formal, standard, informative document that is neat and without errors. In today's business world, a computer-produced resumé is standard (Figs. 11-3 and 11-4).

Your resumé should be on standard-sized ($8\frac{1}{2} \times 11$), white or off-white, good quality paper so that it is easy to handle, file, and read. A resumé that is individually printed (or reproduced well enough so that is appears to be) usually will be more positively received than a carbon copy or a poor-quality photocopy. If you have access to a computer and word processing, you will find it valuable to create a resumé and save it to a disk. In this way, you will be able to easily revise it, and you may even be able to tailor it to an individual job situation. In addition to the capabilities of standard word processing software, there are inexpensive software programs especially designed to facilitate the production of a well-organized and formatted resumé.

To achieve legibility, use wide margins, spacing, indentation, bullets, and numbering to separate different sections and topics. You might want to underline or bold print important items or highlight them with an asterisk or bullet to draw swift attention. When an employer is reviewing many such documents, anything that facilitates review and makes you stand out is an advantage. Ask someone to review the appearance of your resumé and identify those areas that first caught their attention. This helps you to evaluate its appearance.

JAMES R. GOMEZ

1298 Avenida Diaz. • LaQuinta, CA 92253 • Telephone (619) 524-4321 (H)

OBJECTIVE

A beginning REGISTERED NURSE position that will provide the opportunity for professional development and delivery of quality nursing care.

SKILLS

- Work effectively in a multicultural environment.
- Bilingual Spanish/English
- Strong work ethic and experience in working multiple shifts/floating positions.

EDUCATION

COLLEGE OF THE DESERT, PALM DESERT, CA
Associate in Science, June 1995

EXPERIENCE

MANOR CARE CENTER, PALM DESERT, CA
Nursing Assistant, Certified: 1992-Present

MAINTAINED FUNCTION AND DIGNITY OF DEPENDENT ELDERLY ADULTS BY PROVIDING DIRECT CARE, STRONG INTERPERSONAL RELATIONSHIPS, AND EFFECTIVE COLLABORATION WITH NURSING AND ALLIED HEALTH.

NORTHRUP CORPORATION, LOS ANGELES, CA
Machinist: 1982–1992

DIRECTED TEAM IN MEETING TIME AND QUALITY STANDARDS FOR TECHNICAL EQUIPMENT PRODUCTION.

AWARDS

Golden Acorn Award
Cactus Valley Elementary School PTA, LaQuinta, CA

FIGURE 11-3
Resumé of a recent graduate: Example A.

CONTENT

The content of your resumé is critical. It always begins with your name, address, and telephone number (including area code). If you will be moving, indicate the date the move will be effective and provide an alternate method of contacting you after that date. A permanently settled relative or friend who would be willing to forward your mail would be appropriate. Employers are not permitted to ask about age, marital status, and dependents, and you do not need to include this information.

Objective. You should include a personal goal or objective. This may include both a short-term goal such as ''employment as a registered nurse on a general medical unit'' and a longer-term goal such as ''with eventual move to employment in coronary care.'' Be sure

---

WILMA G. EVANS

1625 15th Ave. N.E. • Seattle, WA 98105

RESUMÉ OBJECTIVE
To obtain a position as a REGISTERED NURSE in a perioperative setting where the emphasis is quality care and patient/customer satisfaction.

PROFESSIONAL EXPERIENCE

Dr. Jason Hoeksler	**1989–Present**
Orthopedic surgeon	Surgical Technician: Orthopedic Surgical Technician and
Seattle, WA	Assistant
Seattle Medical Center	**1985–Present**
Seattle, WA	Surgical Technician: General Surgery

SKILLS
- Experienced in perioperative care and management.
- Skilled in all orthopedic procedures.
- Effective manager of equipment and time for fiscal responsibility.
- Team work focused.

EDUCATION

Shoreline Community College	A.A.A.S. in Nursing
Seattle, WA	June, 1996
Seattle Central Community College	Surgical Technician Certificate
Seattle, WA	June, 1985

AWARDS/COMMUNITY SERVICE

Margaret Mallett Memorial Scholarship	1994
Employee of the Year Seattle Medical Center	1988

REFERENCES AVAILABLE

(555) 555-5939
email
mhoskins@scc.edu

FIGURE 11-4
Resumé of a recent graduate: Example B.

that your goal is realistic and does not imply that you are not really interested in a beginning level position. If you state that your goal is to work in an emergency room and you do not have the experience for this kind of position, your application usually will be discarded. If you state that you want to work in maternity nursing and the only position available is in medical–surgical nursing, you may not be considered for the medical–surgical position that you would have accepted although it was not your first choice.

Credentials. You will want to include information regarding your licensure and other credentials. Indicate the date your license will be effective and whether you have a temporary permit to work as a nurse. Indicate when you expect to take your licensing examination and have a license. Your nursing license or permit number should be listed after you have it. If you do not yet have a license, you may choose to put information about when you expect to have your license in your letter of application.

Employment History. Work experience is of critical importance, and you should provide a meaningful employment history. If using a traditional format, for each job you held include address, dates employed, position, and duties. The prospective employer would be especially interested in a previous nursing assistant position or any other position that demonstrates your knowledge of or experience in some area of health care or the assumption of responsibility. Other positions may also be important if you are able to clearly identify skills used in those settings that are transferable to nursing.

If you have had only one or two part-time jobs during your educational program, it would be appropriate to include them in detail. However, if during your educational program you held 15 part-time jobs, it is appropriate to list significant ones that offered valuable experience. In one line write, ''Various part-time jobs to finance schooling: clerk and waitress. Individual names provided on request.'' Include the overall dates for this period.

You may choose a more skill-focused resumé and not include details of all your previous positions. For individuals who are older and have an extensive employment history, a resumé focused on skills and types of positions rather than a chronological list of employers is often the most effective. In order to keep your resumé on one page, you should consider how you can most effectively present employment history. In a skill-focused resumé you can emphasize the responsibilities you have had within positions rather than each specific position. Be sure to include language proficiency if you are fluent in more than English. Computer literacy also may be a valuable skill.

Regardless of the organizational format, we suggest that you focus on accomplishments and use active verbs to describe skills. Words such as supervised, designed, managed, developed, analyzed, coordinated, documented, planned, delegated, created, completed, and operated give life to your resumé and create interest in the reader. See the accompanying display for a list of active verbs you might use (Display 11-3).

Education. Educational background should form another section and cover your nursing education and any specialized courses or postgraduate work you have done. It is appropriate to note any college-level work. Do not include high school information unless you entered your nursing program directly from high school. Then you might indicate your high school and graduation date on one line of your educational information.

In each group of information, list the most recent items first. The most common approach is to group information in the categories just mentioned. See Figures 11-3 and 11-4 for examples of this type of resumé.

If you had educational experiences in an area that especially relates to the position for which you are applying, you might individualize your resumé by briefly identifying these special experiences. For example, you might have had a senior leadership practicum on an orthopedic unit—this would be particularly relevant to an application for a nursing position in orthopedics. If you had a practicum in the facility or agency to which you are applying, indicate this in some way. Your familiarity with their policies and procedures would be a valuable asset. If you attended any special workshops, include those in a separate section.

Additional Experience. Volunteer or community work and awards and honors form two sections when you have these experiences. You might also want to add a section for special

DISPLAY 11-3
Power Verbs for Resumés

- Use of verbs without subjects will be more concise and space conserving.
- Use of words such as ''advanced to'' rather than ''promoted to,'' ''earned'' rather than ''was given'' indicates a person who does things rather than received them.
- Use of ''-ed'' or ''-ing'' as verb endings can both be effective.

accompanied	displayed	inspired	planned
achieved	directed	installed	prepared
acquired	doubled	instructed	presided
activated		insured	procured
administered	earned	integrated	produced
advanced to	educated	intensified	progressed
advised	employed	interviewed	promoted
analyzed	enacted	invented	prompted
arranged	encouraged		proposed
assembled	engineered	keynoted	proved
assisted	established	led licensed	provided
	evaluated	located	
built	executed		reconciled
	exhibited	maintained	reduced
clarified	expanded	managed	regulated
commanded	experienced	manufactured	related
composed		marketed	reorganized
conceived	facilitated	mastered	reported
concluded	formed	mediated	researched
conducted	financed	motivated	satisfied
constructed	formalized		secured
consulted	formulated	negotiated	served
contrived	founded	nominated	serviced
controlled			simplified
converted	generated	obtained	solved
coordinated	governed	officiated	sparked
correlated	graduated	operated	structured
corroborated		ordered	succeeded
created	headed	organized	
		originated	trained
decided	implemented	overcame	transferred
delegated	improved		transformed
demonstrated	improvised	participated	
designed	increased	perceived	unified
detailed	induced	perfected	verified
determined	influenced	performed	
developed	initiated	piloted	won
devised	innovated	pioneered	wrote
discovered		placed	

skills such as computer familiarity or experience with special types of equipment. Choose the items you list under volunteer and community work carefully. If you are 40 years old, the fact that you were student body president in high school would probably be considered irrelevant. However, if you went from high school directly into a nursing program, this information could be important in demonstrating your leadership ability. Your participation in any community organizations, such as the Parent Teacher Association, and service in any leadership roles might also be significant to an employer.

In some instances you may want to list briefly the skills or abilities gained from a particular volunteer activity. For example, if you worked as a volunteer for a Planned Parenthood clinic, you might specify that your duties included individual client counseling in relation to family planning methods. Simply stating that you were a volunteer might not communicate the level of responsibility you assumed. This is an area that you might want to individualize to target the particular skills you think are important to the position for which you are applying.

List awards, honors, and professional associations (such as NSNA) that would demonstrate your competence or leadership ability. You may omit this section if you feel that you have nothing pertinent to enter.

Personal References. References are typed on a separate page and given to the prospective employer if they are requested or copied onto an application form. Be selective in choosing the people you will list as references. Consider the people who know you and would be able to speak positively of you to a future employer, and who would have credibility with the employer.

A primary reference should be an instructor or supervisor from your basic educational program. This person would be able to affirm your ability in the nursing field. Some agencies request two instructor references, so be prepared for that. Another reference should be someone who has employed you and who can describe your work habits and effectiveness as an employee. If you have had any health care work experience, this would be the best work reference. Also look at the position in which you assumed the most responsibility. This should be reasonably recent (within the last 10 years). Again, some employers ask for two work references. You should have available as one reference someone who has known you personally for a relatively long time and who could attest to your ability to relate with others and to such attributes as personal integrity. Not all employers are interested in personal references, but some are. Include full names with titles (if any), addresses, and telephone numbers so that the employer will be able to contact the references easily.

Seek the person's permission before giving an individual's name as a reference. When seeking permission to use someone as a work reference, you might outline what you would like the person to emphasize if contacted—for example: ''If you are contacted, I would particularly like you to provide information about my work habits and effectiveness as an employee.''

Differences of opinion are expressed by employers about the value of a standardized letter of reference addressed ''To Whom It May Concern.'' This may be considered a useful initial presentation of your qualifications by some employers. Other employers want the reference to specifically address their position needs or the qualifications outlined on a reference form. One advantage of the general letter is that you might be able to obtain this reference from a part-time faculty member or supervisor who may no longer be employed by the institution. If you do obtain this type of letter, be sure to carefully preserve the original (perhaps in a clear, plastic sleeve) to show to a potential employer; you would then provide a good quality photocopy for the employer to place in your file. Even when an employer accepts this as an initial reference, your references will most probably be personally contacted as well.

The Interview

The interview should be a two-way conversation in which you will be gaining as well as giving information. Think through the situation before going to the interview and outline information that you want to obtain and questions that you want answered. Writing out your questions so that they are clearly stated, and so that you do not forget items in the tense atmosphere that often exists in an interview situation, is advantageous.

Time spent reflecting on your personal views in advance will be valuable during the interview. Remember that an interview is a chance to sell yourself to an employer, a chance to present yourself as a valuable addition to their nursing staff, and an opportunity to determine how you will fit into that work setting.

When planning for an employment interview, consider your appearance, your attitude and approach, and what the content of the interview will be. Your personal appearance is likely to evoke some type of response from the interviewer. Consider what you would like that response to be and dress appropriately. This means that what you wear when applying for one type of job might be inappropriate when applying for another type of job. For example, if you were applying for a position at a hospital, you would wear businesslike clothing, such as dress pants and shirt, or a suit or dress. Being neat and well-groomed contributes to a businesslike atmosphere. If you were applying for a position in a walk-in health care clinic that offered services to persons who are uncomfortable in a traditional environment, it might be appropriate to wear the casual clothing worn by the workers at the clinic. You need to make a conscious decision about the impression you want to create. Although some may wish that appearances had no effect on the opinions of others, remember that, in reality, appearance often does make a significant difference.

Take a copy of your resumé with you to the interview. In addition, be prepared with the names, addresses, and telephone numbers of all references, and your Social Security number. Take along a black pen to fill out any forms, and a note pad with your questions listed and a place to make personal notes of important information obtained during the interview. This can increase your self-confidence if you have forms to fill out or if questions about statements on your resumé arise during the interview.

Plan to arrive at an interview early. This gives you time to check your appearance and focus your thoughts. When you arrive at an interview, be sensitive to the problems and concerns of the interviewer. If it is apparent that unplanned events are demanding the interviewer's attention, state that you are aware of the difficulty and ask whether it would be more convenient if you made another appointment. Your sensitivity to the interviewer's cues are evidence of your sensitivity to clients' cues.

Your manner in the interview is also important. Although the employer expects an applicant to be nervous, he or she will be interested in whether your nervousness makes you unable to respond appropriately. Follow common rules of courtesy. Wait to be asked to sit down before you take a chair. Avoid any distracting mannerisms, such as chewing gum or fussing with your hair, face, or clothes. Be serious when appropriate, but do not forget to smile and be pleasant. The interviewer is also thinking of your impact on clients, visitors, and other staff members.

When you prepare your responses, try to anticipate possible questions from the interviewer. In order to do this you must know the role of the person interviewing. In large agencies, your first interview might be with a human resources department employee, not a nursing employee; if you are successful at this stage, you might be recommended for an interview in the nursing department.

Role-playing an interview situation with a friend or relative may help you to feel more confident in your responses. Another technique is to visualize the interview situation in your mind and mentally rehearse responses to questions. Some interviewers focus on asking questions about your past experiences and your future plans. Others focus their questions on specific accomplishments and problems encountered in your past nursing experiences. Presenting hypothetical problems for you to consider, and asking you to provide appropriate nursing responses is common. See Display 11-4 for a list of questions you might reflect on as you prepare.

In most instances, be sure to answer questions that are asked rather than skirting them. However, if the interviewer asks a question that is illegal, such as a question regarding age or marital status, you might want to redirect the question to address what appears to be the concern of the interviewer. For example, in response to a question about your age you might say ''Perhaps you believe that I appear to be young and inexperienced. I want to assure you that I have demonstrated my maturity and responsibility both in my nursing education and in my position with (name of employer).'' In response to a question about marital status or children, you could reply ''Perhaps you are concerned about how long I plan to stay in my first position? I want to assure you that whatever my personal situation, professionally, I am looking for a position in an organization where I can be a long-term employee and plan for advancement within the organization.'' Avoid simple yes or no answers, but try to describe or explain in order to give a more complete picture of yourself.

An interview usually covers a wide variety of subjects. The interviewer may direct the flow of topics or may encourage you to bring up the ones that concern you. Applicants who focus initial attention on the issues of wages and benefits may be viewed as more concerned about themselves than about nursing. Therefore, if you are asked to present questions, ask professional questions first. Make sure your questions are appropriate for the interviewer. In the human resources department, you might ask about the overall mission and philosophy of organization, its organizational structure, and how authority and accountability are determined. With a nursing interviewer, demonstrate that you are concerned about how nursing care is given and by whom, where responsibility and authority for nursing care decisions lie, the philosophy underlying care, the availability of continuing education, and where you would be expected to fit into their overall picture. However, before you leave be sure to cover such topics as hours, schedules, pay scales, and benefits.

Some interviews are conducted by a group of interviewers. This might include a person from nursing administration, a unit manager, and a staff development nurse. For an applicant to sit across the table from three to five individuals can be unnerving. You will need to look around the group, being sure to make eye contact with each individual. Make sure that you understand the role of each of the people present. You might actually write down individual names and roles on your notepad and then go back over your list to be sure you

DISPLAY 11-4
Questions to Help You Prepare for a Job Interview

NURSING PHILOSOPHY AND BELIEFS

- What is your philosophy of nursing?
- Is there a nursing theorist that you use as a basis for your nursing practice?
- What do you believe is the most central concept to support excellence in nursing?

PERSONAL GOALS AND PLANNING

- Where do you see yourself in 1 year? 5 years? 10 years?
- Have you developed any professional goals? If so, would you share those with me?
- Why do you want to work here?
- What plans do you have for continuing education in nursing?
- What do you see as your weakest area in nursing?
- What do you see as your strengths in nursing?

YOUR EXPERIENCES

- What experience in your nursing education did you find the most rewarding? Why?
- What experience in your nursing education did you like the least? Why?
- In what kind of settings did you have an opportunity to work as a nursing student?
- What other job experiences have you had? What skill did you develop there that will be useful in nursing?

PROBLEM SOLVING

- Identify a problem in patient care that you encountered as a student and explain how you solved that problem.
- Describe a difficult patient with whom you worked. Include why you found that patient difficult and how you managed the situation.
- Identify a situation in which you were involved in a conflict and describe how you handled that situation. If you had it to do over again, what would you do differently?
- Explain how you would use the nursing process in patient care.
- A problem may be presented to you for your solution. Plan ahead to approach it in a systematic manner.

TECHNICAL SKILLS

- What technical nursing skills do you feel comfortable performing?
- What skills will you require assistance with?
- What do you do when you encounter a technical skill you have not performed before?

THE EMPLOYMENT SETTING

- In what type of unit do you wish to work?
- Why do you want to work here?
- Why do you think we should hire you for this position?

have them correct. This would allow you to direct a question to a specific individual or to use an individual's name when replying to a question. While replying to the person who asks the question, you might also glance at others as you make your point. Be sure that you do not ignore any individual even if one of the interviewers does not seem to ask questions or to be as active in the process as the others. Interviews of this type are often longer than interviews with one person.

Some interviewers are less skilled than others; in these situations the questions may seem less focused and more vague. You may sometimes feel at a loss as to exactly what is being asked. Before proceeding you should seek clarification, but be careful that your manner of asking for clarification does not offend the interviewer. You might ask ''Could you give me an example of the type of situation you were thinking about?'' Another clarifying approach is for you to state clearly what you perceive to be the central question before continuing, ''Let me clarify. You would like me to identify a situation in which I believe I responded effectively to a problem. Is that correct?'' In this situation you may have to take the initiative to be sure that you have an opportunity to present your strengths and skills.

If you are unfamiliar with the interview process, you might benefit from reading several books on the topic. Reading several different books will give you a variety of viewpoints and might provide you with strategies that are comfortable for you.

Follow-up Strategies

Your initial inquiry should always be followed-up. If you were granted an interview, you would follow-up with a letter as described below. If you did not obtain an interview, you should continue to contact the potential employer at intervals in order to learn of other job opportunities and to indicate that you are still seeking a position. When a new position opens, employers do not necessarily go back through previous employment files. They are more likely to interview a person who appears to be currently searching for a position than one who was searching several months previously.

After your interview, you should write a brief thank-you letter to the person who interviewed you. If a group interviewed you, direct the letter to the person who seemed to be in charge. In that letter, thank the individual for the time and attention to your questions and concerns. Restate any agreement you feel was reached. For example, ''I understand that I am to call your office next week to learn whether I have been scheduled for an interview with the maternity unit manager.'' Close your letter with a positive comment about the organization. Even if you are not offered a job or do not choose to work at that facility, you are leaving a positive impression. You can never tell when that will be important to you in the future (Display 11-5).

Do not let this letter be your last contact with that potential employer. Call back as agreed. Even if you do not get a position at this time, you might ask that your application be kept on file because you are still interested in employment with that particular agency. Then continue to call back every two or three weeks to find out if any other positions are available.

Managing a job search is often enhanced by setting up your own record-keeping system. You should have a record of when you contacted an agency, in what manner (letter or telephone call), interviews—including the interviewer's name and the content of the inter-

DISPLAY 11-5
Sample Interview Follow-up Letter

3496 Maple Lane
Sioux City, IA 51103

June 15, 1998

Margery Morris RN
1980 Stone Blvd.
Sioux City, IA 51103

Dear Ms. Morris:

Thank you very much for the time you spent with me in an interview for a Registered Nurse position at St. Luke's Medical Center. I understand that at this time you are unsure of whether you will conduct a new graduate nurse orientation in July. I appreciate your willingness to keep my application on file and notify me at the time you determine your needs. You indicated that I would need to be interviewed by a unit manager for a specific position before being offered employment.

My tour of your facility convinced me that I would be proud to be a member of the St. Luke's staff. The obviously positive morale and the emphasis on continuing education that I saw demonstrated that this is a place where one can grow and develop.

As you directed, I will call your office in four weeks to ascertain the status of my file.

Sincerely,

Constance M. Nichols
Constance M. Nichols

view, and dates and times of any follow-up letters or calls. Have a place to record your own notes or impressions. This will enable you to keep track of details when you manage an extensive job search. By keeping this type of record you will not forget to call an agency to recheck on job availability, or mistakenly send an inquiry letter and resumé twice to the same agency.

Managing A Prolonged Job Search

With the changes in health care, new graduates are sometimes faced with a prolonged job search. Some of the concerns that arise when this happens include: ''What am I doing wrong?'' ''Should I work in health care in another role?'' ''Should I accept a job that I do not feel prepared for?'' ''What happens if my skills get out-of-date?''

Evaluating your own job search strategies and the documents you are producing (your letters and resumé) is critical. You might ask for assistance from a career counselor, from a personal resource, or from friends and family. You might practice your telephone skills and role-play some interview situations. You will want to make sure that you are presenting your very best self to potential employers.

In regard to health care employment, you need to know what the recommendations and opinion of your Board of Nursing are regarding this type of situation. Once you have a registered nurse license, the law usually requires that you function within the expectations of that license in regard to the public. This is true in volunteer or paid work. In many states, the Board has given the opinion that it does not matter what your job title or salary is—if you are a registered nurse you are held to that standard of practice in order to assure the safety of the public. If you take a position as a nursing assistant and are a registered nurse, you could be placed in a no-win situation. The licensing board might hold you to a standard of practice that is closed to you by the employer. This might not become apparent until a problem occurred and you did not respond as a registered nurse, but rather as a nursing assistant.

In order to maintain your knowledge and skills while involved in a prolonged job search, you should plan to attend continuing education events, read journals, and perhaps complete the examinations provided in journal articles to provide yourself with continuing education credits.

You might look for a part-time position in order to work while you continue to search for a full-time position. This would help you to keep skills you have and to grow in proficiency. The experience will also assist you in being a more effective candidate for a full-time position. Volunteer work with any number of agencies might be an avenue for you to maintain and enhance skills and provide further support for obtaining a position. This might be tailored to fit the times available to you while you maintain a non-nursing job in order to continue some type of income.

Do you need to broaden your ideas of what kind of position you will seek and accept? Have you narrowed your search too greatly? Research more extensively the positions available in your community as described above. Consider whether geographic mobility is an option for you. Based on this review, target those types of agencies where positions are more likely to arise. Focus your continuing education and volunteer efforts toward those areas most likely to yield job openings. This might make you a better candidate.

Above all, you will need to maintain a positive attitude and avoid discouragement. Negative attitudes are often translated into your contacts with potential employers and do not present you as a desirable employee. You might form a support group with others who are seeking employment in order to maintain your perspective and give you a forum in which to discuss your feelings.

Resignation

When you decide to leave a nursing position, it is important that you provide the employer with an appropriate amount of time to seek a replacement. The more responsible your position, the more time the employer will need. For a staff nursing position, you should strive to provide a month's notice unless an urgent matter requires that less notice be given. Notice of resignation should be in a letter that is directed to the head of your department, often to the Director of Nursing. Copies should be sent to other supervisory people, such as the head nurse and the supervisor.

The letter of resignation is important in concluding your relationship with the employer on a cordial and positive basis. The feelings left behind when you resign will influence letters of recommendation and future opportunities for employment with that agency. Give a reason for your resignation as well as the exact date when it will be effective. If you have accrued vacation or holiday time and want to take the time off or be paid for it, clearly state that. Comment about positive factors in the employment setting and acknowledge those who have provided special support or assistance in your growth.

If you are resigning because of problems in the work setting and want to note them, do so in a clear, factual, unemotional way. Avoid attacking anyone personally and do not make broad, sweeping negative comments. Try to make the letter a clear and reasonable statement of your position as a professional (Display 11-6).

DISPLAY 11-6
Sample Letter of Resignation

Michael M. Phinney
4210 Center Ave.
Riverdale, IL 60627

June 15, 1998

Ms. Monica Jackson, Director of Nursing
Thornton Medical Center
16630 So. State
Riverdale, IL 60627

Dear Ms. Jackson:

It is with some regret that I notify you of my intent to resign effective August 15, 1998. As you are aware, I have been planning to return to school and continue my education. I have been accepted at the University of Illinois and will be beginning classes this fall.

Although returning to school means that I can move forward in my career, I recognize that this agency has provided me with a firm foundation for the future. The support of the experienced staff, the atmosphere that has encouraged me to develop increased skill, and the friendships I developed here have all contributed to my professional growth.

I wish to thank you and all of the staff for the excellence of the experience I gained here.

Sincerely,

Michael M Phinney

Michael M. Phinney

c: Jennifer Watson RN, Unit Manager 3 West

PROBLEMS EXPERIENCED BY NURSES IN THE WORKPLACE

For many of you, graduating from a nursing program and becoming a registered nurse is the realization of a long-cherished goal. You have spent years preparing for this status and now it is here! What you have viewed as an ideal state, freed from financial pressures that you felt as a student, liberated from the tyranny of the examination, may prove to be quite different from what you had expected. Let us consider some of the problems that may occur as you make this transition from student to professional.

Moving From "Novice to Expert"

The path from novice to expert is a challenging one. Benner's (1984) work in this area has provided a basis for understanding and research into this process. She related this path to the Dreyfus Model of Skill Acquisition (Dreyfus & Dreyfus, 1980) in which the individual moves from novice, to advanced beginner, to competent, to proficient, to expert. Throughout this progression she identified exemplars of nurses performing in six different roles:

1. The helping role
2. The teaching–coaching function
3. The diagnostic and monitoring function
4. Effective management of rapidly changing situations
5. Administering and monitoring therapeutic interventions and regimens
6. Monitoring and ensuring the quality of health care practices and organizational and work-role competencies.

Through interviews with nurses she described the depth of nursing skills and abilities found in the expert nurse. This expertise is forged over time and results from personal experience and personal knowing. One of the challenges for beginning nurses is pressure to function as an expert without this background of growth.

Reality Shock

One problem confronted by the new graduate is the seeming impossibility of delivering quality care within the constraints of the system as it exists. You may feel powerless to effect any changes and may be depressed over your lack of effectiveness in the situation.

Marlene Kramer was the first to call the feelings that result from such a situation *reality shock* (Kramer, 1979). She noted that the new graduate often experiences considerable psychological stress and that this may exacerbate the problem. The person undergoing such stress is less able to perceive the entire situation and to solve problems effectively (Fig. 11-5).

CAUSES OF REALITY SHOCK

With all of the uncertain expectations and demands, the new graduate often feels caught in the middle. As a student, you may think that you are expected to learn a tremendous amount in an alarmingly short time. The expectations may seem high and in some ways unrealistic.

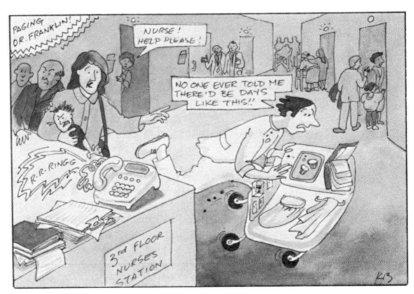

FIGURE 11-5
Some new graduates are disillusioned by the working conditions that they find on their first job.

Then, as a new graduate suddenly thrust into the real world, you may feel insecure and think that your educational program did not adequately prepare you for what is expected of you. On one hand you are expected to function like a nurse who has had 10 years of experience, but on the other hand your new ideas may not be considered because you have so little experience. You may become frustrated because you do not have time to provide the same type of care you gave as a student. For example, you may not have adequate time to deal with a client's psychosocial problems or teaching needs.

As a student, you are taught that the "good nurse" never gives a medication without understanding its actions and side effects, and that evaluating the effectiveness of the drug is essential. As a staff nurse, you may find that the priority is getting the medications passed correctly and on time and that there is little or no time to look up 15 new drugs. As for evaluation, that becomes a dream. How can you evaluate the subtle effects of a medication in the 2 minutes spent passing the medication to a client you do not know? The individually and meticulously planned care that was so important to you as a student may become a luxury when you are a graduate. Often the focus is on accomplishing the required tasks in the time allotted, and it is efficiency in tasks that may earn praise from a supervisor.

Bradby (1990) suggests that reality shock is part of the passage from novice to experienced nurse. She suggests that it be treated as a normal transitional process with a focus on the growth that can occur.

EFFECTS OF REALITY SHOCK

When reality shock occurs, some nurses become disillusioned and leave nursing altogether. Others begin to "job hop" or return to school, searching for the perfect place to practice perfect nursing as it was learned. Some push themselves to the limit, trying to provide ideal care and criticizing the system. This may result in their being labeled nonconformists and troublemakers. Still others give up their values and standards for care and reject ideals as impossibly unrealistic expectations that cannot be fulfilled in the real world. These persons simply mesh with the current framework and become part of the system.

FINDING SOLUTIONS FOR REALITY SHOCK

There is an alternative to these nonproductive coping methods. It is possible to create a role for yourself that blends the ideal with the possible—one in which you do not give up ideals, but see them as goals toward which you will move, however slowly. To do this you need to be realistically prepared for the demands of the real world.

One way of meeting the challenge is to assess yourself as you approach the end of your educational program. Consider what your competencies are. Think about the eight areas of expectation that were discussed earlier in the chapter:

1. Theoretical knowledge for safe practice
2. Use of the nursing process
3. Self-awareness
4. Communication skill
5. Record-keeping
6. Work ethic
7. Skill proficiency
8. Speed of functioning

Second, gain information about what the employers in your community expect from new graduates. This can be done by talking with experienced nurses, requesting interviews with nursing administrators, meeting with faculty, and contacting recent graduates who are currently employed. Try to get specific information. If you have a nursing student organization, setting up a forum for speakers from various agencies might be one avenue to gaining this insight.

After you have gathered this information, try to correlate it with a realistic appraisal of your own ability to function in accordance with an employer's expectations. If you identify any shortcomings, the time to try to remedy them is before graduation. If you identify a lack in certain technical skills, you might register for extra time in the nursing practice laboratory to increase your proficiency. You could even time yourself and work to increase speed as well as skill. You might consult with your clinical instructor to arrange for experiences that would help you gain increased competence. If you recognize that you consistently have difficulty functioning within a time frame, you might obtain employment in a hospital or other health care facility while still in school; this will give you more experience in organizing work within the time limits that the employer sees as reasonable.

As you plan for your first job, you can examine the psychological challenges to be met. Understanding that you are not alone in your feelings of frustration is often helpful. It may be useful to form a support group of other new graduates who meet regularly to discuss problems and concerns and seek solutions jointly. You can also gain valuable reinforcement from other nurses in your work setting. Many have successfully dealt with the problems you face and are able to provide support and help. This ''mentor'' relationship is an important one and needs to be cultivated.

When confronted with areas of practice that you would like to see changed, weigh the importance of an issue. Use your energies wisely. The "politics of the possible" is important to you. Learn how the system in which you are employed functions and how to use that system for effective change. You, as a person, are important to nursing, so it is important that you neither burn yourself out nor abandon the quest for higher-quality nursing care; you should be able to continue to work toward improving nursing and bringing it closer to its ideals.

Some hospitals attempt to help new graduates deal with reality shock by making orientation programs more comprehensive and by providing an experienced nurse to work as a preceptor to the new graduate. Nurse internships or residencies in some settings have been created to provide a planned and organized transition time during which the new graduate participates in a formal program, including classes, seminars, and rotations to various units of the hospital. Unfortunately, restructuring in many health care agencies has greatly limited orientation time and decreased the support available to the new graduate. The new graduate is required to be more self-directed in identifying needs and the ways that those might be met within the constraints of the system.

Some hospitals provide an opportunity for nursing students to work during the summer before the last year of their basic program to become familiar with the hospital and the nursing role. In this type of program the nursing student may be employed as a nursing assistant, but participate in a planned program that introduces the role of the registered nurse. In other instances, nursing students work as nursing assistants and the orientation to the nursing role in the agency depends upon the initiative the individual takes. You may wish to inquire whether hospitals in your area have developed any of these or other programs to assist you when you are a new graduate.

Burnout

Burnout is a form of chronic stress related to one's job. This problem arises after you have been in practice for a period of time. It can be identified by feelings of hopelessness and powerlessness, and accompanied by a decreased ability to function both on the job and in personal life. Burnout primarily occurs in nurses who work in particularly stressful areas of nursing, such as critical care, oncology, or burn units. It also occurs in other areas when staffing is inadequate or interpersonal relationships are strained. The downsizing of nursing staff and the rapid changes in the health care environment have contributed to burnout in some settings.

SYMPTOMS OF BURNOUT

Symptoms of burnout include both physical changes and psychological distress. Exhaustion and fatigue, frequent colds, headaches, backaches, and insomnia all may occur. There may be changes in disposition, such as being quick to anger or exhibiting all feelings excessively. As burnout progresses, ability to solve problems and make decisions decreases. This frequently results in an unwillingness to face change and a tendency to block new ideas. There may be feelings of guilt, anger, and depression because one cannot meet the expectations for doing a "perfect job."

In response to these feelings, some nurses quit their jobs and move on to other settings.

These other settings may not even be in nursing. Others remain in their jobs, but develop a personal shell that tends to separate them from real contact with clients and coworkers; they may become cynical about the possibility of anyone doing a good job and may function at a minimal level. A few become more and more unable to function and find themselves in jeopardy of losing their positions.

CAUSES OF BURNOUT

Many causes of burnout have been discussed in the literature. Prominent among them is the conflict between ideals and reality. Just as this is a problem for the new graduate, it is also a problem for the experienced nurse. In trying to achieve the ideal, the nurse drives harder and harder and becomes critical of the environment and of himself or herself. Nurses see themselves as being responsible for all things to all people and often take on more and more responsibility, thus increasing their own stress level.

Another cause of burnout is the high level of stress that results from practicing nursing in areas that have high mortality rates. Continually investing oneself in clients who die can take a tremendous toll on personal resources. In addition, the demand is constant for optimal functioning.

Inadequately staffed institutions may also place great stress on nurses. The clients are in need of care, the nurse has the skills to provide the care, and yet the clients do not receive good care. The nurse typically tries to accomplish more, staying overtime, skipping breaks and lunch, and running throughout the shift. Despite this effort, there is little job satisfaction because the things that are left undone or that are not done well seem to be more apparent than all the good that is accomplished.

PREVENTING BURNOUT

Burnout can best be prevented by mounting a stress-reduction effort involving the nursing staff, supervisory personnel, the hospital administration, and other health care workers. The most important objective seems to be bringing burnout into the open and acknowledging the existence of the problems. This alone helps the individual nurse move away from the feelings of separation and alienation that often accompany burnout. Whatever the problems, they seem less frightening if they are defined as ''normal'' and if the individual nurse does not see himself or herself as the only person not performing as the ''perfect nurse.''

A second step is to provide for group discussions during which nurses can share feelings and specific concerns in an accepting atmosphere. This sharing may lead to concrete plans to reduce the stress created by the setting. For example, if one source of stress is conflicting orders between two sets of physicians involved in care, a plan might be developed whereby the nurses no longer take responsibility for the conflict, but refer the problem to some authority within the medical hierarchy. This type of resolution is possible only when the problem of burnout is being addressed by the whole health care team. However, it also requires that nurses give up trying to control ''everything.''

Giving nurses more control over their own practice often decreases stress. Assuming more control is limited by the constraints of the setting, but it may involve flexible scheduling, volunteering for specific assignments, and participating in committees that determine policies and procedures.

As an individual nurse, you also can take actions to prevent burnout. These are the same general actions that are designed to control stress in any aspect of life. Paying attention to your own physical health is an important preventive measure; this includes maintaining a balanced program of rest, nutrition, and exercise. Another important point is not to subject yourself to excessive changes over short periods of time, because changes increase stress. You may decide, for example, not to move at the same time you change to a different shift. A period of ''wind down'' or ''decompression'' after work helps you to avoid carrying the stress of the workplace into your private life; this period may involve physical exercise, reading, meditation, or any different activity. The activity you choose should not create more demands and increase stress. An important resource is someone who is willing to listen while you ventilate your feelings and talk about your problems. Sometimes this is a family member or personal friend, but it may be more appropriate for this to be a coworker or counselor.

Rotating out of a high-stress area, such as a burn unit or pediatric oncology, before you become ''burned out'' may allow you to rebuild resources and return to the job with enthusiasm. This can be done only if there is no stigma or blame attached to the need to rotate and if other nurses are available for replacement. In client care areas that are known to be stressful, it is helpful to have a counselor available for nurses. Consulting with this counselor should be viewed by the staff as a positive step and not as an admission of some lack or fault. The counselor needs to be someone who understands the setting and who has the skills to assist people in coping with stress.

Burnout is a serious concern in the nursing profession, but there are strategies for managing it. If you are in a high-stress situation, you need to plan for prevention before you become burned out.

SEX DISCRIMINATION IN NURSING

The three major areas in which there is concern about sex discrimination in nursing are the issues of comparable worth, discrimination against men in nursing, and sexual harassment.

Comparable Worth

Nursing has been, and still is, a profession dominated by women. Laws exist in many states that prohibit explicit sex discrimination in salary for a given job. For example, if both men and women are hired by a health care provider as registered nurses, they must be compensated on the same basis. This principle has been expanded to encompass jobs that involve essentially the same work, although the titles may differ. The janitor and the maid may have different titles, but if they have essentially the same tasks, then they must be paid on the same basis. In one case, nurse practitioners (who were primarily women) in an agency argued that they should receive the same compensation as the physician's assistants (who were primarily men) because they performed basically the same tasks. The difference in the salaries was seen by these nurses as a form of sex discrimination.

The next step that many women would like to see accepted is the principle of compensation based on comparable worth. Jobs may be studied and assigned points or rank based on educational requirements, skills required, level of responsibility, and authority.

Those with the same points or rank are considered to be of comparable worth although the actual substance of the work may differ. Alaska has a law barring discrimination in pay for work of comparable character.

Many women believe that different jobs of comparable worth are not compensated equally because of sex discrimination. Most jobs that are found to score high in education requirements, skill, and responsibility, and yet have low salaries, are jobs that historically have been held by women. Nursing is one example of such a job. For example, physicians' assistants are primarily men and nurse practitioners are primarily women. The average salaries for physicians' assistants have tended to be higher than the average salaries for nurse practitioners in many areas. Where different job descriptions exist for these two groups, equity would need to be based upon determining some type of comparable worth. Groups of women have brought suit against employers charging sex discrimination based on failure to provide equal pay for jobs of comparable worth.

Currently, the political climate does not support positive responses to claims of discrimination based on comparable worth; the argument against this premise is that jobs requiring comparable education and skills commonly have different wages based on market forces. When these jobs are held primarily by men or primarily by women, this does not constitute discrimination but simply reflects the realities of the marketplace. This will continue to be an issue in the field of nursing.

Discrimination Against Men

Men in nursing also have expressed concern about sex discrimination. Their concern is not monetary, but is related to being allowed to practice in all areas of nursing and being accepted within the profession. Anti-male sexism in the United States was discussed by Kus (1985), who pointed out that society stereotypes men just as feminists have criticized that it stereotypes women. He makes a strong case for the importance of nurses examining the stereotypes they hold about men. Stereotypes narrow our thinking and interfere with people being able to develop to their fullest potential. It is appropriate for women in nursing to examine their own behavior and identify whether they have been guilty of perpetuating outmoded stereotypes of the nurse and supporting a type of discrimination toward men that they would fight to eliminate for women.

In some facilities or areas men are not allowed to care for women clients, or if they are allowed to care for women, restrictions are placed on them in terms of obtaining consent for care from each client. Those who support the limitations on the practice of men in nursing state that it is a matter of providing for the modesty and privacy of female clients. This position was upheld by a court decision in favor of a hospital that refused to assign a man to a nursing position in labor and delivery (Arkansas judge . . . , 1981). The argument was made that the client did not have free choice of a nurse but rather was assigned a nurse for care, and therefore the restrictions were appropriate.

In an article in the *American Nurse*, Ketter (1994) presents the situations of men who have felt discrimination in the workplace based on their gender. One of these men has filed three complaints with Equal Employment Opportunities Commission (EEOC) regarding discrimination in employment in obstetric/gynecologic settings in the 3 years he has been in nursing. His case is expected to end up in federal court.

Those who oppose limitations on the practice of men in nursing state that, as a professional, a nurse (whether a man or woman) should always consider the privacy and modesty of a client of either gender. This can be done without excluding anyone from providing care in any area. By careful assessment, the nurse can determine the true needs of the client and plan for appropriate avenues to deliver that care. Furthermore, the point has been made that men as physicians have not been excluded from any branch of medicine and this has not created problems. Physicians are not always chosen by the client either. House staff are assigned, referrals are made to specialty physicians, and many group plans designate a physician to provide care. Female nurses care for male clients in all situations. This has been accepted because women are seen in a nurturing, mothering role that the public associates with nursing.

The American Assembly for Men in Nursing (see Appendix B) provides a forum for the concerns of men in nursing and those who are concerned about the problems of sex discrimination. This organization seeks to educate people and opposes any limitations on opportunities available to men.

Sexual Harassment

Sexual harassment has been identified as behavior of a sexual nature that creates a work environment that is perceived as hostile and unduly stressful. Sexual harassment may take the form of comments about an individual's body, persistent unwanted attempts to initiate a personal relationship, the ongoing use of suggestive or obscene language, unwanted touching, or direct sexual advances. Both men and women may be the objects of sexual harassment. Issues of sexual harassment have come into the news in many ways in the last few years. This is an issue that has been a concern in nursing. Because nurses are involved with personal care of individuals of the opposite sex, there is sometimes the unspoken assumption that they will not be offended by sexual comments, jokes, or innuendo.

Harassers in the health care workplace may be clients, coworkers, or physicians. According to Kaye (1996) and Williams (1995), most harassers in the health care workplace are physicians; this follows the general data that shows that sexual harassment is a demonstration of personal power over others. Historically, physicians have had the most power in health care environments. Temper tantrums, verbal abuse, and inappropriate sexual remarks were often tolerated from physicians because other health professionals knew that they did not have the power to change these behaviors. While recognizing the problem, it is important not to stereotype physicians, because the majority of physicians are professional and appropriate in their relationships.

Individuals should take steps to stop sexual harassment by giving clear, direct verbal messages that indicate that the behavior in question is unwanted, unpleasant, and must stop. Sometimes this alone stops inappropriate behaviors. If clear, direct messages are not successful, the individual should then report the matter in writing to an immediate supervisor. Any individual who believes that he or she has been the victim of sexual harassment would be wise to keep records of the behavior and of all attempts to stop the behavior in question. If you belong to a collective bargaining group, that is also a resource to assist you if you believe yourself to be the victim of sexual harassment.

Employers have a legal and ethical responsibility to have clear policies that prohibit sexual harassment, and to provide an appropriate working environment. These policies should be publicized so that everyone is aware of them. The courts support the responsibility of the employer to maintain the work environment free of sexual harassment (Neuhs, 1994; Wolfe, 1996).

WORKPLACE SAFETY AND HEALTH FOR NURSES

Nurses have expressed concern regarding safety in the working environment for many years. Employees have a right to expect their employers to provide the safest working environment possible. Some hospitals employ an occupational health nurse to examine the working environment, and use employment practices to promote health and safety on the job. Nurses themselves, however, often have been lax in recognizing on-the-job hazards and acting for self-protection; this can be likened to the response of those who continue to smoke despite their knowledge of the health hazards of smoking, or those who fail to wear seatbelts even though statistics show fewer fatalities in automobile accidents when seatbelts are worn. Some people continue to do those things that they know are detrimental to their health and well-being. Unfortunately, nurses are no exception (Fig. 11-6).

The Bureau of Labor Statistics tracks and reports data related to occupational hazards. In recent reports they have identified that hospitals have an incidence of work-related illness or injury of 11.8 per 100 full-time workers. Nursing homes are even more hazardous with an incidence of 17.3 per 100 workers. Nurse aides were even more at risk than registered nurses (RNs Facing . . . , 1995). Personal awareness is the first step in attempting to control this growing problem.

Infection as an Occupational Hazard

Transmission of infection is a major concern when caring for infected clients. The presence of resistant organisms causes extra concern and makes treatment difficult. All hospitals have an infection control officer, usually a registered nurse, who has the expertise to guide the staff in planning appropriate infection control procedures. Staff in other settings may not have access to such an expert.

The hidden danger for nurses lies in those clients who have not been diagnosed as having an infection and for whom specific infection control measures have therefore not been prescribed. Universal precautions have been mandated by OSHA for use with all clients in all settings (that is, universally) to protect staff from blood-borne pathogens. These precautions prevent the spread of HIV, hepatitis B, and other such blood-borne pathogens. Nurses who have frequent contact with blood and blood products, and those engaged in intravenous therapy, have a special risk for exposure to hepatitis B. Although a vaccine exists to protect against this disease, the vaccine itself is not without side effects; therefore, a discussion with a physician regarding risks versus benefits for you as an individual is appropriate before undertaking immunization. The Occupational Safety and Health Administration (OSHA) has developed standards that require employers to pay for hepatitis B immunization for those employees with significant exposure to blood and body fluids that can transmit blood-borne organisms.

The acquired immunodeficiency syndrome (AIDS) has created a reevaluation of all approaches to infection control and of health care workers' obligations to provide care for those with communicable diseases. AIDS remains a serious concern for all health care

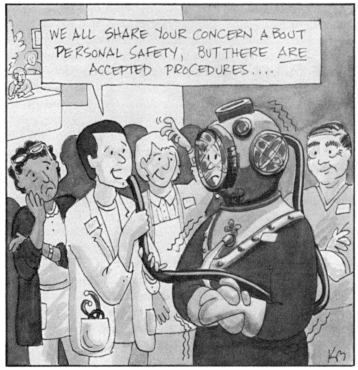

FIGURE 11-6
Personal safety and health in the work environment are important concerns for nurses.

workers. One of the first employer actions toward preventing AIDS and other blood-borne diseases was the provision of ''sharps'' containers wherever needles were used. Another important employer responsibility is the provision of a supply of gloves and protective eyewear for employee use. These measures are mandated by OSHA as part of universal precautions. However, not all cases of transmission of blood-borne pathogens can be prevented by universal precautions. Needle-stick injuries—especially those with large-bore needles (such as bone marrow aspiration needles)—continue to be the most frequent transmission source. These injuries are not prevented by wearing gloves.

More attention is now being given to designing needles and other sharp devices in new ways that provide greater protection. For example, a needle with a protective plastic housing is available for injections. These needles are unlikely to injure an individual even if they are not handled properly. Needleless intravenous connections are also available. Syringes are available that have a protective cover that the needle retracts into immediately after use. These safer devices are more expensive; therefore, some employers have been reluctant to make the change, because they are not required to do so. Nurses have a legitimate interest in requesting that hospitals provide safer equipment; one nurse is launching a nationwide campaign for the use of such equipment (An HIV-infected RN . . . , 1996).

Blood-borne pathogens are not the only pathogens of concern in the health care environment. The new Standard Precautions recommended by the Centers for Disease Control and Prevention (CDC, 1996), often referred to as Body Substance Precautions, are used in many places—but they are not required. These precautions protect clients and staff from infections that might be transmitted by *any* body substance. When these new Standard Precautions were being formulated, OSHA indicated that regulations would likely be changed from the current requirement for Universal Precautions to a requirement for the more extensive Standard Precautions. Because of the anti-regulatory stance of the 103rd Congress, OSHA did not proceed with formulating new regulations. This may occur in the future.

The incidence of tuberculosis is again on the rise, with drug-resistant strains of the organism. Although rooms with special ventilation and special masks that are impervious to the tuberculosis organism are available, individuals may be in contact with health care providers long before they are clearly diagnosed. Should nurses in high-risk areas such as the emergency room wear special masks during all client contact, or is this unrealistic? These are important questions to consider.

Although the details of infection control are beyond the scope of this text, we remind you that you hold the key to protecting yourself in many ways. Often health care workers become lax in their attention to the use of gloves or eye protection because these measures are inconvenient. It is your responsibility to use the very best techniques for self-protection. Nurses must assume responsibility for their own protection through conscientiously carrying out appropriate measures at all times. Employers must be held accountable for providing the supplies and environment to make this possible.

Hazardous Chemical Agents

Anesthetic gases can increase the risk of fetal malformation and spontaneous abortion in pregnant women who are exposed to them on a regular basis. Standards exist for waste-gas retrieval systems and the allowable level of these gases in the air. Nurses working in operating rooms should seek information on the subject and expect that hospitals will provide a safe environment.

Chemotherapeutic agents used in the treatment of cancer are extremely toxic, and nurses who work in settings where such agents are prepared and administered should seek additional education regarding their administration, not only in relation to the client's safety but also in relation to personal safety. The employer is responsible for providing the equipment needed to maintain safety when handling these agents. In many settings, protocols now require the routine use of personal protective equipment when handling chemotherapeutic agents.

Contact with many medications, especially antibiotics, during preparation and administration may cause the nurse to develop sensitivity. This may not only create transitory problems, such as a hand rash, but may also be a threat if treatment for a serious infection is compromised at some later date. Other medications are absorbed through the skin and may produce an undesirable effect. Nurses must take personal responsibility for their own safety in regard to these agents. Nurses who understand these hazards will handle all drugs with discretion and be careful not to expose themselves to these agents.

Cleaning agents and disinfectants used in the hospital may also be hazardous if used improperly. Employers are now required by OSHA to maintain a list of all chemicals used in the work environment, along with information on their possible effects, and the appropriate treatment if individuals are accidentally exposed to them. If you work with these agents, you should seek out this information and be sure that you handle chemicals correctly.

Back Injuries

Because nursing includes providing direct care to incapacitated individuals, back injuries are a common occupational hazard. Back injuries in general are a serious concern because they interfere with the working life of people in their most productive years. Nursing assistants in long-term care facilities have the highest incidence of back injuries. As staff numbers are reduced, remaining staff often feel pressure to move and lift people and equipment without essential assistance. Back injuries then increase (RNs facing . . . , 1995).

Some institutions provide instruction in lifting, transfer, posture, body mechanics, other back-saving strategies to help prevent injury. Mechanical lifting devices provide a means of moving clients without danger to staff. More types of lifting devices are now available and more employers are open to purchasing equipment to prevent these costly injuries. You need to be aware of the potential for back injury and examine your own work habits. Some nurses feel that they must accomplish certain tasks even if the necessary assistance is not available, and therefore carry out actions of danger to themselves. Nurses must learn to be assertive in regard to their own safety.

Violence in the Workplace

Most nursing students think of hospitals as places where victims of violence are helped. Rarely do they think of themselves as victims of violence in their own workplace. According to OSHA, two-thirds of nonfatal workplace assaults happen in health and social services facilities. The majority of these are assaults by clients on nursing staff, and more occur in psychiatric mental health settings than in other settings. Assaults on staff by visitors and outsiders also occur; most of these take place in emergency rooms. In addition to assaults, 18 RNs and 88 other health care workers died in workplace homicides between 1980 and 1990 (Violence is still . . . , 1996).

OSHA has issued guidelines that can be used by facilities trying to establish a safer workplace. These are not enforceable rules, but may represent what is termed the ''General Duty'' clause in the OSHA Act. The guidelines call for clear programs designed to protect workers. These programs would include an assessment and analysis of the workplace for hazards and a plan for prevention of problems. One form of prevention is training employees in the management of hostile and violent behavior. Ways of identifying hostile and assaultive clients should be developed so that staff can be warned to take extra personal safety precautions. Other important environmental safeguards include the use of such devices as metal detectors, panic buttons, and bullet proof glass where appropriate. Adequate staff to manage potentially violent behavior is of particular concern in psychiatric/mental health settings. The addition of security personnel is important in some environments. There should be an attitude throughout the institution of zero tolerance for abusive or assaultive behavior.

In addition to preventing and managing problem situations, there should be clear guidelines for reporting both verbal and physical abuse and following through on all complaints. Health care institutions should work with law enforcement professionals when abusive or assaultive behavior occurs to assure that legal procedures are carried out correctly.

Those who report incidents should receive support and assistance and be assured that there will be no reprisals or blaming. Some nurses have been reluctant to report verbal and physical abuse or assault because of personal and institutional beliefs that health care staff should be able to handle these behaviors independently. Another common belief in health care environments is that all behavior has meaning for the individual and therefore mandates that inappropriate behaviors on the part of clients should be accepted by staff. Social constraints and adverse consequences related to inappropriate behavior are a valuable ally in redirecting the behaviors of those who are cognitively impaired, mentally ill or developmentally delayed. Nurses need support from their work environments in accessing these avenues to protect themselves.

Workers' Compensation

If you believe that you have a work-related injury or illness, you must follow the policies and procedures prescribed by your facility or by state regulation (Injured . . . , 1994). This includes reporting the injury as soon as possible after it happens. In most institutions this is done on an incident or quality assurance report. A common error is to delay reporting in the belief that you should only report something if you know it will be serious or require medical care. By the time you know this, it may be much more difficult to prove that the problem was work-related.

Employers may seek to have workers' compensation claims disallowed to limit their financial liability. Because back injuries are the most common work-related injuries, and often there is no clear objective evidence of damage even when pain is present, stigma frequently is attached to those who have back injuries. While HIV and Hepatitis B are transmitted through needle-stick injuries, they are also transmitted through other unsafe behaviors. These factors may underlie attempts by an employer to disallow claims for care and time lost from work due to these work-related illnesses or injuries. Prompt, thorough reporting is essential to future claims.

You should also have any injury assessed by an appropriate health care provider. If your agency has an occupational health nurse, you may be required to be seen there for initial screening. One concern is whether you may receive care from the provider of your choice or whether you must receive care from a designated provider. This varies based on the regulations governing work-related injury and illness in your state. You should ask this question of your employer and then research it through your state workers' compensation office. If the laws allow the employer or a state agency to designate the provider and you go to another of your choice, you may not be reimbursed for expenses incurred.

Compensation for time off work is another concern when a work-related problem occurs; you usually are required to use your sick leave, but additional time may be available through the workers' compensation program. In general these programs do not match your working salary, so your income will be lessened. This is one of the reasons that many individuals choose to have private disability insurance that assists in providing replacement income when you cannot work because of illness or disability.

The Americans With Disabilities Act requires that employers seek ways to provide reasonable accommodation for individuals with disability in order that they can continue to work. This might include transferring an individual to a different position or modifying the work environment to provide a setting in which the individual can function. Employers have been known to refuse to make accommodations and to try to terminate an individual who has an ongoing disability. Those with work-related illness and disability do have legal rights within the system. Sometimes it requires considerable effort to sustain those rights.

KEY CONCEPTS

- Throughout the history of nursing there have been changing employment patterns, moving from a focus on the home and the community in the first part of this century to a focus on acute care institutions.
- In today's health care world the percentage of nurses employed in hospital inpatient settings is diminishing as more outpatient, home care, long-term care, and community settings are established for the delivery of care.
- Competencies needed by the newly licensed registered nurse can be categorized by criticality and by frequency.
- Employers have expectations in eight basic areas: theoretical knowledge for safe practice and decision making, ability to use the nursing process, self-awareness, communication skills, understanding the importance of documentation, commitment to a work ethic, proficiency in specified technical skills, and speed of functioning.
- Developing a successful career pathway involves setting personal short- and long-term goals and developing a plan for maintaining and enhancing your own competence.
- To obtain a nursing position you will need to identify potential employers, develop a professional resumé, write appropriate letters to employers, and interview effectively.
- Reality shock occurs when an idealistic new graduate enters the real world of practice and has difficulty with the expectations and demands found there. You can prepare for this transition by attending to your own expectations and developing personal strategies for coping.
- Burnout is a stress response experienced by nurses and others who work in occupations that make many emotional demands. Burnout may be alleviated by planned actions, but it may be necessary to change job settings when stress accumulates.
- Nurses see sex discrimination in the workplace manifested as wage discrimination against women, job opportunity discrimination against men, and sexual harassment in the workplace.
- Occupational safety and health are special concerns for nurses because of the infectious nature of the illnesses with which they come in contact, the toxicity of some chemicals in the nursing environment, and the potential for back injury and violence.
- Nurses who experience a work-related injury must carefully follow all relevant rules and regulations regarding reporting the injury, completing appropriate forms, and seeking care in order to assure that they receive assistance for any medical care and lost wages.

Critical Thinking Activities

1. Write out your short- and long-term professional goals with a brief plan on how you can achieve these goals. Think critically about the obstacles you will

text continued

Critical Thinking Activities (continued)

need to overcome to reach these goals. How will you deal with the obstacles?

2. Create an effective resumé and samples of letters to employers that present you as a positive addition to their staff.

3. With a group of nursing students, develop personal strategies for managing reality shock. Discuss your rationale for any strategy you propose.

4. Compare burnout with the stress response you have studied in relation to client care. Compare the strategies that you have taught clients with those suggested for preventing burnout.

5. Review the advertisements for nursing positions in three current journals and analyze them for gender bias.

6. Research the occupational health program offered by a local employer of nurses. Evaluate that program in relation to health hazards in the workplace of which you are aware.

7. Formulate an appropriate response to experiencing sexual harassment in the workplace. Include specific statements you would use and each step you would take if the harassment continued.

REFERENCES

An HIV-infected RN finds a cause: Universal use of safer needles. Am J Nurs 96(4):69–70, 1996

Arkansas judge rules male nurse out of labor/delivery. Am J Nurs 81(7):1253, 1981

Benner P. From Novice to Expert. Menlo Part, CA: Addison-Wesley, 1984

Bradby M. Status passage into nursing: Another view of the process of socialization into nursing. J Adv Nurs 15(10):1220–1225, 1990

Chornick N, Yocom CJ, Jacobson J. 1992–1993 Job Analysis Study of Newly Licensed, Entry-Level Registered Nurses. Chicago: National Council of State Boards of Nursing, 1993

Dreyfus SE, Dreyfus HL. A five-stage model of the mental activities involved in directed skill acquisition. Unpublished report supported by the Air Force Office of Scientific Research (AFSC), USAF (Contract F49620-79-C-0063), University of California at Berkeley, 1980 (as reported in Benner P, Novice to Expert, Menlo Park, CA: 1984)

Injured on the job? Nursing 24(6):28, 1994

Kaye J. Sexual harassment and hostile environments in the perioperative area. AORN J 63(2): 443–446, 448–449, 1996

Kaye J, Donald CG, Merker S. Sexual harassment of critical care nurses: A costly workplace issue. Am J Crit Care 3(6):409–415, 1994

Ketter J. Sex discrimination targets men in some hospitals. Am Nurse 26(4):3, 24, 1994

Kramer M. Reality Shock. St. Louis: CV Mosby, 1979

Kus RJ. Stages of coming out: An ethnographic approach. West J Nurs Res 7(2):177–194, 1985

National League for Nursing. Educational Outcomes of Associate Degree Nursing Programs: Roles and Competencies. Publication No. 23-2348. New York: National League for Nursing, 1991

Neuhs HP. Sexual harassment: A concern for nursing administrators. J Nurs Admin 24(5):47–52, 1994

RNs facing new danger at work. Am J Nurs 95(10):78, 81, 1995

Williams M. The prevalence and impact of violence and sexual harassment of registered nurses in the workplace. Chart 92(4):5–6, 1995

Wolfe S. Legally speaking: If you're sexually harassed. RN 59(2):61–64, 1996

FURTHER READING

Alward R, Monk T. The Nurse's Shift Work Handbook. Washington, DC: American Nurses Publishing Co., 1993

A guide to national/international, travel, and home health nursing opportunities. Am J Nurs 94(1):72, 1994

Brady B. How I was sexually harassed. Nursing 24(5):52–56, 1994

Brady J. Memoirs of a traveling nurse. Am J Nurs 94(1):74, 76, 1994

Buerhaus PI, Dang D, Lehman DL, et al. Analysis of state and local hospital employed RN labor markets. Nurs Econ 11(4):223–228, 258, 1993

Busy nurses need stressbusters. Am Nurse 26(2):5–6, 1994

Butts BJ, Witmer DM. New graduates: What does my manager expect? Nurs Management 23(8): 46–48, 1992

''Career Guide.'' Nursing, monthly feature

Career Planning Guide. New York: National Student Nurses Association, annual publication

Coleman S, Hansen S. Reducing work-related back injuries. Nurs Management 25(11):58, 60–61, 1994

Foley ME. Change signals need for career security versus job security. Am Nurse 26(2):1, 3, 1994

Fulmer H, Cashman S, Bushnell K. Community-oriented primary care: A model for the future. Am Nurse 26(2):19, 1994

Job Focus. American Journal of Nursing, monthly feature

Johnson C. Coping with compassion fatigue. Nursing 22(4):116, 118–119, 120, 1992

Kairns DM. Protect yourself: Set boundaries. RN 55(3):19–22, 1992

Ketter J. Nurses, HIV exposure and the burden of proof. Am Nurse 26(5):14, 21, 1994

Ketter J. Retraining programs benefit staff nurses. Am Nurse 26(4):1, 3, 1994

Libbus MK, Bowman KG. Sexual harassment of female registered nurses in hospitals. J Nurs Admin 24(6):26–31, 1994

Lovejoy RL. When are you entitled to worker's compensation? RN 53(3):81–83, 1990

Miya PA. Ethical dilemmas: Touchy subject . . . sexual harassment. Am J Nurs 94(9):56, 1994

RN Nursing Opportunities. RN Magazine, annual publication

Schmidt PL, Schoville R, Williams M. From expert to novice. Am J Nurs 93(9):53–56, 1993

Serow WJ, Cowart ME, Chen Y, Speake DL. Health care corporatization and the employment conditions of nurses. Nurs Economics 11(5):279–291, 1993

Sullivan P. Stress and burnout in psychiatric nursing. Nurs Standards 8(2):36–39, 1993

Survival Skills in the Workplace: What Every Nurse Should Know. Washington, DC: American Nurses Publishing Co., 1990

Tammelleo AD. Hurt at work? Who dictates where you get care? RN 57(12):64, 1994

Travel nursing: Get up and go! Nursing '93 23(12):60–62, 1993

Preparing for Workplace Participation

We are born in organizations, educated by organizations, and most of us spend much of our lives working for organizations.
(Etzioni, 1964)

Objectives

After completing this chapter, you should be able to:

1. Discuss the purpose of mission statements.

2. Analyze the relationships among organizational charts, chains of command, and channels of communication within organizations.

3. Delineate the characteristics of shared governance and the advantages of a shared governance approach.

4. Describe various patterns of nursing care delivery, identifying the major characteristics of each.

5. Discuss the history of collective bargaining as it applies to nursing.

6. Analyze the processes through which resolution is achieved in collective bargaining issues.

7. Identify at least four professional concerns that should be addressed in a contract for nurses.

8. Discuss the concerns nurses have regarding membership in a collective bargaining group and the reasons for each of these concerns.

9. Outline the advantages and disadvantages of having the state nurses' association serve as a bargaining agent for nurses.

10. Compare and contrast the characteristics of a grievance and a complaint.

KEY TERMS

Accountability	Authority	Bargain in good faith
Agency shop	Authoritative mandate	Binding arbitration

Broad span of control
Case method
Chain of command
Channels of communication
Clinical ladder
Collective action division
Collective bargaining
Common interest bargaining
Concession bargaining
Contract
Cross-training
Deadlock
Division of labor
Final offer
Flat organization
Functional method

Government seizure
Grievance process
Injunction
Impasse
Job description
Informational picketing
Lock out
Mediation
Mission statement
Narrow span of control
National Labor Relations Act
National Labor Relations Board
Negotiate–negotiation
Organization
Organizational chart

Organizational hierarchy
Policy
Professional collectivism
Protocol
Ratify
Reinstatement privilege
Role transition
Shared governance
Span of control
Standards of care
Tall organization
Team nursing
Total patient care
Unfair labor practice
Unions
Union busting

Most new graduates begin their practice as employees of health care organizations. This may be in an acute care hospital, a long-term care facility, an intermediate care facility, or a variety of other organizations that offer challenging opportunities. Accepting employment in a health care organization requires that you adapt to the policies and procedures established by that organization. You will go through what we refer to as *role transition,* the process of assuming and developing a new role. This process occurs most easily when you have a basic understanding of the organization, how it operates and functions, and how you can participate effectively in the activities of that workplace. It is also helpful to be able to anticipate some of the frustrations you may encounter.

This chapter presents content that we believe will assist you in your transition from student to employee. We begin with a brief discussion of the structure of organizations and some of the most common conditions of employment, and then present the most common avenues through which employees participate in workplace decisions. Because we can only touch on these topics, students are encouraged to gain greater depth in this area by reading books devoted to this topic.

ORGANIZATIONAL STRUCTURE

An *organization* may be defined as a formally constituted group of people, with identified tasks, who work together to achieve a specific purpose defined by the organization. All organizations have structure and purpose. Organizations that have the delivery of health care as their primary objective usually are considered bureaucratic organizations—because they operate and are administered through a number of departments and subdivisions, with designated individuals who have responsibility for carrying out various functions. Some would attribute the bureaucracy we see in health care to the militaristic and religious aspects of its history.

All organizations have a purpose, or a reason for existing. This purpose is typically expressed in the form of a *mission statement*, which outlines what the organization plans to accomplish. Sometimes mission statements incorporate statements of philosophy (beliefs), purpose, and goals or objectives into a single statement; other times the philosophy, purposes and goals are addressed in addition to the mission statement. These statements serve as a benchmark against which an organization's performance can be evaluated.

In order to survive, any organization must make enough money to meet expenses and to improve and develop; some also seek to provide a profit return to investors. This is as true in health care as it is in Wall Street businesses. A central goal of most organizations is to seek an organizational structure that is efficient while providing maximum effectiveness. As the values and priorities of our society change, and as new technology becomes available, health care organizations must also make adaptations. Thus, today we encounter a health care system experiencing tremendous transformation (see Chapters 1 and 2).

In organizational theory, the concept of management is associated with structure. The structure of an organization may be defined as "the sum total of the ways its labor is divided into distinct tasks and then coordination is achieved among these tasks (Huber, 1996, p. 226); in other words, it is the way it is "put together" in order to accomplish its goals. Breaking work into pieces or tasks which are assigned to various individuals or groups is known as *division of labor*. The structure of an organization is influenced by its size, age, services, technical components, and environment. There are a number of elements that comprise, describe, and outline the structure of any organization and how it functions, each reflecting a slightly different aspect of the whole. These include organizational charts, chains of command, channels of communication, job descriptions, and policies and procedures.

The Organizational Chart

The structure of any large group comprises both a formal and an informal organization. The formal organization is what can be seen on an *organizational chart*. The organizational chart is a graphic, pictorial means of portraying various roles and patterns of interaction among parts of a system. It identifies formal chains of command, communication channels, and the authority for decision making. In most groups we also find an informal organization, sometimes called the "grapevine," which represents informal or social relationships; it is not depicted on an organizational chart or formally acknowledged in any specific manner, but it can often have a profound effect on how an organization functions.

The organizational chart is typically represented by boxes stacked in a pyramid-shaped chart. The greatest authority exists at the top of the chart (often a single box), and authority declines as you move toward the base (many boxes). Persons occupying jobs that are located at the top of the organizational chart are considered administrators, executives, or "the management," and those closer to the base are considered employees or staff. Located between these two levels is an area known as "middle management," comprising a group of individuals who coordinate and control activities of specified groups of workers.

The organizational chart may take one of several forms, reflecting the type of administration operating within that organization. One of the terms used to describe these forms is *span of control*, which refers to the number of employees supervised by a manager. An organization is said to have a *narrow span of control* when the activities of the organization rest in the hands of a few individuals. If, however, the organization has chosen to have a *broad span of control*, it places authority and responsibility for decision making in the hands of a larger number of individuals. Today, most health care organizations are moving toward a broader span of control; of course, there are many variations of this classical picture.

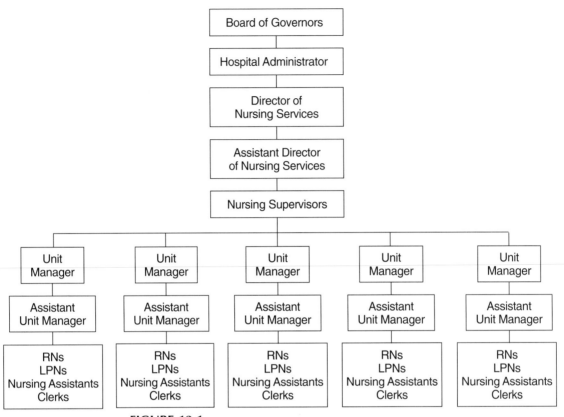

FIGURE 12-1
Centralized (tall) organizational structure of nursing service.

The power to make decisions is a key factor in the structure and function of any organization. With regard to the decision-making process, organizations may also be described as having a centralized (or tall) or a decentralized (or flat) structure. An organization is said to be *centralized* when the authority to make decisions is vested in a few individuals (Fig. 12-1). Conversely, when the decision making involves a number of individuals, and filters down to the individual employee, the organization is said to operate in a *decentralized* fashion. Later in this chapter we will discuss the concept of shared governance, which embraces a decentralized structure and function (Fig. 12-2).

The Chain of Command

All organizations have a *chain of command*. The chain of command represents the path of authority and accountability from individuals at the top of the organization to those at the base of the organization. It is often referred to as the *organizational hierarchy*. Thus, in hospitals we typically find that the nursing administrator gives directions to and evaluates the performance of the assistant administrator, who in turn gives direction to and evaluates

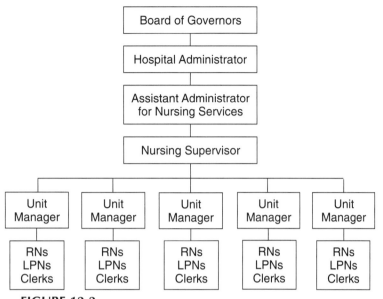

FIGURE 12-2
Decentralized (flat) organizational structure of nursing sevice.

the performance of the nursing manager, and so forth. When we are looking at this process from the base of the organization to the top, we frequently use the language ''reports to''—which indicates that the nursing manager is accountable for her activities to the assistant administrator, and the assistant administrator is accountable to the nursing administrator. Similarly, we will find the registered nurse giving direction to and overseeing the activities of the practical (vocational) nurse and the nursing assistant. The length of the chain of command will vary depending on the size of the organization.

Almost without exception, the salaries commanded by persons at the top of the organizational hierarchy are greater than those of persons close to the base. Likewise, the experience, educational requirements, hours worked, and responsibilities are greater for persons with positions near the top of the organizational chart.

Channels of Communication

Channels of communication are, as their name implies, the patterns of message-giving within an organization. The channels of communication usually reflect the chain of command. Thus, the nurse manager communicates concerns and information to the assistant administrator, who may have the authority and responsibility to deal with the problem, or who will relay the concern to the nursing administrator. The nursing assistant will report her concerns to the staff nurse, who may have the authority to deal with the issue, or who will report it to the head nurse or manager. For a nurse manager to report a concern directly to the administrator is referred to as ''looping'' the system; it is generally considered improper and inappropriate to skip or bypass any of the levels in the communication system. For example, if a staff nurse disagrees with a pharmacy technician who delivers medications to the unit, and takes this problem directly to the supervisor of the medical unit on which she works without first discussing it with her head nurse, this is considered "looping" the system. You readily can see how this would put the head nurse of the unit at a distinct disadvantage, should the supervisor ask her about the incident.

Channels of communication run up and down the organizational chart, moving from one level of responsibility and authority to the next.

Authority, Responsibility, and Accountability

Authority, responsibility and accountability are three terms frequently used when discussing the ways that various groups or organizations operate. *Authority* can be defined as the right to act or to command the action of others. It is based on one's position in the hierarchy of the organization. For example, the team leader has the authority to determine which team members will provide care to which patients. The team leader might also assign a nursing assistant to work with you.

Responsibility refers to the distribution and acceptance of a task or job, or the obligation to take on and accomplish an assignment. For example, the team leader assigns you the care of four patients and you agree to that assignment; therefore, their care is your responsibility. You have an obligation to secure the desired outcome with regard to that care.

Accountability involves a liability factor and can be defined as the liability for task performance. Accountability flows upward in the organizational hierarchy and can be interpreted to mean "the buck stops here." For example, if you delegate to the nursing assistant the responsibility for checking the vital signs of your four patients, you are still accountable for that activity. You will need to be sure that the vital signs are taken, that they are accurate, and that they are reported and documented. Accountability cannot be delegated; you must answer for the care you give and also for the care you ask others to complete. This has become a very sensitive issue for nurses as more unlicensed assistive personnel are hired to replace licensed staff in an effort to contain costs.

Job Descriptions

Another important aspect of any organization is its *job descriptions*. Job descriptions are written statements, usually found in policy manuals, that describe the duties and functions of the various jobs within the organization, and the scope of authority, responsibility and accountability involved in each position. Job descriptions should explain the role of each individual working for the company or organization from the president to the janitor.

Sometimes job descriptions are very specific; other times they are more broadly stated. If broadly stated, procedure manuals may help to specify a task or responsibility. Job descriptions provide the foundation for performance standards for each position, and should provide the basis for evaluation. Job descriptions may also include competencies expected of employees, and can provide the basis for Competency-Based Orientation (CBO)—a program used especially for new graduates and for cross-training. *Cross-training* involves teaching one member of the health care team to perform functions usually associated with another position. For example, a respiratory therapist might learn to perform basic patient care skills and, when not needed for respiratory therapy treatments, be available to answer lights and respond to patient needs.

Job descriptions may also be in the form of *clinical ladders*. A clinical ladder differentiates and defines the skills and performance expected of nurses in terms of levels. Typically three or four levels of performance are defined, with each higher level having greater responsibility and authority than the previous one. A new graduate usually enters the system as a Clinical Nurse One (or similar title), and moves to Clinical Nurse Two and Three as the nurse becomes more proficient. Salary increases typically accompany movement from one level to another. Sometimes additional formal education or continuing education is required for advancement. Through this process the nurse is supported and encouraged to develop greater clinical expertise. The clinical ladder also serves as a mechanism for recognizing and rewarding nurses who wish to remain in direct care positions rather than seek administrative positions.

Policies and Procedures

A *policy* is a designated plan or course of action for a specific situation. In organizations, the responsibility and authority for assuring that appropriate policies are adopted rests with the governing board. The governing board usually delegates the development of policies to the chief administrative officer. The development of policies for a specific department is usually delegated by the administrator to individuals or groups in the department that will be most affected by the policy. Once their work is completed, the policy is returned to the governing board for review, possible revision, and adoption. The management within the organization has the responsibility for assuring that the policies are followed and that more specific policies are developed if necessary.

Written copies of all policies are usually placed in a policy manual that is available in each department. Depending on the area in which you are employed, you will find varying needs for referring to the policy manual in your role as a new employee. As you might anticipate, the need for special policies related to occurrences in an emergency department, delivery room, or a critical care unit is greater than in a general medical or surgical unit in a hospital. Special unit policies are sometimes termed *protocols*. For example, the protocol for dealing with a patient seen in the emergency department suffering from a dog bite determines which local authorities should be notified, who is responsible for seeing that they are notified, and perhaps general management of the wound.

Procedure manuals are also found in each unit or department. Procedure manuals spell out how a particular nursing activity is to be completed, often describing it in a number of steps. For example, you may find a procedure for changing the dressing on a central intravenous line, for administering oncologic agents, and for doing a host of other procedures such as catheterizations.

Nurses have been given more responsibility for affecting and developing institutional policies and procedures, and serving as representatives to various committees that monitor, review and update policies and procedures. As hospitals move to broader spans of control and to greater involvement of all employees in decision making, grassroots participation in policy formation is becoming more commonplace. The nature of a policy and the breadth of its scope will determine whether it needs further review within the organization.

Similar to policies, procedures and protocols are *standards of care*. Standards of care are authoritative statements that describe a common or acceptable level of client care or performance. Thus, standards of care define professional practice. The American Nurses

Association (1991) has formulated general standards and guidelines for nursing practice. These apply across the nation and are broad and general in nature. Similarly, state practice acts contain language that describes the standard of practice that applies to all nurses licensed in that state. Each agency may also develop standards of care for patients with selected health care problems. The standards may take the form of generalized nursing care plans, with which you are already familiar. Some standards are being incorporated into documents termed *care pathways* or *critical pathways.* These identify both outcomes and care activities that are expected to be appropriate for each 24-hour period of hospitalization. These standards of care become the basis for evaluation of care and for quality improvement within the organization.

SHARED GOVERNANCE

Few industries have felt the impact of technology as much as health care. Ranging from new systems of information and communication to different administrative structures, to changing approaches to systems of evaluation, the health care delivery system has seen a radical acceleration in all forms of technology. In the realm of administrative structure, one of the more important of these has been the recent move to a pattern of *shared governance* within health care agencies.

Shared governance is a form of a professional practice model that involves shared decision making by nursing staff and nursing management, as opposed to the administrative decision area being controlled by management. This structure allows nursing staff to make major decisions within the organization; it attempts to get the decision-making process as close to where the action is occurring as possible. Often this pattern of organization is paired with the concept of total quality improvement (TQI), which has as its hallmark emphasis on the customer. Alexander, Bourgeois, and Goodman (1994, p. 283) state "TQI and shared governance (1) empower all employees, (2) encourage decision making at the appropriate level within the organization, (3) promote teamwork with consensus and shared responsibility, (4) encourage and recognize employee contributions, and (5) provide opportunities for personal growth."

The shared governance format may take a number of approaches, including a councilar model in which committees and councils have defined authority and functions, a congressional model that involves an elected representative system, or an administrative model comprising committees or forums in which people communicate and share ideas (Porter-O'Grady, 1987). The committees or councils result in staff actively participating in management, and, as a consequence, gaining autonomy, control over the work environment, and greater job satisfaction. Often councils will report to a nursing executive board that serves as a coordinating and approval body. Within this framework, the nurse is held to greater accountability within the context of peer-defined and peer-operated parameters (Porter-O'Grady, 1990). The traditional role of the supervisor as one who hires, evaluates, promotes, and fires has become a thing of the past. Peer evaluations may have taken its place.

The shared governance model has become widespread in hospitals. Its implementation requires that staff nurses participate in professional development sessions that increase nurses' understanding of the decision-making process, team building, group dynamics, leadership, and budgeting (Jacoby & Terpstra, 1990).

The continuance of shared governance models in today's health care system has been questioned by many. The reengineering and restructuring of the health care delivery system demonstrated through multi-hospital systems, consolidations, mergers, and the use of nurses as primary care providers and case managers may result in the demise of shared governance, or in its assuming a different format. It is a time of much change.

PATTERNS OF NURSING CARE DELIVERY

The nursing department of any health care institution carries major responsibility for the quality of nursing care delivered. Throughout the years, the structure of the delivery of care has taken a number of different formats. The astute student will note that the particular pattern of care that was in vogue changed about every 20 years; among the factors influencing the delivery pattern selected were the types of patients served, the type of care provided, the cost of the care, and the number and education of potential employees. Perhaps a wider variety of patterns of care is being used today than at any other time in nursing's history. In the following section we describe the typical implementation of several patterns of care delivery. However, it is important to remember that you might find a particular pattern of care practiced a little differently in different settings.

The Case Method

The *case method* was the first system used for the delivery of nursing care in the United States (used around the change of the century) and should not be confused with the term ''case management'' used today (discussed later). With the case method, the nurse worked with one patient (or case) only, and was expected to meet all of that patient's needs. The nurse often lived in the patient's home, and was expected to assume other household duties, such as cooking for the patient and family, and light housekeeping when not busy with the patient. Nurses worked long hours and were poorly paid. Advancing technology and increasing costs made this type of care delivery impractical, but vestiges of its structure can be seen in today's home health nursing, where the nurse is assigned to various cases. However, the role of the registered nurse in home health care is typically one of assessment, planning, skilled intervention, supervision of the care provided by a home health aide, and evaluation of progress.

The Functional Method

The *functional method* of care delivery emerged during the Great Depression of the 1930s. This method allowed for the care of greater numbers of patients in hospitals and for the advancing technology. Typically, nursing tasks were assigned by the head nurse to the various persons employed on the unit, according to the level of skills required for performance. One nurse might take all temperatures, another do all dressings, while yet another administered all medications, charted them, and provided a list of replacement needs to the head nurse. Assignments varied depending on the size of the unit, the number of personnel available, and their skill levels. The head nurse gave a report to the next shift. Although economical and efficient, this system of care delivery had the disadvantage of fragmenting care—no single individual was responsible for the planning of the care. Patients were confused about who was caring for them, and communication among caregivers was lacking. Nursing care came to be viewed as procedures and tasks. This pattern of care still may be used in long-term care facilities or sub-acute units, largely due to the educational preparation of the care providers. Some nurses are concerned that the economic push in today's health care institutions may see many hospitals returning to functional approaches to care.

Team Nursing

The concept of *team nursing* was introduced in the early 1950s, and promised to result in more patient-centered care. This approach to care was based on the premise that each unit would have at least two teams composed of variously educated care providers. For example, a team might be composed of two nurse aides, an orderly, a licensed practical (vocational) nurse, and a registered nurse, and led by a "team leader" who was a more experienced registered nurse. Team members worked together, each performing those tasks for which they were best prepared. The team leader made assignments, had overall responsibility for the care of patients on her unit, might give all medications, and gave a report to the team that followed on the next shift. An important part of this form of nursing was the "team conference," at which members of the team joined together to communicate about the needs of their patients and to plan for care. Without the conference and the communication, team nursing might be little different from functional nursing. Today, as we see more health care facilities decreasing the number of registered nurses and adding more unlicensed assistive personnel, team nursing may again become a prevalent method of care delivery (Fig. 12-3).

Total Patient Care

During the late 1970s and early 1980s, many hospitals returned to a *total patient care* type of assignment, in which a registered nurse or licensed practical (vocational) nurse is assigned for all care needs. A nurse is assigned to the care of a group of four to six patients, depending on how acutely ill each patient is, and depending on patient needs. This returns a greater sense of control to nurses, giving them a greater sense of autonomy, and fostering a greater sense of involvement in the whole spectrum of care and in patient outcomes. This type of care focuses on the total person (from which its name is derived) rather than on a collection of tasks or procedures.

Primary Care Nursing

In a pattern of *primary care*, which came into popular application in the 1980s, one nurse is assigned the responsibility for the care of each patient from the time the patient is admitted to the hospital until that patient's discharge. The primary nurse is responsible for initiating and updating the nursing care plan, patient teaching, and discharge planning. An associate nurse works with this same patient on other shifts and on the primary nurse's day off, carrying out the plan of care developed by the primary nurse. Obvious benefits of this

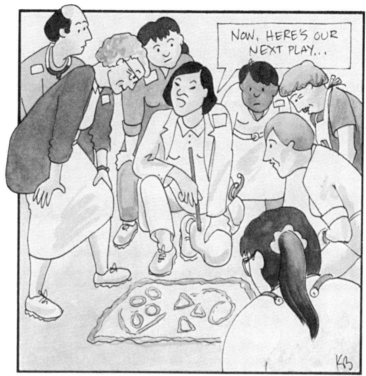

FIGURE 12-3
Team conference, planning, and communiation are critical elements of team nursing.

method include the continuity of care for the patient, and job satisfaction for the nurses because they have more autonomy and control. However, because it requires more nurses, it is also more expensive than other methods. Under this system every nurse is a primary nurse for a few patients and an associate nurse for others. Sometimes the nurse functioning in an associate role has difficulty following the plan of the primary nurse, or may disagree with the established plan of care. The patient's condition may also change rapidly, requiring the plan to be changed without consulting the primary nurse. Another concern is the level of expertise and commitment required of all nurses and the fact that nurses who work autonomously with patients soon forget how to delegate responsibilities.

Case Management

Case management is a process of monitoring an individual patient's health care for the purpose of maximizing positive outcomes and containing costs. A key to case management is the identification of a critical pathway for care and treatment that includes specific time-lines and protocols. The case manager typically follows the patient from the diagnostic phase through hospitalization, rehabilitation, and back to home care, ensuring that plans are made in advance and that the patient receives care that will achieve the most positive

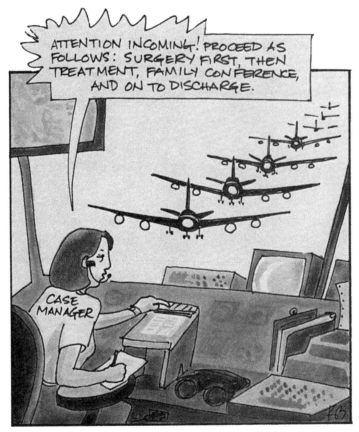

FIGURE 12-4
The case manager may follow the patient from the diagnostic phase through hospitalization, rehabilitation, and back to home care.

outcomes. It goes beyond primary nursing to responsibility for managing the patient's interaction with the entire health care system, and may not include the provision of any direct care (Fig. 12-4).

Registered nurses are the group of health care professionals who most often act as case managers. In some settings social workers also act as case managers. Case managers may be employed by third-party payers (such as insurance companies) or by health care agencies such as hospitals or long-term care facilities. Case managers employed by a particular institution might also be involved in wellness programs such as blood pressure management, stress management, smoking cessation programs, and exercise classes.

Some objections to this form of care delivery come from physicians, who see the role of the case manager as an infringement on their historical rights of autonomy in decision making. Providers may also believe that the case manager is more concerned with cost factors than with what is best for the individual, arguing that quality is sacrificed to cost containment.

DELEGATION

Delegation in nursing can be defined as assigning to a competent individual the responsibility of performing a particular nursing task in a selected situation. In so doing, you authorize another person to act in your stead, but you retain the accountability for the activities performed. The appropriate and effective assignment of work to others is a part of all organizations and work groups.

The delegation of responsibilities to others has become a greater issue in nursing within recent years. As hospitals strive toward restructuring and cost containment, more categories of caregivers who have minimal nursing education and experience have been hired to assist in the provision of nursing care, and are viewed as nurse extenders; in most instances this has resulted in fewer registered nurses working on a unit. These unlicensed assistive personnel have a variety of titles, and in all instances have less formal education than the registered nurse; in some instances it may be minimal.

As a beginning staff nurse, you may have had little experience in delegating tasks to others. However, this skill, like many others, can be learned. It requires some critical thinking and analysis on your part. You must know the level of competence of each of your team members, including each individual's strengths and weaknesses; the requirements of the tasks you plan to delegate (that is, the degree of complexity they involve); and the amount of time available to supervise the tasks. You should be knowledgeable about the nurse practice act of the state and any practice limitations that might exist. You also must possess good communication skills which are critical to communicating assignments, setting down your expectations, and providing ongoing follow-up and evaluation.

It is important that you assign the right task to the right person. This is where your knowledge of your workers and the job descriptions of the institution is critical; this will help you know how closely you must supervise an individual. Generally speaking, the tasks that have the highest level of predictive outcome (those that are routine and standard) are the best ones to delegate to others. For example, if you delegate to a nursing assistant the responsibility for getting a patient into a wheelchair, you can anticipate that the assistant will be able to carry out this task. However, you would not want to delegate a task requiring a high level of nursing judgment and evaluation. You will also want to consider the potential for harm and how difficult a task is to perform. Remember, in all instances you remain accountable for the care you have delegated.

Once you have decided which tasks can be delegated to which team members, it is important that you give clear and complete directions to those responsible for completing the assignments. After giving instructions, ask questions that will provide an indication of whether your directions have been clearly understood.

It is also necessary to provide to your team members the authority to complete the assigned work once it has been delegated. When you first learn to delegate, there may be a tendency to want to do everything yourself, or to "hold on" to all responsibilities. This response may be due to a lack of confidence in the abilities of others, concern that to be done correctly something must be done by yourself, or even concern that someone else may do it better. However, constraints on your own time will be such that many tasks must be delegated, and you will need to accomplish some of your responsibilities by using the skills of others.

In all instances you will want to monitor the outcomes of the care that has been delegated. You also will want to provide your team members with feedback regarding their performance, emphasizing the things done well and offering constructive assistance to those who have not met reasonable expectations.

Nurses, as a group, have been concerned about the use of nurse extenders because of the effect on patient care and the legal responsibility that nurses must assume for tasks performed by others. As a result of this apprehension, many state boards are issuing statements regarding the use of unlicensed assistive personnel. Be certain that you know whether such a statement is in effect in your state and, if it is, the nature of the content and guidelines.

COLLECTIVE BARGAINING

Collective bargaining is a process that allows employees who are members of the union to participate in management decisions with regard to terms of employment, salaries, benefits, working conditions and similar issues. Because of nursing's long history as a profession of dedication, altruism, and service, initially collective bargaining was a controversial issue within nursing. Some saw this process as detracting from the professional role of the nurse. Today, however, nurses are vitally concerned about contracts, services, third-party payers, comparable worth, patients' rights, shared governance, and a host of issues that can be discussed at the bargaining table. Nurses believe that people who choose nursing as a career should have the opportunity to have some voice in patient care assignments, length of the work day and week, fringe benefits, and wages, without losing face with the public at large, members of the medical profession, or other colleagues. This thinking was succinctly outlined in a statement by Janet Muff (1988, p. 245):

We are not in this business out of charity, as altruists and nightingalists would have us believe. We are here to make money, to use our minds and our skills, to provide services to patients on our own terms. We need no longer apologize and feel guilty.

History of Collective Bargaining

As early as the 1850s, Horace Greeley, a reformer, publisher, and politician, was generating interest in and giving impetus to collective bargaining issues in his editorial columns in the *New York Tribune*. During the early part of the 20th century, efforts by workers to organize were met with opposition from employers, governmental officials, and some members of the public. After the Great Depression that immobilized the United States in the late 1920s and early 1930s, several laws were enacted to help improve workers' conditions. Franklin D. Roosevelt was elected president in 1932, and his New Deal administration saw the passage of the National Industrial Recovery Act. One result of this act was the creation of the National Recovery Administration, whose purpose was to administer codes of fair practice within given industries. The nation was called on to accept an interim blanket code that established a 35- to 40-hour work week for workers, minimum pay of 30 to 40 cents an hour, and prohibition of child labor—all issues that had long been advocated by nurses.

On July 5, 1935, the National Labor Relations Act (NLRA) became the national labor policy of the United States. Also known as the Wagner Act, for Senator Robert F. Wagner (who introduced the legislation), the NLRA gave workers federal protection in their efforts to form unions and organize for better working conditions. It listed as unfair practice any actions on the part of employers that would interfere with this process. Senator Wagner wanted management and labor to resolve their mutual problems through a system of self-government. This act also created the National Labor Relations Board (NLRB), a quasi-judicial body that was to ensure that the conditions of that legislation were properly enforced.

The NLRB has the responsibility for administering the NLRA. In addition, it has two primary functions: to conduct secret-ballot elections that will determine that the majority of employees of a unit desire the representation of a given union in collective bargaining procedures, and to prevent and rectify unfair labor practices committed by employers or unions. It also has the responsibility for determining into which bargaining units, of the eight established for health care workers in acute care facilities, various employees will be assigned. This is important to nurses because it enables them to have a separate unit and, therefore, to deal with issues important to their role in health care delivery. Of interest is recent discussion regarding to which unit nursing practitioners and advance practice nurses should be assigned (O'Meara & O'Meara, 1995).

The original NLRA used the term labor organization, which was defined in language that could be interpreted to exclude nursing and several other professions, such as teaching and medicine, that were organized through professional organizations. These early labor unions often were viewed negatively by the public—an image that was reinforced in movies, in newspapers, and on radio. Often portrayed as rowdy, aggressive, and hostile, unions did not seem to fit well in nursing.

In 1947, the original NLRA was amended through the Taft-Hartley Act (also known as the Labor Management Relations Act). Because of heavy lobbying on the part of hospital management, the act was written in such a way as to specifically exclude nonprofit hospitals from the legal obligation of bargaining with their employees. Although the administrations of some hospitals chose to negotiate salaries and working conditions with their employees, many did not, and no legal action could be taken to force the process.

By 1931, the American Nurses Association (ANA) was publicly recognizing its obligation with regard to the general welfare of its members, and developed within its organization a legislative policy addressing this concern. Some suggest that this effort was spurred by the fact that other groups, particularly the Service Employees International Union (SEIU), an affiliate of the American Federation of Labor/Congress of Industrial Organizations (AFL/CIO), were actively working to organize health care workers. Other factors also were important. Before 1930, most nurses were employed in public health, visiting nurse, or private duty positions. Much of the care within hospitals was delivered by students, aides, and orderlies, under the direction of a head nurse. As more care was delivered in the hospital setting, the number of nurses employed by these facilities grew. The existing working conditions affected more people.

In 1945, a committee was appointed by the ANA to study employment conditions. This study culminated in the creation of an ANA Economic Security Program in 1946. This action was followed by the enactment of a resolution that would encourage state nurses' associations to act as exclusive bargaining agents for their respective memberships in the important areas of economic security and collective bargaining. Also in 1946, the SEIU formed its first RN Guild in New York City.

The concept of professional collectivism, which emphasizes that good care is dependent on satisfactory working conditions and satisfaction with nursing itself, began to take shape. However, concern for the image of the nurse and nursing prompted a no-strike policy to be officially adopted by the ANA in 1950, and it remained in effect until it was rescinded in 1968.

By 1947, with the impetus provided by the Economic Security Program of ANA, collective bargaining between nurses and hospital administrations had been implemented in several states, and negotiated contracts were in effect. Many hospital employers were voluntarily developing contracts with employees and were showing genuine concern about working conditions. Some states were mandating that state hospitals negotiate with all employees, but there was no federal requirement for this process.

Federal legislation passed in 1962 enabled employees of federal health care institutions to participate in collective bargaining. In 1967, investor-owned hospitals and nursing homes were also included, and the ANA was identified as the bargaining agent for the nurses of the Veterans Administration hospitals. Legislation passed in 1970 saw the inclusion of non-profit nursing homes in the collective bargaining process. Concurrently, SEIU and other labor-related organizations were also bargaining for nurses.

Finally, on August 25, 1974, Public Law 93-360 was put into effect; it amended the Taft-Hartley Act to provide economic security programs for those employed in nonprofit hospitals, and brought health care facilities and their employees under the jurisdiction of the NLRB. Nonprofit hospitals were legally required to bargain with nurses for better wages, hours, staffing conditions, patient–nurse ratios, and a voice in hospital governance. To ensure that the public would be protected from strikes or work stoppage, several amendments were attached to the NLRA passed in 1974, including the requirement of longer notification periods and provisions mandating participation in mediation.

Understanding the Basic Language

Intelligent bargaining begins with an awareness of the process itself. It involves a formal negotiation process. As the word ''bargaining'' implies, collective bargaining consists of a set of procedures by which employee representatives and employer representatives negotiate to obtain a signed agreement (contract) that spells out wages, hours, and conditions of employment that are acceptable to both. A key word in this definition is *negotiate.*

BARGAINING AND NEGOTIATING

To negotiate means to bargain or confer with another party or parties to reach an agreement. *Bargaining* implies a discussion of the terms of the agreement and suggests that there will be give and take—that neither party will obtain all items asked for in the contract. Ideally, negotiations would proceed in a somewhat philosophical vein, moving toward reasonable compromises that would allow each side to achieve many of the conditions it requested, but this does not always occur.

Common interest bargaining refers to a process in which the employer and employee representatives begin by identifying those areas in which they agree and those goals or values held by both parties. Based on shared values and goals, the two parties then begin to work out their differences in regard to specific policies and conditions. Although relatively new as an approach to collective bargaining, common interest bargaining is gaining attention as a less adversarial process that may preserve effective working relationships and lessen feelings of alienation between supervisory personnel and employees involved in the union.

UNIONS AND COLLECTIVE ACTION

Collective bargaining allows employees working together as an organized unit to negotiate. A *union* is a legally authorized organized group of employees that negotiates and enforces labor agreements. Its major concern is improvement in the wages, hours, and working conditions of its members. Collective bargaining units tend to become organized when a group of persons in an institution identifies common problems and concerns and becomes interested in forming a unit (Flanagan, 1992). When a branch or part of a professional association assumes this responsibility, as often occurs in nursing, the negotiating group may be known as a *collective action division*. The activity of the group may be referred to as *professional collectivism*, which supports the premise that the quality of patient care is directly tied to working conditions and that collective action is a professional responsibility. A professional organization must work under the same legal constraints as a union. It provides legal counsel and representatives to assist with negotiations, may lobby on behalf of issues, or may participate in other activities that would further the economic welfare of nurses. It oversees the development of the contract.

THE CONTRACT

The conclusion of the bargaining process should result in a signed contract that converts to writing the agreements that have been reached. A *contract* is ''an agreement between two or more people to do something, especially one formally set forth in writing and enforceable by law'' (Neufeldt, 1996 [Webster's], p. 302). In most instances a contract need not be in writing, but it is much easier to implement if it is written and signed by all involved. The contract remains in effect until breached or terminated. Most negotiated contracts define the period of time—usually 2 or 3 years—during which the established conditions are effective.

Before being put into effect, a contract must be *ratified*. This means that the terms of the contract must be accepted by the members of the bargaining group. This is usually done by a vote of the membership.

RULES GOVERNING LABOR RELATIONS

When two parties agree to begin the negotiation process, it is understood that both will *bargain in good faith.* Bargaining in good faith is a poorly understood concept, but generally it means that the parties will meet at regular times to discuss (with the intent to resolve) any differences over wages, hours, and other employment conditions. Failure to carry out these activities could lead to an unfair labor practice.

An *unfair labor practice* is any action that interferes with the rights of employees or employers as described in the amended NLRA. It is not possible to discuss all of these in detail; however, some examples follow. An employer must not interfere with the employee's right to form a union or other organized bargaining group, join the group, or participate in the group's activities. The employer may not attempt to control a group, once organized, or to discriminate against its members in regard to hiring or tenure. Most important, the employer must bargain collectively and in good faith with representatives of the employees.

Likewise, labor organizations have constraints placed on their activities. They, too, must bargain in good faith. They must not restrain or coerce employees in selecting a bargaining group to bargain collectively. They may not pressure an employer to discriminate against employees who do not belong to the labor organization.

One of the issues frequently brought up in negotiations that usually results in a dispute is that of *agency shop*. When an agency shop clause is in effect, all employees are required to pay dues for membership. The obvious advantage of this requirement, from the workers' point of view, is encouraging membership in the union. The union is required to represent all employees, members or not. Negotiating a contract, monitoring compliance with its provisions, and facilitating the grievance process may be costly. The union, therefore, desires to have a greater percentage of paying members to support these activities. There are several variations in provisions related to agency shop. If, because of religious or philosophical beliefs, employees are unwilling to pay dues to the bargaining group, provisions may be made to pay the same sum to a nonprofit group such as a church or foundation. In some instances, those who are already members of the union are required to remain members for the life of the contract, although no one is required to become a member. In some states, laws referred to as ''right to work laws'' forbid the establishment of an agency shop.

Settling Labor Disputes

When labor disputes arise, several actions can be taken to help resolve the differences. Initially, of course, the parties continue to negotiate, and may agree to extend the negotiation period if progress in settling differences is being made.

When the two parties doing the negotiating cannot come to agreement on an issue, they are considered to be *at impasse*, or are *deadlocked* on the issue.

MEDIATION AND ARBITRATION

Perhaps the most commonly used method of seeking agreement between parties is through *mediation* and *arbitration*. A *mediator* is a third person who may join the bargainers in early sessions to assist the parties in reconciling differences and arriving at a peaceful agreement. Mediation involves finding compromises, and the mediator assists with this. He or she must gain the respect of both parties and must remain neutral to the issues presented.

An *arbitrator* is technically defined as a person chosen by agreement of both parties to decide a dispute between them. The primary difference between a mediator and an arbitrator is that the mediator assists the parties in reaching their own decision, whereas the arbitrator has the authority to actually make the decision for the parties if necessary. However, the terms mediator and arbitrator and mediation and arbitration often are used interchangeably; in fact, a mediator may also serve as an arbitrator (Fig. 12-5).

Arbitration may take several forms. It may be mediation–arbitration, in which a third person joins the parties in the negotiation process before any serious disputes arise. This person's role is to act as a mediator who will attempt to keep the parties talking, suggest compromises, and help establish priorities. If an agreement is not reached by a specified

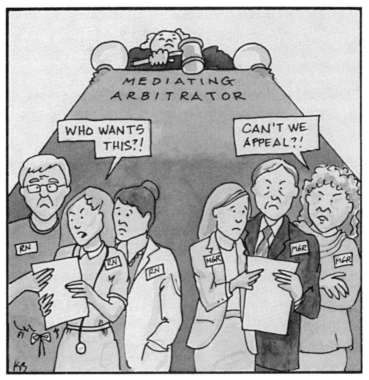

FIGURE 12-5
The arbitrator's decision may not really please either side.

date, or if it appears that the issue is deadlocked with neither party willing to compromise, the mediator then assumes the role of an arbitrator and makes a decision based on the information gained in the role of mediator.

Another form of arbitration is called *binding arbitration*. This means that both parties are obligated to abide by the decision of the arbitrator. Some people see this as the least desirable alternative in settling disputes because it may result in a decision that is not satisfactory to either side, but one by which both must abide. It has been suggested, in instances in which binding arbitration is used, that the parties spell out exactly which of the issues are to be decided by the arbitrator. Binding arbitration has the advantage of resolving deadlocked issues without a strike. It also encourages both parties, knowing that the arbitrator's decision may not please either side, to reach a compromise on their own.

The *final offer* approach is a type of binding arbitration. Employer and employee bargaining representatives reach agreement on as many issues as possible. The deadlocked issues and a final position from each side are then presented to the arbitrator, who is obligated to select only the most reasonable package. The arbitrator may not develop a third alternative, which would "split the difference." The final offer approach encourages both sides to come up with a fairly realistic package and serves to close the gap on issues.

One criticism of any type of arbitration is the expense involved. Arbitrators must be paid for their services. Arbitration is also criticized because it undermines voluntary collective bargaining and allows parties to avoid unpleasant confrontation with their own difficulties by shifting that responsibility to a public authority. However, it is useful in preventing the disruption of services.

Arbitration may be requested from the American Arbitration Association or from available state, public and private mediation and conciliation services. The American Arbitration Association is a nonprofit, nonpartisan organization that, for a nominal fee, will provide a list of qualified arbitrators. Most states also have available groups such as the Public Employees Relations Commission that also can provide a list of mediators and arbitrators.

STRIKES AND LOCKOUTS

When the negotiation process breaks down, lockouts and strikes are likely to occur. A *lockout* occurs when an employer closes a factory or other place of business to make employees agree to terms. One can readily see how undesirable this would be in the health care system, but it has occurred in some instances.

A *strike* occurs when workers refuse to work, thus imposing economic hardship and pressure on the employer. When the negotiation process breaks down, employees use the strike to emphasize their position. Workers may be striving to improve their own working conditions, salaries, and benefits. The most recent strikes by nurses, however, have been over issues related to patient care rather than those related to the economic status of the nurses. Striking places a serious economic hardship on employees and therefore is not undertaken lightly. Sometimes a strike is used to gain public attention to the labor dispute and to create public pressure for a settlement. This is only successful if the public agrees with the position of the striking workers.

Strikes in nursing are undertaken only with advance notice—to enable patients to be transferred to another facility. Typically, arrangements are made with another hospital to admit patients during the strike. The striking nurses may also agree to provide staffing to critical care, labor and delivery, and emergency departments of the facility in which the strike is occurring.

REINSTATEMENT PRIVILEGE

A *reinstatement privilege* is a guarantee offered to striking employees that they will be rehired after the strike, provided that they have not engaged in any unfair labor practices during the strike, and provided that the strike itself is lawful. The hospital may replace a striking nurse during the strike. If strikers agree unconditionally to return to work, the employer is not required to rehire a striking nurse at that time. However, recall lists are developed, and if the nurse cannot find regular and equivalent employment, he or she is privileged to recall and preference on jobs before new employees may be given employment.

Nurses may lose their reinstatement privileges because of misconduct during a lawful strike. For example, strikers may not physically block other nurses and personnel from entering or leaving a struck hospital. Strikers may not threaten nonstriking employees and may not attack management representatives. These types of activities usually do not occur in strikes conducted by nurses, but are not outside the realm of possibility.

OTHER METHODS OF INFLUENCING SETTLEMENT

There are a wide variety of methods by which solutions can be reached in the negotiating process. The following discussion addresses the more formal and far-reaching of these activities.

One method of reaching solution is to employ an *authoritative mandate*, in which a peaceful settlement is encouraged by a president, secretary of labor, or other high-ranking or influential person. This is usually employed when the situation becomes critical and when continuance of a strike would cause problems for a great number of people.

Another technique is *informational picketing*, which involves employees carrying informational signs outside of the institution. Informational picketing is not designed to stop work, but rather to inform the public of the concerns under dispute. This tactic is designed to create public pressure on behalf of the union and the employees, and is seen frequently.

In some instances, an *injunction* may be requested. This results in a court order that requires the party or parties involved to take a specific action or, more commonly, to refrain from taking a specific action. Employers may use this measure to forestall or end a strike. Unions may use this measure to stop a lock-out.

In still other instances an institution or company may be subjected to *government seizure and operation*. Government employees are then used to run the plant, firm, or industry in question. This is seldom seen in the health care industry, for obvious reasons. However, this option was used in Montana in 1991, when state employees decided to strike. The National Guard was called in to replace striking state patrolmen.

What to Look for in a Contract

The negotiation process should ultimately conclude in the development of a written contract that is signed by both bargaining groups and management representatives. The contract establishes guidelines for working conditions such as overtime, floating, work schedules, job security, and retention and recruitment of staff (Boisvert, 1991). It usually spells out certain other privileges to be provided to employees such as in-service education, leaves, health and safety provisions, committee participation, and tuition reimbursement (Flanagan, 1992). The contract may also provide guidelines for the grievance process.

A contract must meet certain specified criteria to be legally binding. It must result from mutually agreed-on items arrived at through a ''meeting of minds.'' Something of value must be given for a reciprocal promise, that is, professional duties for an agreed-on sum. Contracts can be enforceable whether written or oral, but it is easier to work with those that are written (Rothman & Rothman, 1977).

Although each agreement will differ, most contracts have a fairly general format that includes:

- A preamble stating the objectives of each party
- A statement recognizing the official bargaining groups
- A section dealing with financial remuneration, including wages and salaries, overtime rates, holiday pay, and shift differentials
- A section dealing with nonfinancial rewards, that is, fringe benefits such as retirement programs, types of insurance available, free parking, and other services provided by the employer

- A section dealing with seniority in respect to promotions, transfers, work schedules, and layoffs
- A section establishing guidelines for disciplinary problems
- A section describing grievance procedures
- A section that may explicitly state codes of conduct or professional standards

Several other areas that are negotiable are important and should be incorporated into a contract for nurses. These may be included in the section dealing with professional standards or nursing care. The following are generally accepted as items that should be considered in a contract involving professional nurses.

First, the contract should provide for shared governance—that is, professional policy decisions should be developed by professional staff and administration who work jointly on the policy. This often takes the form of a nursing practice council or a professional performance committee. The committees should be identified, duties described, and benefits and rights clarified.

Second, the contract should provide for individual professional accountability. It establishes the guidelines for such issues as floating, overtime, and scheduling. It should include areas related to evaluation, such as peer evaluation of a practitioner's competence. It also should assure job security, stipulate retention and recruitment efforts, and deal with issues of promotion or dismissal.

Third, the contract should define the collective professional role. This spells out the responsibility of registered nurses as professional practitioners and describes their part in the planning of patient care. The purpose of this is to strengthen nurses' influence on the quality of care. It should discourage the encroachment of non-nursing staff into nursing practice and might include guidelines for staffing ratios.

Other items that should be included in contracts relate to health and safety provisions, in-service education or continuing education, tuition reimbursement, and leaves of absence. All of these will affect the quality of the work experience (Fig. 12-6).

It is important that, as a new graduate, you know whether there is a contract in effect in the institution in which you seek employment or in the community in which you plan to work. You should also be knowledgeable about the terms of the existing contract so that you might best fulfill your obligations, and recognize and benefit from the provisions to which you are entitled. The organization to which you are applying for employment can provide you with a copy of the current contract. The state nurses' associations can be contacted for information regarding the organization that represents nurses in a particular hospital or facility. They can also provide a copy of any contracts that have been negotiated for which they represented the nurses.

The Grievance Process

Effective contracts will include, in addition to wages, hours, working conditions, and other items, a section that spells out the grievance procedure. A *grievance* is a circumstance or action believed to be unjust and in violation of a contract (or of policies if a contract is not in place). The *grievance process* represents an established and orderly method to be used in the adjustment of grievances between parties. In this sense, it represents a problem-solving mechanism.

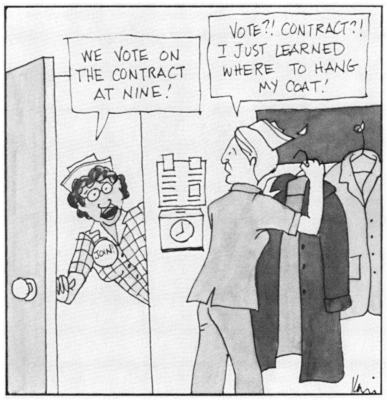

FIGURE 12-6
As a new graduate, you may find yourself poorly prepared to make decisions that are involved in bargaining issues.

The steps to be used in mediating grievances are usually included in the collective bargaining contract. Some organizations that lack formal collective bargaining agreements have developed internal policies that outline grievance procedures. Perhaps you are aware of grievance processes from your students' handbook, where the processes in place in an educational program are shared with students.

Grievances are usually related to interpretations of a contract. They generally occur as a result of a misunderstanding or difference of opinion about the contract or its language, or as a result of direct violations of the contract. Although grievances can be filed by either the management or an employee, most cases are filed by an employee.

The grievance process spells out in writing in the contract a series of steps to be taken to resolve the area of dissension. Initially the employee and the immediate supervisor attempt to resolve the disagreement through informal talk. If no resolution occurs, the discussion moves to the steps of the grievance process. These steps involve others within the organization, and include notifications and responses in writing, strict time lines for action, and eventually the involvement of people at higher levels within the organization (such as representatives from the bargaining unit, a grievance chairman, the personnel director, and

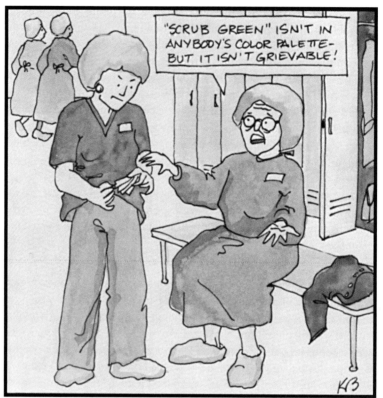

FIGURE 12-7
It is important to discriminate between complaints and grievances.

administrative representatives), and perhaps the services of an arbitrator toward the end of the dispute. Failure to comply with the time lines that are in effect results in the discussion coming to a halt. If an arbitrator is involved, that person's decision is usually binding (Fig 12-7).

It is important to discriminate between complaints and grievances. Employees may have complaints that are not violations of the contract. For example, Nurse No. 1 may object that she was required to float from the postpartum unit to the nursery; she had been oriented to the nursery but preferred to work in the postpartum unit. Nurse No. 2 was required to float from a medical unit to a surgical unit to which she had not been oriented. If the contract in this hospital stipulates that no one would be floated to a unit to which he or she had not been oriented, Nurse No. 1 had a complaint, whereas Nurse No. 2 had a grievance.

The absence of grievances may not be the best indicator of the health of an organization. It is entirely possible that problems are not being addressed. On the other hand, a high number of grievances is an indication of problems within the organization. These problems often relate to the language of the contract or the education of the employee to the conditions of the contract. Another barometer of the health of an organization is the level at which the grievances are resolved. It is most desirable to settle most grievances at the informal level, without the involvement of an arbitrator.

The grievance procedure may sound like many steps that take a great deal of time, and indeed this is true. Although most grievances are settled short of arbitration, they are still time and energy consuming. Grievances can best be avoided if everyone has a good understanding of the terms of the contract and if sound personnel policies are developed and applied consistently and equitably. Open discussions between the employees and management to review mutual concerns and share information help reduce the number of grievances. Mutual respect is a critical element in any organization.

Issues Related to Collective Bargaining and Nursing

Four major issues of collective bargaining affect the nursing profession. The first of these relates to the fact that some nurses see collective bargaining as unprofessional. The second is the issue of which bargaining group will represent nursing if nurses do participate in collective bargaining. The third issue is an individual one and relates to the question of whether to join a union when one exists; the fourth deals with the role of the supervisor.

At one time, the issue of whether nurses should participate in strike activities was of much concern. Many nurses found the withholding of services from patients to be unprofessional, and therefore, personally unacceptable. Others viewed the strike as a final method for bringing attention to the needs of the nurse as a citizen. Fortunately, as bargaining groups representing nurses became more knowledgeable and skilled in the process, strikes occurred less frequently. Disagreements at the bargaining table are more commonly resolved through mediation and arbitration, much to the relief of many professionals.

These issues may take on greater or lesser importance depending on the area of country involved, the length of time the nurses in that area have been participating in collective bargaining, and the group chosen to represent the nurses at the bargaining table. As a staff nurse you may, at some time, have to make a decision regarding whether to strike. In making this decision, you will want to be well-grounded in the issues at hand, and the arrangements that have been made for continuing to provide services in emergency situations and in special hospital areas such as labor and delivery.

PROFESSIONALISM AND COLLECTIVE ACTION

The strain that exists between professionalism and collective action has probably received more space in recent nursing literature than any other issue related to collective bargaining.

The argument against unionism has its roots in the history of nursing itself. Nursing was perceived by many, including nurses, as a selfless, all-serving, altruistic calling. The act of caring for others, even if that meant subordination of the individual to the goals of that care, was to be compensation enough for the services rendered. The strong religious influence that pervaded the early development of nursing added to this concept of the profession. Early leaders in nursing espoused this dedication to its arts. In 1893, Lavinia Dock stated:

Absolute and unquestioning obedience must be the foundation of the nurse's work, and to this end complete subordination of the individual to the work as a whole is as necessary for her as for the soldier. (Cited in Bullough & Bullough, 1966)

Another factor that has hampered the strong development of unionization in nursing is the fact that nursing is primarily a woman's profession. Although more men now enter nursing, only about 3% of the registered nurses in the United States are male.

Early social beliefs that woman's role should be submissive, supportive, and obedient were extremely compatible with the expectations that our society placed on nurses. The paternalism that has existed in the health care delivery system has also made the process of collective bargaining for nurses a slow one (see Chapters 4 and 5). The combination of the role of women and the role of the nurse under earlier paternalistic practices had the nurse caring for the "hospital family," looking out for the needs of all (from patient to physician) and being responsible for keeping everyone happy (Ashley, 1976). The tendency to see the physician as the father figure in the health care system, the nurse as the corresponding mother figure, and the patients as the children has done little to promote the autonomy of nursing as a profession. A quote by Campbell (1980, p 1286) demonstrates the use of the family concept in health care: "If we are to keep unions out of the profession we, as nurses, must make every effort to build loyalty and a family feeling among our fellow nurses."

Despite the fact that nursing has a history of ambivalence toward union negotiations, today we see nurses involved in collective bargaining in greater numbers than ever before. Several factors are responsible for this change. Wilson and colleagues (1990) have identified these as: the focus on the continued high cost of health care and the need to examine this rise; the scrutiny that has been placed on employee's salaries as part of this process; the fact that nurses comprise the largest number of employees in hospitals (nearly half); and changes in the NLRA allowing nurses to bargain collectively. Various sources differ with regard to whether unionization of hospital employees results in higher hospital costs.

In the early years of collective bargaining by nurses, there was some reticence to use the term "unionism." Much of the nursing literature surrounding the issue used appropriate and less emotionally charged synonyms. Today the term "unionism" is used with increasing frequency, reflecting a change in sentiment supporting the belief that nurses should be involved in collective bargaining, and also reflecting the general acceptance of the process by the public at large.

Many have come to believe that the collective action of nurses provides one of the best avenues for achieving professional goals and exercising control over nursing practice. As nurses are called on to assume greater responsibility for complicated decisions, collective bargaining through a professional organization may provide the means to implement the concept of collective professional responsibility.

Certainly the way that collective bargaining will be perceived by the nurse, and by the public that is served, will be determined by the manner in which the bargaining is conducted. Nurses as a group need to develop the skills necessary to communicate to the public the importance of their role in health care delivery. They must be able to handle conflicts and work toward resolution while maintaining integrity and dignity. Nurses need to become enlightened and informed, and they need more than a superficial understanding of the process of collective bargaining.

Nurses may benefit from broadening their perceptions. This applies to many issues in nursing practice—particularly bioethical issues—in addition to collective bargaining (see Chapter 10). Many nurses dichotomize issues into categories such as good/bad, right/wrong, best/worst. Nurses need to work toward understanding and accommodating different points of view and acknowledging that areas of compromise do exist.

REPRESENTATION FOR NURSES

Of far greater controversy than whether nurses should unionize is the issue of which organization should represent nurses at the bargaining table. This is determined by elections that are supervised by the NLRB. To become the certified collective bargaining representative of a group of employees, the organization in question must receive 50% of the votes cast, plus one.

When nurses first began to organize, the ANA, through the state nurses' associations, was the bargaining representative. This group still represents more nurses than all other organizations combined. In 1991, across the country, state associations represented more than 139,000 registered nurses through more than 840 bargain units (Fuller-Jonap, 1994). However, there has been a strong movement on the part of other organizations to vie for the representative position. It has been estimated that more than 30 labor organizations represent health care workers (Miller, 1980). The ANA has been representing nurses since 1946. The National Union of Hospital and Health Care Employees (representing nurses since 1977) and the SEIU have voted to unite, creating something of a "super union" for health care workers. The Federation of Nurses and Health Professionals began organizing nurses in 1978. Other groups representing nurses in various parts of the country include the United Food and Commercial Workers, the Teamsters Union, and the American Federation of Teachers.

Nurses face a difficult decision when trying to decide which group can represent them best. In recent years, this decision has occupied perhaps more time and effort on the part of nurses than has the actual bargaining. Those who have strong allegiance to the ANA contend that only registered nurses should bargain for registered nurses. One of the reasons given for this position is that in collective bargaining, nurses face different issues than other workers. In addition to concerns about salary, benefits, working conditions, and the like, nurses also want to negotiate questions pertaining to staffing, patient care concerns, and participation on joint hospital committees. Many believe that only nurses can effectively negotiate such items. These people contend that hospital administrations, fearing the power of labor unions, will bargain more constructively and positively with nurses themselves. They also believe that the ANA will be a stronger, more united organization if it serves as both the professional association and the bargaining agent.

Others believe that nurses compromise their collective bargaining powers when the recognized union is a group other than the state nurses' association. They think that when nurses do not bargain for themselves, the "organization shrivels and their influence on health care weakens" (Mallison, 1985, p. 943).

Some parts of the country are experiencing a trend toward having an organization other than the professional nurses' association represent nurses. Chief among the arguments for bargaining conducted by another group is the issue of supervisor membership in the professional association (discussed later in this chapter). Proponents of this position would also contend that it is not realistic for one group (ie, the ANA) to work with the professionalism aspect of nursing as well as with the issues of wages, benefits, and working conditions.

Some would argue for two organizations—one to represent issues related to professionalism, and another to negotiate salaries. If nurses choose to have one group involved in professional concerns (eg, codes of ethics, standards of care, and updating skills required in the practice of the profession) and a second group representing them at the bargaining table, there are some obvious drawbacks. First and foremost is the matter of cost, because both organizations would be collecting dues. Many consider the cost of belonging to the ANA and to the state association to be very high, with dues of approximately $350.00 per year. Additional membership dues in another organization, which are equally as expensive, might be prohibitive. Second, many believe that the union would become the dominant force between the two groups, because money and working environment issues both speak strongly. There are no easy answers to this question, and it will certainly be one of the biggest issues facing nurses in the future.

TO JOIN OR NOT TO JOIN

Once an individual nurse has gained an understanding of collective bargaining and has developed a personal philosophy about the professional role of the nurse, he or she will be ready to make a decision regarding membership in the bargaining unit.

In working with students who are soon to embark on professional careers, we find that it is easier for them to decide whether to bargain collectively than it is to decide to part with the money that is required for membership. Many nurses want better working conditions and higher salaries, but are all too willing to let someone else fund these endeavors and work to achieve them.

It is in response to these concerns that many ''agency shop'' clauses have been added to contracts. Those who are members and are active in the negotiation process believe it is inappropriate for some to benefit from the labors of the bargaining process without having contributed, at least financially, to the effort. The presence of agency shop clauses may serve as either an asset or a deterrent to recruitment, depending on the applicant's viewpoint.

THE SUPERVISOR AND COLLECTIVE BARGAINING

In 1994, a nursing home argued before the Supreme Court that the licensed practical nurses in its employ were supervisors (because of their role in directing nursing assistants in patient care) and, therefore, were not protected by the National Labor Relations Act. The Supreme Court, in a 5 to 4 decision, ruled in favor of the nursing home. Nursing organizations engaged in collective bargaining have expressed serious concern regarding the implications of this ruling for all nurses. Labor groups expect to lobby for legislation that would alter this interpretation of the NLRB (''Striking at Bargaining,'' 1994).

This issue was again addressed in February of 1996, when the National Labor Relations Board ended nearly 2 years of deliberation by ruling that charge nurses at Alaska's Providence Medical Center could not be called ''supervisors'' simply because the role requires some direction of other workers. The Board stated that the essence of the nurse's role was ''judgment,'' and went on to explain that authority that arises from professional knowledge is distinct from the authority of a front-line manager (NLRB to the Supreme Court, 1996).

Changing Trends With Regard to Collective Bargaining

At one time economic concerns and working conditions may have been the principal motivators for collective action. However, by the mid-1980s subtle, and at times not so subtle, changes were occurring throughout the United States with regard to collective bargaining, unionism, and labor–management relations. Some working in the area of contract management reported a shift from the adversarial relationship that had historically existed between the employee and the employer (which focused on salaries, work hours, and the like) to one that placed greater emphasis on the quality of work life.

CONCESSION BARGAINING

Concession bargaining is a process in which there is an explicit exchange of reduced labor costs for improvements in job security. This has been occurring with increasing frequency. An example would be a shift in emphasis from one that asks for increases in salary to one that focuses on eliminating the practice of calling nurses and telling them not to report for work because the census has dropped (on these days the nurses do not receive salary). These changes have been seen in industry more than in nursing, although the strike of 6000 Minnesota nurses was triggered by hospital practices related to the layoff of staff and the involuntary reduction of hours (6,000 Minnesota RNs, 1984).

"UNION BUSTING"

A trend seen in health care institutions during the 1980s, and persisting in some areas today, is an effort toward "union busting." Although technically illegal when referring to methods used to get rid of an existing union, the term *union busting* has been expanded to include a wide range of legal activities that slow down collective bargaining. Pressured by rapidly escalating health care costs, and influenced by the changing attitudes toward work, hospital administrators have hired consultants and law firms to assist and advise in discouraging and impeding organizational activities. This is also a counteraction to the courting by unions of the expanding groups of previously unorganized professionals, such as physicians and nurses. Antiunion organizing campaigns are usually aimed at strategies that will delay and thus drag down the momentum of organizing efforts. This could include challenging union membership, attempting to decertify elections, and failing to bargain in good faith—thus drawing out the negotiating process (Ballman, 1985).

ISSUES OF DISCRIMINATION

As nurses have become more comfortable and knowledgeable about the bargaining process, their energies have been directed toward a variety of issues. These include such concerns as pay equity, discrimination against female employees, comparable worth, and the rights of employees to know the hazards within a work environment (see Chapter 11). In some instances, discriminatory practices against male nurses have also been an issue.

CHANGES IN THE NUMBER OF BARGAINING UNITS

Within hospitals there are many different positions and job titles ranging from professional staff through office staff to those responsible for hospital maintenance. In nursing alone, there are groups of registered nurses, licensed practical nurses, and nursing assistants. As these various groups have been granted authority to organize into bargaining units, concern has been expressed about the number of unions with which any hospital administration must bargain at any given time. Some fairly elaborate estimates have been made regarding the amount of time demanded by the collective bargaining process.

When the NLRA was first passed in 1974, the NLRB specified that seven employee bargaining units would exist within the health care industry (Wilson, Hamilton, and Murphy, 1990, p. 37). Those seven groups were registered nurses, physicians, other professional employees, technical employees, business office and/or clerical employees, and skilled maintenance employees.

In 1984, the NLRB determined that bargaining units would be decided on a case-by-case basis. This resulted in the number of bargaining units being reduced to three: all professionals, all nonprofessionals, and guards.

In 1989, the NLRB once again proposed a new rule that resulted in the establishment of eight collective bargaining units. At this time it was also determined that the rule would apply to all hospitals of all sizes. In response, the American Hospital Association (AHA) sought and obtained a permanent injunction against the rule. Subsequently, ''all-RN'' units were legally approved. As might be expected, the AHA and the ANA occupied opposite points of view with regard to this issue.

The latest activity regarding this issue occurred in April, 1991. The U.S. Supreme Court upheld the NLRB in its authority to define bargaining units for health care workers in acute care hospitals, and allowed for all-RN bargaining units (Supreme Court, 1991).

THE WORKPLACE ADVOCACY INITIATIVE

One of the most recent activities has been a move on the part of the ANA to improve the work environment and allow nurses to gain control over nursing practice. Ideally this would assure that patients would receive the best possible nursing care.

In 1991, the ANA selected 16 states to receive grants to initiate or improve the workplace advocacy programs. Two grants focused on exploring new methods of ensuring that nurses are involved in decisions affecting the quality of their work environments in states where the state nurses association does not represent them at the bargaining table. The other grants were used to mount organizing campaigns that would result in strengthening the bargaining programs of the state association.

Other aspects of the ANA Workplace Advocacy Initiative included providing data about salaries and related economic and employment issues; providing information related to health, safety, and other workplace concerns; developing systems of analysis of compensation packages; consultation; and supporting networks for sharing information and providing mutual support.

The Impact of Shared Governance on Collective Bargaining

The greater involvement of staff nurses in health care agency decision making may have a significant impact on the collective bargaining process. Many of the issues that historically were resolved at the bargaining table, such as the use of agency nurses, work load, and policies regarding floating from one unit to another, are now resolved at the committee or council level. Each nurse has greater accountability for participation in decision making outside of the bargaining process and for implementing decisions that have been made. With mechanisms for change built into the operational pattern of the health care agency, nurses may find less to negotiate at the bargaining table and, in reality, the processes may provide some duplication of one another.

KEY CONCEPTS

- One of the critical elements of any organization is its mission statements. Mission statements explicitly outline the purpose of the organization and may also contain the philosophy and goals of the group.
- Organizations may be structured a number of different ways. Some are tall and centralized, while others are flat and decentralized.
- All organizations have chains of command, channels of communication, and spans of control that describe lines of authority and accountability. These can be depicted in organizational charts that represent the formal organization. An informal organization also exists within organizations.
- Organizations have developed job descriptions that outline the responsibilities of all employees, and policies and protocols to guide the activities of the employees.
- Many hospitals are now using a shared governance process, a form of practice model which involves shared decision making by nursing staff and management. It results in a decentralized organization and often results in greater job satisfaction for nurses.
- A number of patterns of nursing care delivery have existed over the years. These include the case method, the functional method, team nursing, total patient care, primary nursing, and case management.
- Since 1974, it has been possible for nurses to bargain collectively for salaries, working conditions, and fringe benefits. This process also allows for their participation in committees focused on improving patient care and patient care standards.
- The collective bargaining process culminates in a contract that places in writing the decisions reached at the bargaining table. As a new graduate, you should know whether the health care agency at which you are seeking employment has a contract in effect.
- A contract usually includes a section that spells out the process to be used in a grievance. Should a grievance arise, it is essential that all steps be followed as outlined in the contract. Nurses need to be able to distinguish between issues that are grievances and those that are simply complaints.
- One of the issues surrounding nurses and collective bargaining is related to which group should do the bargaining for nurses. Many believe this process is best conducted by a professional nursing organization; others believe they will be served best by an organization that has collective bargaining as its major focus.
- Trends with regard to the collective bargaining process include concession bargaining, ''union busting,'' issues of discrimination, and changes in the number of bargaining units.

Critical Thinking Activities

1. Based on your perception of the needs in your community, write a mission statement for a hospital that would serve the needs of the area.
2. Compare the various patterns of nursing care delivery with the pattern being used in a facility where you currently receive clinical experience. Analyze the pattern in current use and evaluate whether another pattern of care delivery would be more or less effective. Provide a rationale for your answer.
3. If possible, interview some nurses who are working in a shared governance environment. Identify what they find satisfying about shared governance. How would they like to see it changed?
4. Do you support the concept of nurses becoming members of a union? If so, should all employees of an organization be required to pay membership fees? Give the rationale to support your views.
5. Outline the major disadvantages of unions in nursing and give examples to demonstrate the disadvantages you perceive.
6. If the collective bargaining agent in the hospital in which you worked was other than the state nurses' association, would you belong to both organizations? What factors would you use to support your decision?
7. What are the reasons that grievance processes need to be spelled out in a contract?

REFERENCES

Alexander MK, Bourgeois A, Goodman LR. Total quality improvement: Bridging the gap between education and service. *In* Strickland OL, Fishman DJ: Nursing Issues in the 1990s. Albany, NY: Delmar Publishers, 1994:280–289

Ashley JA. Hospitals, Paternalism and the Role of the Nurse. New York: Teachers' College Press, 1976

Ballman CS. Union busters. Am J Nurs 85(9):963–966, 1985

Boisvert SC. Collective bargaining: Another view. Maine Nurse 78(4):5, 1991

Bullough V, Bullough B: Issues in Nursing: Readings Selected From Books and Periodicals to Form a Basis for Discussion of Problems in Nursing Today. New York: Springer-Verlag, 1966:96

Campbell GJ. *In* Opinions: Is bargaining unprofessional for nurses? AORN J 31(6):1289, 1980

Etzioni A. Modern Organizations. Englewood Cliffs, NJ: Prentice-Hall, Inc., 1964:1a

Flanagan L. How collective bargaining benefits nurses. Directions: American Nurse Supplement. October:8–9, 22, 1992

Fuller-Jonap F. Collective bargaining in nursing: Benefits, issues, and problems. *In* Strickland OL, Fishman DJ: Nursing Issues in the 1990s. Albany, NY: Delmar Publishers, 1994:33–45

Huber D. Leadership and Nursing Management. Philadelphia: WB Saunders Co., 1996

Jacoby J, Terpstra M. Collaborative governance: Model for professional autonomy. Nurs Management 21(2):423–444, 1990

Mallison MB. Weathering the economic climate. Am J Nurs 85(9):943, 1985

Miller RU. Collective bargaining: A nursing dilemma. AORN J 31(6):1197, 1980

Muff J. Altruism, socialism and nightingalism: The compassion traps. *In* Muff J: Women's Issues in

Nursing: Socialization, Sexism, and Stereotyping. Prospect Heights, IL: Waveland Press, 1988:234–247

NLRB to the Supreme Court: Labor law protects nurses. Am J Nurs 96(4):67,72, 1996

Neufeldt V. (Ed.). Webster's New World Dictionary (3rd ed.). New York: Macmillan, 1996

O'Meara SM, O'Meara DP. NLRB to issue landmark decision on nurse practitioners. Nurse Practitioner 20(12):14, 16, 24, 1995

Porter-O'Grady T. Nursing governance in a transitional era. *In* Chaska NL: The Nursing Profession: Turning Points. St. Louis: CV Mosby, 1990:432–439

Porter-O'Grady T. Shared governance and new organizational models. Nursing Economics 5(6): 281–286

Rothman DA, Rothman NL. The Professional Nurse and the Law. Boston: Little Brown, 1977

6,000 Minnesota RNs strike back at layoff trend. Am J Nurs 84(7):941, 948, 1984

Striking at bargaining rights, court says RNs are supervisors. Am J Nurs 94(7):67, 70–71, 1994

Supreme Court okays all-RN unit. Am Nurse, June: 1, 1991

Wilson CN, Hamilton CL, Murphy E. Union dynamics in nursing. J Nurs Admin 20(2):35–39, 1990

FURTHER READING

Beletz E, Meng MT. The grievance process. Am J Nurs 77(2):256–260, 1977

Browne MN, et al. Litigation and collective bargaining: Two pay equity strategies. A D Nurse 3(6): 18–20, 1988

Castrey BG, Castrey RT. Mediation: What it is, what it does. J Nurs Admin 10(9):18–21, 1980

Eldridge I, Levi J. Collective bargaining as a power resource for professional goals. Nurs Admin Q Winter:29–40, 1982

Flanagan L. All-RN rule to have major impact. Am Nurse March:26, 1982

Gross JA. Conflicting statutory purposes: Another look at fifty years of NLRB law making. Indust Labor Rel Rev 39(10):7–18, 1985

Hudacek SS. Collective bargaining—not a dinosaur of the past. Adv Clin Care 5(1):27–28, 1990

Ketter J. Staff nurses celebrate 20 years of NLRB protection. Am Nurse 26(6):3, 9, 1994

McCarty P. ANA launches workplace initiative—SNAs get grants for RN advocacy, new organizing. Am Nurse 22:1, 7, April 1991

Pettengill MM. Collective bargaining: Impact on nursing. *In* Chaska NL: The Nursing Profession: Turning Points. St. Louis: CV Mosby, 1990:454–463

Pettengill MM. Multilateral collective bargaining and the health care industry: Implications for nursing. J Prof Nurs 1(5):275–282, 1985

Scott K. SNA representation means increased job satisfaction. Am Nurse 25:24, January, 1993

Smith GR. Unionization for nurses: An issue for the 1980s. J Prof Nurs 1(4):192–201, 1985

Stickler KB. Union organizing will be divisive and costly. Hospitals 64(13):68–70, 1990

Targeting charge nurses, hospitals move to prove RN "supervisors." Am J Nurs 94(9):75, 1994

Nursing Licensing Authorities (Boards of Nursing) United States and U.S. Territories

Note: For specific information regarding licensure requirements, regulations, and fees, contact the specific licensing authority. Current addresses, telephone numbers, and directors can also be obtained on the internet through the National Council of State Boards of Nursing at http://www.ncsbn.org/pfiles/mbdirect.html

ALABAMA

Alabama Board of Nursing
P.O. Box 303900   Phone: (334) 242-4060
Montgomery, AL 36130   FAX: (334) 242-4360
Executive Director: Judi Crume, Executive Officer

ALASKA

Alaska Board of Nursing
Dept. of Comm. & Econ. Development
Div. of Occupational Licensing   Phone: (907) 269-8161
3601 C Street, Suite 722   FAX: (907) 562-5781
Anchorage, AK 99503
Executive Director: Dorothy Fulton, Executive Director

AMERICAN SAMOA

American Samoa Health Services
Regulatory Board
LBJ Tropical Medical Center   Phone: (684) 633-1222
Pago Pago, AS 96799   FAX: (684) 633-1027
Executive Director: Marie Ma'o, Director, Nursing Services

ARIZONA

Arizona State Board of Nursing
1651 E. Morten Avenue, Suite 150   Phone: (602) 255-5092
Phoenix, AZ 85020   FAX: (602) 255-5130
Executive Director: Joey Ridenour, Executive Director

ARKANSAS

Arkansas State Board of Nursing
University Tower Building
1123 S. University, Suite 800   Phone: (501) 686-2700
Little Rock, AR 72204   FAX: (501) 686-2714
Executive Director: Faith Fields, Executive Director

CALIFORNIA

California Board of Registered Nursing
P.O. Box 944210   Phone: (916) 322-3350
Sacramento, CA 94244   FAX: (916) 327-4402
Executive Director: Ruth Ann Terry, Executive Officer

California Board of Vocational Nurse and
Psychiatric Technician Examiners
2535 Capitol Oaks Drive, Suite 205   Phone: (916) 263-7800
Sacramento C 95833   FAX: (916) 263-7859
Executive Director: Teresa Bello-Jones, Executive Officer

COLORADO

Colorado Board of Nursing
1560 Broadway, Suit 670   Phone: (303) 894-2430
Denver, CO 80202   FAX: (303) 894-2821
Executive Director: Karen Brumley, Program Administrator

CONNECTICUT

Connecticut Department of Public Health
Board of Examiners for Nursing
410 Capitol Avenue, MS 12NUR   Phone: (860) 509-7624
P.O. Box 340308   FAX: (860) 509-7650
Hartford, CT 06134
Executive Director: Marie Hilliard, Executive Officer

DELAWARE

Delaware Board of Nursing
Cannon Building, Suite 203   Phone: (302) 739-4522
P.O. Box 1401   FAX: (302) 739-2711
Dover, DE 19903
Executive Director: Iva Boardman, Executive Director

DISTRICT OF COLUMBIA

District of Columbia Board of Nursing
614 H. Street, N.W.   Phone: (202) 727-7468
Washington, DC 20001   FAX: (202) 727-7662
Executive Director: Barbara Hagans, Contact Person

FLORIDA

Florida Board of Nursing
4080 Woodcock Drive, Suit 202   Phone: (904) 858-6940
Jacksonville, FL 32207   FAX: (904) 858-6964
Executive Director: Marilyn Bloss, Executive Director

GEORGIA

Georgia Board of Nursing
166 Pryor Street, S.W.   Phone: (404) 656-3943
Atlanta, GA 30303   FAX: (404) 657-7489
Executive Director: Shirley Camp, Executive Director

Georgia State Board of Licensed
Practical Nurses
166 Pryor Street, S.W.   Phone: (404) 656-3921
Atlanta, GA 30303   FAX: (404) 651-9532
Executive Director: Patricia Swann, Executive Director

GUAM

Guam Board of Nurse Examiners
P.O. Box 2816   Phone: (671) 475-0251
Agana, GU 96910   FAX: (671) 477-4733
Executive Director: Teofila Cruz, Nurse Examiner Administrator

HAWAII

Hawaii Board of Nursing
P.O. Box 3469   Phone: (808) 586-2695
Honolulu, HI 96801   FAX: (808) 586-2689
Executive Director: Kathleen Yokouchi, Executive Officer

IDAHO

Idaho Board of Nursing
P.O. Box 83720   Phone: (208) 334-3110
Boise, ID 83720   FAX: (208) 334-3262
Executive Director: Sandra Evans, Executive Director

ILLINOIS

Illinois Department of Professional Regulation
James R. Thompson Center   Phone: (312) 814-2715
100 West Randolph, Suite 9-300   FAX: (312) 814-3145
Chicago, IL 60601
Executive Director: Jacqueline Waggoner, Nursing Act Coordinator

Illinois Department of Professional Regulation
320 W. Washington St., 3rd Floor   Phone: (217) 785-9465
Springfield, IL 62786   FAX: (217) 782-7645
Executive Director: Mary Jo Southard,
Chief Testing Officer

INDIANA

Indiana State Board of Nursing
Health Professions Bureau
402 W. Washington St., Suite 041   Phone: (317) 232-2960
Indianapolis, IN 46204   FAX: (317) 233-4236
Executive Director: Laura Langford, Executive Director

IOWA

Iowa Board of Nursing
State Capitol Complex   Phone: (515) 281-3255
Des Moines, IA 50319   FAX: (515) 281-4825
Executive Director: Lorinda Inman, Executive Director

KANSAS

Kansas State Board of Nursing
Landon State Office Building
900 S.W. Jackson, Suite 551   Phone: (913) 296-4929
Topeka, KS 66612   FAX: (913) 296-3929
Executive Director: Patsy Johnson, Executive Administrator

KENTUCKY

Kentucky Board of Nursing
312 Wittington Parkway, Suite 300   Phone: (502) 329-7000
Louisville, KY 40222   FAX: (502) 329-7011
Executive Director: Sharon Weisenbeck, Executive Director

LOUISIANA

Louisiana State Board of Nursing
3510 N. Causeway Blvd., Suite 501   Phone: (504) 838-5332
Metairie, LA 70002   FAX: (504) 838-5349
Executive Director: Barbara Morvant, Executive Director

Louisiana State Board of Practical Nurse Examiners
3421 N. Causeway Blvd., Suite 203   Phone: (504) 838-5791
Metairie, LA 70002   FAX: (504) 838-5279
Executive Director: Terry DeMarcay, Executive Director

MAINE

Maine State Board of Nursing
24 Stone Street   Phone: (207) 287-1133
State House Station #158   FAX: (207) 287-1149
Augusta, ME 04333
Executive Director: Jean Caron, Executive Director

MARYLAND

Maryland Board of Nursing
4140 Patterson Avenue   Phone: (410) 764-5124
Baltimore, MD 21215   FAX: (410) 358-3530
Executive Director: Donna Dorsey, Executive Director

MASSACHUSETTS

Massachusetts Board of Registration in Nursing
Leverett Saltonstall Building   Phone: (617) 727-9961
100 Cambridge Street, Room 1519   FAX: (617) 727-2197
Boston, MA 02202
Executive Director: Theresa Bonanno, Executive Director

MICHIGAN

Bureau of Occupational and Professional Regulation
Michigan Department of Consumer and Industry Services
Ottawa Towers N., 611 W. Ottawa   Phone: (517) 373-9102
Lansing, MI 48933   FAX: (517) 373-2179
Executive Director: Carol Johnson, Licensing Administrator (Board Support Section)

Office of Testing Services
Michigan Department of Commerce
P.O. Box 30018   Phone: (517) 373-3877
Lansing, MI 48909   FAX: (517) 335-6696
Executive Director: Kara Schmitt, Director, OTS

MINNESOTA

Minnesota Board of Nursing
2700 University Avenue, Wes #108   Phone: (612) 642-0567
St. Paul, MN 55114   FAX: (612) 642-0574
Executive Director: Joyce Schowalter, Executive Director

MISSISSIPPI

Mississippi Board of Nursing
239 N. Lamar Street, Suite 401   Phone: (601) 359-6170
Jackson, MS 39201   FAX: (601) 359-6185
Executive Director: Marcia Rachel, Executive Director

MISSOURI

Missouri State Board of Nursing
P.O. Box 656   Phone: (573) 751-0681
Jefferson City, MO 65102   FAX: (573) 751-0075
Executive Director: Florence Stillman, Executive Director

MONTANA

Montana State Board of Nursing
111 North Jackson   Phone: (406) 444-2071
P.O. Box 20051   FAX: (406) 444-7759
Helena, MT 59620
Executive Director: Dianna Wickham, Executive Director

NEBRASKA

Professional and Occupational Licensure Division
Nebraska Department of Health
P.O. Box 94986   Phone: (402) 471-4376
Lincoln, NE 68509   FAX: (402) 471-3577
Executive Director: Charlene Kelly, Section Administrator

NEVADA

Nevada State Board of Nursing
P.O. Box 46886   Phone: (702) 739-1575
Las Vegas, NV 89114   FAX: (702) 739-0298
Executive Director: Lonna Burress, Executive Director

NEW HAMPSHIRE

New Hampshire Board of Nursing
Health & Welfare Building
6 Hazen Drive   Phone: (603) 271-2323
Concord, NH 03301   FAX: (603) 271-6605
Executive Director: Doris Nuttelman, Executive Director

NEW JERSEY

New Jersey Board of Nursing
P.O. Box 45010   Phone: (201) 504-6586
Newark, NJ 07101   FAX: (201) 648-3481
Executive Director: Vacant Position, Executive Director

NEW MEXICO

New Mexico Board of Nursing
4206 Louisiana Boulevard, NE   Phone: (505) 841-8340
Suite A   FAX: (505) 841-8347
Albuquerque, NM 87109
Executive Director: Nancy Twigg, Executive Director

NEW YORK

New York State Board of Nursing
State Education Department
Cultural Education Center, Room 3023   Phone: (518) 474-3843
Albany, NY 12230   FAX: (518) 473-0578
Executive Director: Milene Sower, Executive Secretary

NORTHERN MARIANA ISLANDS

Commonwealth Board of Nurse Examiners
Public Health Center
P.O. Box 1458   Phone: (670) 234-8950
Saipan, MP 96950   FAX: (670) 234-8930
Executive Director: Elizabeth Torres-Untalan, Chairperson

NORTH CAROLINA

North Carolina Board of Nursing
P.O. Box 2129   Phone: (919) 782-3211
Raleigh, NC 27602   FAX: (919) 781-9461
Executive Director: Carol Osman, Executive Director

NORTH DAKOTA

North Dakota Board of Nursing
919 South 7th Street, Suite 504   Phone: (701) 328-9777
Bismarck, ND 58504   FAX: (701) 328-9785
Executive Director: Ida Rigley, Executive Director

OHIO

Ohio Board of Nursing
77 South High Street, 7th Floor   Phone: (614) 466-3947
Columbus, OH 43266   FAX: (614) 466-0388
Executive Director: Dorothy Fiorino, Executive Director

OKLAHOMA

Oklahoma Board of Nursing
2915 N. Classen Blvd., Suite 524   Phone: (405) 525-2076
Oklahoma City, OK 73106   FAX: (405) 521-6089
Executive Director: Sulinda Moffett, Executive Director

OREGON

Oregon State Board of Nursing
800 NE Oregon Street, Box 25   Phone: (503) 731-4745
Suite 465   FAX: (503) 731-4755
Portland, OR 97232
Executive Director: Joan Bouchard, Executive Director

PENNSYLVANIA

Pennsylvania State Board of Nursing
P.O. Box 2649   Phone: (717) 783-7142
Harrisburg, PA 17105   FAX: (717) 787-0250
Executive Director: Miriam Limo, Executive Secretary

PUERTO RICO

Commonwealth of Puerto Rico
Board of Nurse Examiners
Call Box 10200   Phone: (787) 725-8161
Santurce, PR 00908   FAX: (787) 725-7903
Executive Director: Luisa Colom, Executive Director

RHODE ISLAND

Rhode Island Board of Nurse
Registration and Nursing Education
Cannon Health Building   Phone: (401) 277-2827
Three Capitol Hill, Room 104   FAX: (401) 277-1272
Providence, RI 02908
Executive Director: Carol Lietar, Executive Officer

SOUTH CAROLINA

South Carolina State Board of Nursing
Executive Center Drive, Suite 220   Phone: (803) 731-1648
Columbia, SC 29210   FAX: (803) 731-1647
Executive Director: Margaret Johnson, Interim Executive Director

SOUTH DAKOTA

South Dakota Board of Nursing
3307 South Lincoln Avenue   Phone: (605) 367-5940
Sioux Falls, SD 57105   FAX: (605) 367-5945
Executive Director: Diana Vander Woude, Executive Secretary

TENNESSEE

Tennessee State Board of Nursing
426 Fifth Avenue North   Phone: (615) 532-5166
1st Floor—Cordell Hull Building   FAX: (615) 741-7899
Nashville, TN 37247
Executive Director: Elizabeth Lund, Executive Director

TEXAS

Texas Board of Nurse Examiners
P.O. Box 140466   Phone: (512) 305-7400
Austin, TX 78714   FAX: (512) 305-7401
Executive Director: Katherine Thomas, Executive Director

Texas Board of Vocational Nurse Examiners
William P. Hobby Bldg., Tower 3   Phone: (512) 305-8100
333 Guadalupe Street, Suite 3-400   FAX: (512) 305-8101
Austin, TX 78701
Executive Director: Marjorie Bronk, Executive Director

UTAH

Utah State Board of Nursing
Division of Occupational and Professional Licensing
P.O. Box 45805   Phone: (801) 530-6628
Salt Lake City, UT 84145   FAX: (801) 530-6511
Executive Director: Laura Poe, Executive Administrator

VERMONT

Vermont State Board of Nursing
109 State Street   Phone: (802) 828-2396
Montpelier, VT 05609   FAX: (802) 828-2484
Executive Director: Anita Ristau, Executive Director

VIRGIN ISLANDS

Virgin Islands Board of Nurse Licensure
P.O. Box 4247   Phone: (809) 776-7397
Veterans Drive Station   FAX: (809) 777-4003
St. Thomas, VI 00803
Executive Director: Winifred Garfield, Executive Secretary

VIRGINIA

Virginia Board of Nursing
6606 W. Broad Street, 4th Floor   Phone: (804) 662-9909
Richmond, VA 23230   FAX: (804) 662-9943
Executive Director: Nancy Durrett, Executive Director

WASHINGTON

Washington State Nursing Care Quality Assurance Commission
Department of Health   Phone: (360) 753-2686
P.O. Box 47864   FAX: (360) 586-5935
Olympia, WA 98504
Executive Director: Patty Hayes, Executive Director

WEST VIRGINIA

West Virginia State Board of Examiners for Practical Nurses
101 Dee Drive   Phone: (304) 558-3572
Charleston, WV 25311   FAX: (304) 558-4367
Executive Director: Nancy Wilson, Executive Secretary

West Virginia Board of Examiners for Registered Professional
Nurses
101 Dee Drive   Phone: (304) 558-3596
Charleston, WV 25311   FAX: (304) 558-3666
Executive Director: Laura Skidmore Rhodes, Executive Secretary

WISCONSIN

Wisconsin Department of Regulation
and Licensing
1400 E. Washington Avenue   Phone: (608) 266-2112
P.O. Box 8935   FAX: (608) 267-0644
Madison, WI 53708
Executive Director: Thomas Neumann, Administrative Officer

WYOMING

Wyoming State Board of Nursing
2020 Carey Avenue, Suite 110   Phone: (307) 777-7601
Cheyenne, WY 82002   FAX: (307) 777-3519
Executive Director: Toma Nisbet, Executive Director

Nursing-Related Organization

	Year Established	Membership Eligibility	Publications (monthly unless otherwise noted)
Overall Professional Organizations			
American Nurses Association (ANA) 600 Maryland Ave. SW Suite 100 West Washington, DC 20024-2571	1896	RNs only	*American Journal of Nursing,* *The American Nurse* (for others, write for list)
International Council of Nurses (ICN) 3, Place Jean Marteau 1201 Geneva 20, Switzerland	1900	National professional nurse organizations	*International Nursing Review*
National Federation of Licensed Practical Nurses, Inc. 1418 Aversboro Rd. Garner, NC 27529		All LPNs or LVNs	
National Federation of Specialty Nursing Organizations (NFSNO) 875 Kings Highway West Deptford, NJ 08096		Specialty nursing organizations	
National League for Nursing (NLN) 350 Hudson Street New York, NY 10014	1952	Individuals and agencies interested in the profession of nursing and delivery of nursing care	*Nursing and Health Care Perspectives* (for others, write for list)
National Student Nurse Association (NSNA) 555 West 57th Street Suite 1327 New York, NY 10019	1953	Officially enrolled students of RN and RN baccalaureate programs	*Imprint* (5 times/yr)

	Year Established	Membership Eligibility	Publications (monthly unless otherwise noted)
Organizations Related to Scholarship and Leadership in Nursing			
Alpha Tau Delta 5207 Mesada St. Alta Loma, CA 91737	1921	Students in baccalaureate programs in nursing	*Captions of Alpha Tau Delta* (biennial)
American Academy of Nursing (AAN) c/o American Nurses Association 600 Maryland Ave., SW Suite 100 West Washington, DC 20024-2571	1973	Members elected by current members, based on contribution to nursing Use title "Fellow" (FAAN)	*Nursing Outlook* (bimonthly)
Sigma Theta Tau International 550 West North Street Indianapolis, IN 46202-3163	1922	High achievers: senior students in baccalaureate, master's and doctoral programs; outstanding RNs with baccalaureate or higher degree	*Image, Reflections* (newsletters, both quarterly)
Groups Related to Ethnic/Racial Origin			
American Indian Nurses Association (AINA) PO Box 1588 Norman, OK 73071	1972	Student nurses and RNs of American Indian ancestry	*Newsletter of the AINA* (bimonthly)
Association of Black Nursing Faculty (ABNF) Inc. 1708 N. Roxboro Rd. Durham, NC 27701		Nursing faculty members of African-American background and those interested in their issues	
National Association of Hispanic Nurses 1501 Sixteenth St., NW Washington, DC 20036	1976	Hispanic nurses, associate/all nurses	Newsletter (quarterly)
National Black Nurses Association, Inc. 1012 Tenth Street, NW Washington, DC 20001-4492	1971	African-American RNs	*Journal of National Black Nurses' Association* (twice yearly)
Phillipine Nurses Association of America, Inc. P.O. Box 10200 San Diego, CA 92120		Filipino nurses and those interested in their issues	
Educationally Oriented Associations			
American Association of Colleges of Nursing (AACN) One Dupont Circle, NW Suite 530 Washington, DC 20036-1110	1969	Collegiate program with upper-division major in nursing	*Journal of Professional Nursing* (bimonthly) *AACN Newsletter* (10 times/yr) (for others, write for list)
Commission on Graduates of Foreign Nursing Schools (CGFNS) 3600 Market St., Suite 400 Philadelphia, PA 19104-2651			

	Year Established	Membership Eligibility	Publications (monthly unless otherwise noted)

Council on Collegiate Education for Nursing for the Southern Regional Education Board (SREB)
  1340 Spring Street, NW
  Atlanta, GA 30309
	1963	Colleges and universities in the southern states that have nursing programs	Write for list

Mid-Atlantic Regional Nursing Association (MARNA)
  350 Hudson Street
  New York, NY 10014
	1981	Agencies preparing persons in health care and that deliver health care	*Marnagram* (quarterly)

Midwest Alliance in Nursing, Inc. (MAIN)
  2511 East 46th Street, Suite E-3
  Indianapolis, IN 46205
	1979	Agencies engaged in providing direct nursing care or teaching persons to provide direct care	*MAINlines* (bimonthly newsletter)

National Association for Practical Nurse Education and Service, Inc. (NAPNES)
  1400 Spring Street, Suite 310
  Silver Springs, MD 20910
	1941	All persons interested in LPN/ LVN education	*Journal of Practical Nursing* (quarterly)
			NAPNES Forum

National Council of State Boards of Nursing (NCSBN)
  676 N. St. Clair
  Suite 550
  Chicago, IL 60611-2921
	1978	State/territorial licensing boards	*Issues*

National Organization for Associate Degree Nursing (NOADN)
  1730 N. Lynn St.
  Suite 502
  Arlington, VA 22209-2004
	1985	Open	*Advancing Clinical Care*

North American Nursing Diagnosis Association (NANDA)
  1211 Locust St.
  Philadelphia, PA 19107
	1976	RNs	*Nursing Diagnoses*

New England Organization for Nursing (NEON)
  Hewitt Hall, University of New Hampshire
  Durham, NH 03824
	1964	Colleges and universities in the New England states that have nursing programs	Write for list

Western Institute of Nursing (WIN)
  PO Drawer P
  Boulder, CO 80302
	1957	Colleges and universities in the western states that have nursing programs	Write for list

Occupational or Specialty-Related Organizations			

Academy of Medical Surgical Nurses
  East Holly Ave., Box 56
  Pitman, NJ 08071			

American Academy of Ambulatory Care Nursing
  East Holly Ave., Box 56
  Pitman, NJ 08071
	1974	RNs in administration of ambulatory nursing	

	Year Established	Membership Eligibility	Publications (monthly unless otherwise noted)
American Academy of Nurse Practitioners Capitol Station LBJ Bldg. PO Box 12846 Austin, TX 78711		Registered nurses in advanced practice as nurse practitioners	
American Association for the History of Nursing, Inc. PO Box 90803 Washington, DC 20003	1980	Anyone interested in the history of nursing	*The Bulletin* (4 times/yr)
American Association of Critical Care Nurses (AACN) 101 Columbia Aliso Viejo, CA 92656-1491	1969	RNs, LPNs, student nurses	*Critical Care Nursing* *Focus on Critical Care* (bimonthly)
American Association of Diabetes Educators 600 N. Michigan Ave. Suite 1400 Chicago, IL 60661		Individuals engaged in educating those with diabetes	
American Association of Legal Nurse Consultants 4700 West Lake Ave. Glenview, IL 60025			
American Association of Office Nurses 109 Kinderkamack Rd. Montvale, NJ 07645			
American Association of Spinal-Cord Injury Nurses 75-20 Astoria Blvd Jackson Heights, NY 11370-1178	1983	RNs and LPNs who practice in diverse SPCI settings	*SCI Nursing* (quarterly journal) Also educational and practice guidelines
American Burn Association Burn Treatment Center Crozier-Chester Medical Center 15th and Upland Avenue Chester, PA 19013		Professionals working with burn patients	
American College of Nurse Midwives (ACNM) 818 Connecticut Avenue NW Suite 900 Washington, DC 20006	1955	RNs who are certified Nurse Midwives or students in accredited programs	*Journal of Nurse Midwifery* *Quickening* (newsletter)
American Holistic Nurses Association 401 Lake Boone Trail, Suite 201 Raleigh, NC 27607	1981	Active: RN, LPN/LVN Contributing: all others	*Journal of Holistic Nursing* (annual) *Beginnings* (newsletter)
American Association of Neuroscience Nurses (AANN) 224 N. Des Plaines Suite 601 Chicago, IL 60661	1968	RNs	*Journal of Neuroscience Nursing* (bimonthly)

	Year Established	Membership Eligibility	Publications (monthly unless otherwise noted)
American Association of Nurse Anesthetists (AANA) 222 South Prospect Ave. Park Ridge, IL 60068-4001	1931	RNs who are certified registered nurse anesthetists (CRNAs)	*American Association of Nurse Anesthetists Journal* (bimonthly) *AANA Bulletin* (bimonthly)
The American Association of Nurse Attorneys (TAANA) 720 Light Street Baltimore, MD 21230-3826	1982	Nurses who are attorneys or are in law school and attorneys in nursing schools	*Inside TAANA* (newsletter, quarterly)
American Association of Occupational Health Nurses (AAOHN), Inc. 50 Lenox Pointe Atlanta, GA 30324-3176	1942	RNs practicing in an occupational health setting	*AAOHN Journal* *AAOH News*
American Nephrology Nurses Association (AANA) North Woodbury Road, Box 56 East Holly Avenue Pitman, NJ 08071	1969	RNs, LVNs employed in the field	*Journal of AANA* (6 times/yr) *AANA Update* (newsletter)
American Organization of Nurse Executives (AONE) 325 Seventh St NW Suite 700 Washington, DC 20036		RNs in administrative positions	
American Psychiatric Nurses' Association 1200 Nineteenth St NW Suite 300 Washington, CD 20036			
American Public Health Association (APHA) Public Health Nursing Section 1015 15th Street, NW Washington, DC 20005	1972	All persons interested in Public Health Various categories of membership available	*American Journal of Public Health* *The Nation's Health*
American Radiological Nurses Association 2021 Spring Rd Suite 600 Oakbrook, IL 60521	1981	Active: RNs employed in radiologic nursing Associate: other RNs and LPNs in radiologic nursing	*ARNA Images* (4 times/yr)
American Society for Long-Term Care Nurses 660 Lonely Cottage Drive Upper Black Eddy, PA 18972-9313	1990	Anyone interested in supporting long-term care	*ASLTCN Journal* (bimonthly)
American Society of Ophthalmic Registered Nurses (ASORN), Inc. PO Box 193030 San Francisco, CA 94119	1976	RNs working in ophthalmology	*Insight* (newsletter)

	Year Established	Membership Eligibility	Publications (monthly unless otherwise noted)
American Society of Pain Management Nurses 1550 So. Coast Highway Suite 201 Laguna Beach, CA 92651		Student and corporate memberships available	*ASPMN Pathways* (quarterly newsletter)
American Society for Parenteral and Enteral Nutrition—Nurses' Committee 8630 Fenton Street, Suite 412 Silver Springs, MD 20910-3803	1975	Multidisciplinary: professionals working with parenteral and enteral nutrition	
American Society of Plastic and Reconstructive Surgical Nurses, Inc. East Holly Rd, Box 56 Pitman, NJ 08071	1975	Active: RNs, LPNs working in the field Associate: RNs, LPNs interested in the field	*Journal of Plastic and Reconstructive Surgical Nursing*
American Society of Post-Anesthesia Nurses 6900 Grove Rd. Thorofare, NJ 08086	1980	RNs, LPNs, Anesthesiologists, CRNAs	*Breathline Journal of Post Anesthesia Nursing* (quarterly)
American Urological Association Allied 11512 Allecingie Parkway, Suite C Richmond, VA 23235	1972	Active: RNs, LPNs, PAs, technicians Associate: industry, physicians	*AUAA Journal* (quarterly) *Urogram* (newsletter)
Association for Practitioners in Infection Control 505 E. Hawley St. Mundelein, IL 60060			
Association of Nurses in AIDS Care (ANAC) 704 Stoney Hill Road, Suite 106 Yardley, PA 19067 (215) 321-2371 http://www.mc.vanderbilt.edu/adl/pathfinders/missions/anac.html	1988	Nurse, industry, and affiliates interested in promoting health, welfare, and rights of HIV-infected persons	*Journal of the Association of Nurses in AIDS Care (JANAC)* *ANACdotes* (quarterly newsletter)
Association for Professionals in Infection Control and Epidemiology 1016 16th Street NW Washington, DC 20036	1972	Active: professionals in infection control Associate: other	*AJIC* (bimonthly) (for others, write for list)
Association for the Care of Children's Health 3615 Wisconsin Avenue, NW Washington, DC 20016	1965	All individuals interested in children's health	*Children's Health Care* (for others, write for list)
Association of Operating Room Nurses (AORN) 2170 S. Parker Road, Suite 300 Denver, CO 80231-5711	1949	Active: RNs employed in OR or in a related educational program or in research	*AORN Journal*
Association of Pediatric Oncology Nurses 4700 West Lake Rd. Glenview, IL 60025-1485	1976	RNs	*APON Newsletter* (quarterly) (for others, write for list)

	Year Established	Membership Eligibility	Publications (monthly unless otherwise noted)
Association of Rehabilitation Nurses 4700 West Lake Rd. Glenview, IL 60025-1485	1974	Regular: RNs Associate: all interested persons	*Rehabilitation Nursing* (bimonthly journal) Pamphlets
Association of Women's Health, Obstetric, and Neonatal Nurses (AWHONN) (formerly NAACOG) 700 14th Street NW Suite 600 Washington, DC 20005 (202) 662-1600	1969	RNs and allied health individuals in OGN nursing	*Journal of Obstetric Gynecologic, and Neonatal Nurse (JOGN)* (bimonthly) *AWHONN Newsletter*
Coalition of Nurse Practitioners, Inc. PO Box 123 East Greenbush, NY 12061	1980	Nurse practitioners and students in nurse practitioner programs	*Coalition Communique* (quarterly)
Department of School Nurses of the National Education Association (NEA) 1201 Sixteenth Street, NW Washington, DC 20036	1968	School nurse members of the NEA	*The School Nurse*
Dermatology Nurses' Association East Holly Avenue, Box 56 Pitman, NJ 08071-0056	1981	Active: RNs, LPNs/LVNs involved in dermatology	*DNA Focus* (bimonthly newsletter)
Developmental Disabilities Nurses' Association 1720 Willow Creek Circle, Suite 515 Eugene, OR 97402			
Drug and Alcohol Nursing Association 660 Lonely Cottage Dr. Upper Black Eddy, PA 18972	1979	Active: nurses caring for clients with drug- and alcohol-related disorders Associate: all others	*DANA Newsletter* (quarterly)
Emergency Nurses Association (ENA) 216 Higgins Rd. Park Ridge, IL 60068	1970	RNs	*The Journal of Emergency Nursing* *Emergency Nursing Care Curriculum*
Flight Nurse Section Aerospace Medical Association Washington National Airport Washington, DC 20001	1964	Designated flight nurses and RNs who are members of Aerospace Medical Association	*Aviation Space, and Environmental Medicine*
Hospice Nurses Association 5512 No. Umberland St. Pittsburgh, PA 15217-1131			
International Association for Enterostomal Therapy (IAET), Inc. 2081 Business Center Drive Suite 290 Irvine CA 92715	1968	Active: graduates of accredited IAET program	*Journal of Enterostomal Therapy*
Intravenous Nurses' Society, Inc. 2 Brighton Street Belmont, MA 02178	1973	Nurses interested in intravenous therapy	*Journal of Intravenous Therapy*

	Year Established	Membership Eligibility	Publications (monthly unless otherwise noted)
National Alliance of Nurse Practitioners 325 Pennsylvania Ave, SE Washington, DC 20003-1100		DONS in long-term care agencies	
National Association of Directors of Nursing Administration in Long Term Care (NADONA/LTC) 10999 Reed Hartman Hwy., Suite 229 Cincinnati, OH 45242			
National Association for Health Care Recruitment PO Box 5769 Akron, OH 44372	1975	Active: health care recruiters	*Recruitment Directions* (10 times/yr)
National Association of Neonatal Nurses 1304 Southpoint Blvd. Suite 280 Petaluma, CA 94954	1984	Regular: RNs Associate: all others	*Neonatal Network: The Journal of Neonatal Nursing* (bimonthly)
National Association of Orthopaedic Nurses East Holly Avenue, Box 56 Pitman, NJ 08071	1980	RNs, LPNs, LVNs	*Orthopaedic Nursing* (for others, write for list)
National Association of Nurse Practitioners in Reproductive Health 325 Pennsylvania Ave. S.E. Washington, DC 20003			
National Association of Pediatric Nurse Associates/Practitioners (NAPNAP) 1101 Kings Highway North, Suite 206 Cherry Hill, NJ 08034	1973	RNs with advanced education who are primary care practitioners in pediatrics	*The Pediatric Nurse Practitioner* (newsletter) *The Journal of Pediatric Health Care*
National Association of Physicians Nurses 900 South Washington St. Suite G-13 Falls Church, VA 22046			
National Association of School Nurses Lamplighter Lane, PO Box 1300 Scarborough ME 04074	1969	Active: RNs employed by educational institutions Other categories for students, retirees, organizations	*School Nurse Journal NAS Newsletter* (quarterly)
National Flight Nurses Association 6900 Grove Road Thorofare, NJ 08086-9447	1981		*Aeromedical Journal* (bimonthly) *Across the Board* (quarterly)
National Gerontological Nurses Association 7250 Parkway Dr., Suite 510 Hanover, MD 21076		Other categories for students, retirees, organizations	

	Year Established	Membership Eligibility	Publications (monthly unless otherwise noted)
National Nurses Society on Addiction 4101 Lake Boone Trail Suite 201 Raleigh, NC 27607	1983	Regular: RNs Associate: all others	*Annual Review of Nursing and the Addictions* Quarterly newsletter
Nurse Consultants Association, Inc. 414 Plaza Drive, Suite 209 Westmont, IL 60559	1979	RNs with 60% of income from consultant-type sources	Quarterly newsletter Annual membership directory
Nurses Organization of Veteran's Affairs 1726 M Street NW Suite 1101 Washington, DC 20034			
Oncology Nursing Society 501 Holiday Drive Pittsburgh, PA 15220		Nurses interested in oncology	
Respiratory Nursing Society 4700 West Lake Ave. Glenview, IL 60025-1485			
Society for Vascular Nursing (SVN) 309 Winter Street Norwood, MA 02062	1982	Active: currently licensed nurses	*SVN Journal* (quarterly)
Society of Gastroenterology Nurses and Associates, Inc. 401 N. Michigan Ave. Chicago, IL 60611	1974	Individuals employed as gastrointestinal nurses or assistants	*Gastroenterology Nursing* (bimonthly)
Society of Otorhinolaryngology and Head-Neck Nurses, Inc. 116 Canal St., Suite A New Smyrna Beach, FL 32168	1976	RNs actively working in ORL/head-neck nursing	*ORL-Head and Neck Nursing* (4 times/yr) *Update* (quarterly newsletter)
Transcultural Nursing Society College of Nursing Madonna University 36600 Schoolcraft Rd. Livonia, MI 48150	1979	Nurses and nonnurses	Biannual newsletter
Society of Pediatric Nurses 7250 Parkway Drive Suite 510 Hanover, MD 21076			
World Federation of Neuroscience Nurses PO Box 3703 Parramotta, NSW 2150 Australia		Professional nurses working in neuroscience	
Miscellaneous			
American Assembly for Men in Nursing 437 Twin Bay Drive Pensacola, FL 32534-1350	1971	All those supportive of the concerns of men in nursing	*Interaction*

	Year Established	Membership Eligibility	Publications (monthly unless otherwise noted)
National Nurses for Life 1998 Menold Allison Park, PA 15104			
Nurses Christian Fellowship 6400 Schroeder Road PO Box 7895 Madison, WI 53707	1948	Christian students and RNs	*Journal of Christian Nursing* (quarterly)
Nurses Educational Funds 555 West 57th Street New York, NY 10019	1911	Donors welcome	Semiannual newsletter
Nurses' House, Inc. 350 Hudson Street New York, NY 10014	1925	Payment of annual contribution	

Index

Note: Page numbers in *italics* indicate illustrations; those followed by t indicate tables; those followed by d indicate display material.